An Introduction to Global Health Delivery

An Introduction to Global Health Delivery

Practice, Equity, Human Rights

JOIA S. MUKHERJEE

Associate Professor

Division of Global Health Equity, Brigham and Women's Hospital

Department of Global Health and Social Medicine, Harvard Medical School

Chief Medical Officer, Partners in Health

OXFORD
UNIVERSITY PRESS

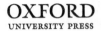

OXFORD
UNIVERSITY PRESS

Oxford University Press is a department of the University of Oxford. It furthers
the University's objective of excellence in research, scholarship, and education
by publishing worldwide. Oxford is a registered trade mark of Oxford University
Press in the UK and certain other countries.

Published in the United States of America by Oxford University Press
198 Madison Avenue, New York, NY 10016, United States of America.

Library of Congress Cataloging-in-Publication Data
Names: Mukherjee, Joia S., author.
Title: An introduction to global health delivery : practice,
equity, human rights / Joia S. Mukherjee.
Description: Oxford ; New York : Oxford University Press, [2018] |
Includes bibliographical references.
Identifiers: LCCN 2017029611 | ISBN 9780190662455 (pbk. : alk. paper)
Subjects: | MESH: Global Health | Health Equity | Human Rights | Health Policy
Classification: LCC RA441 | NLM WA 530.1 | DDC 362.1—dc23
LC record available at https://lccn.loc.gov/2017029611

9 8 7 6 5 4 3 2

Printed by Sheridan Books, Inc., United States of America

Contents

Foreword

This book was written by an academic physician who has dedicated her life to improving access to comprehensive health services to people facing both poverty and disease in more than a dozen countries. *An Introduction to Global Health Delivery* is, quite simply, the best introduction to an emerging field of study and pragmatic action known as global health equity, which has injected new resources and new enthusiasm into the tired arena of international public health. But this book is more than an introduction, and Joia Mukherjee is more than an academic doctor. This volume is a concise summary of a century marked by stunning scientific discovery. But Mukherjee, an infectious disease specialist who is both a pediatrician and an internist, has dedicated her life to addressing the dark side of medical progress: the always uneven and usually dismal failures to deliver the fruits of science to the poor.

Dr. Mukherjee's has not been the life of a short-term expert consultant, helicoptering in and out of troubled regions to offer advice and criticism, but the long-term commitment to expanding teams of Haitians, Rwandans, Malawians, Peruvians, and fellow Americans who are themselves committed to building robust care-delivery systems able to address the needs of their neighbors. As in the parable of the Good Samaritan, she and her colleagues have helped to redefine the very notion of neighbor—and to instantiate the concept of pragmatic solidarity. But this work is not the topic of *An Introduction to Global Health Delivery*, even though Mukherjee's long tenure as Chief Medical Officer of Partners In Health informs her analysis, and she draws on it often to illustrate key lessons. What she attempts, and succeeds in doing, is to offer what many students—undergraduates as well as students of medicine, nursing, and public health—have long clamored for: a primer not only of recent developments in global health, including its successes, but also a patient dissection of what has worked less well—and what hasn't worked at all.

From the points of view of the bottom billion, progress in access to basic health has been slow. In the course of considering well known epidemics of AIDS, tuberculosis, malaria, cholera, and Ebola, Mukherjee offers what most clinicians cannot: an analysis of how and why the delivery of medical care for the sick and injured must be linked to an analysis of how and why policy decisions make care delivery a commodity out of reach for many in greatest need of it. To take one of several examples, consider the paradigm of *selective primary care* proposed as an "interim strategy for disease control in developing countries." This is the paradigm that held sway as Mukherjee began her own medical studies, which took place in America's elite universities. The estimated cost for such a strategy was then held to be about 25 cents per person per year.

Since the medical school and teaching hospitals in which she trained are on the same planet as the developing countries in question, any physician or nurse in training might wish to know what sort of medical care could be delivered with such meager financing? The answer is none at all, which is why disease control—and not even the most selective of primary care—was the objective of this and related schemes. Medical care, in this view, was not on the policy agenda for the unfortunate beneficiaries. Even though medical students learned next to nothing about healthcare policy, insurance, or financing, one needn't be a math whiz or the parent of a child with leukemia to figure this out. Even a full schedule of vaccines that might make disease control possible costs more than was advocated for public budgets during these grim years. They lasted right up until the beginning of this century.

AIDS and AIDS activism upended these hangdog strategies, and Mukherjee leads with this example for good reason. It's a story she knows well, since she was and is deeply involved not only in providing clinical care—I've had the great privilege to practice alongside her for the past two decades—but in working with activists and policy makers to roll out some of the first AIDS treatment programs in poor and rural reaches of Haiti and several countries on the most heavily burdened continent. Most of the other case studies of past global health interventions pale in comparison. But many of them have borne fruit nonetheless.

So why have some global health interventions worked while others have not? Answering this question is, Mukherjee argues, the topic matter of a veritable science of delivery, which is why this book also includes a concise history of the regional and global institutions tasked with controlling epidemics that transcended shifting international borders—as spheres of influence became empires, and then colonies became nations. The contrasting fates of two contemporaneous campaigns, one ambitious and one patterned in an anemic version of selective primary care, are well described in Mukherjee's brief account. Many nations were independent in name only after the world came to be divided in three; and the rise of what we now consider modern and worldwide bureaucracies addressing the grotesquely unequal burdens of disease as the first, second, and third worlds were transformed into constituent groups of least developed, middle-income, and developed nations.

During all these transformations, the world's poorest remained shut out of human progress, including advances in medicine and public health, and now, as Mukherjee shows us, the real work of addressing health disparities must begin. If a new generation is to shoulder this burden along with the excluded, hers is the perfect guidebook for the way forward. Mukherjee's experience as a teacher, whether at Harvard or in Haiti, and her close attention to a large body of knowledge cited in this book's reference materials, have afforded her the ability to lay out clearly and without jargon some of the most vexing problems faced by students and practitioners alike.

I noted above that Joia Mukherjee is not your average academic doctor. "The world is not OK," she observes. But far from being a catalogue of misery, this excellent survey is fired by a belief that activism works, or can, for those still shut out of modernity. It's fueled, too, by the conviction—born of experience on four continents and over a quarter of a century—that the road to universal health care is the one we are now traveling. It's a road with bumps, pitfalls, dead-end diversions, and other traps. But Mukherjee knows, as did nineteenth century abolitionists, that the arc of history bends slowly towards justice.

Paul Farmer
Kono, Sierra Leone
August 2017

Acknowledgments

In stunned silence, I watched Lovely die in front of me. Her bloated belly, red hair, and swollen feet screamed the medical diagnosis—kwashiorkor, protein calorie malnutrition. Starvation. The heartache, anguish, and even shame on her mother's face pierced my psyche. Cynthia, Lovely's mother, took her child to every weigh-in. Lovely's vaccinations were all up to date. The little girl died under the watchful eye of a child survival program—the only health care available to children in impoverished countries throughout most of the late 20th century. These twice-yearly campaigns provided growth monitoring, vaccinations, deworming, oral rehydration salts, and vitamin A to children under five years of age. I once volunteered in such a child survival program—I weighed Lovely, recorded her weight on a growth chart. I held the multicolored chart of the four food groups in my hands and educated Cynthia about the proper weaning foods to give her children—beans, meat, eggs. But Cynthia, I knew, didn't have food. She didn't own land. She didn't have money. Children do not die of starvation because of their mothers' ignorance. Mothers know when their kids are hungry from their ceaseless cries. They know when their children are dying of starvation when the crying stops. More than 25 years ago, I first witnessed death from starvation. In my youth, ignorance, and relative solitude I delivered the prescribed health education to Cynthia and other mothers but I could not make sense of a world where a starving child was not offered food. I felt ashamed then and now at the gross inequity of a world with enormous wealth—and starving children. Health disparities are a thermometer of this injustice.

The world in which I once lived was one focused only of health education and prevention. Treatment was not given. Providers blamed Lovely's death on her mother's ignorance of the proper weaning food to give Lovely. By the same standards, Sarah was blamed for contracting human immunodeficiency virus (HIV) because she didn't demand condom use from her sexual partners. Yet the money she got for sex allowed her to feed her children for another day. Pedro was blamed for developing drug-resistant tuberculosis. Yet daily transportation to the clinic cost him a day's wages making his adherence to the prescribed treatment erratic. This book is for Lovely, Cynthia, Sarah, and Pedro. It is for the thousands of patients I have cared for who are destitute and struggle daily to survive. Their destitution is not a choice, it is not a product of bad behavior or ignorance. It is deeply structural, related to historical and present-day forces of racism, wealth disparity, militarism, gender inequality. Their social and medical conditions are severe and very often lethal. Their illnesses are costly, often catastrophically so. These patients—who have lived and died on my watch—deserve more than prevention, more than health education, more than what is sustainable on the meager budget of the countries in which they live in. People like Lovely, Cynthia, Sarah, and Pedro deserve quality, modern health care—care that is delivered with compassion and respect for human dignity. Indeed, the destitute have a right to health. We all do.

That prevention-only world burst open because of the brave fight of those who demanded AIDS treatment access for all at the turn of the millennium. Among whom I am personally indebted to the example set by my friends including Eric Sawyer, Gregg Gonsalves, Mark Harrington and the many activists that people the movement for health care as a human right. The new possibility of delivering curative medical care even in the world's poorest places was born from their fight for health care as a human right. It is my hope that this book, "An Introduction to Global Health Delivery: Practice, Equity, Human Rights," continues that struggle and may serve as a call to action to those who want to learn about or even join the movement to provide health care to all as a human right.

Of the many people who have supported the writing of this book, I must first extend my deepest gratitude to Paul Farmer, Ophelia Dahl, Jim Kim, and Todd McCormack, the founders of Partners in Health (PIH) the American medical charity they created in 1987 to make a preferential option for the poor in health care. PIH is where I have found my home and my inspiration since 1999. Before I knew PIH, I was broken by the chasm of inequity I experienced as I worked in East Africa and watched friends die of HIV and children die of starvation only to return to the jarring glitter of the American shopping mall. That fractured psyche that can only be repaired with a radical vision of social justice and the constant work needed to achieve that vision. Operationalizing the vision of global health—delivery, equity, and justice—continues to be the most difficult work I know. It is work, however, that is immensely joyful because of the many amazing friends with whom I engage daily in this struggle.

Social justice is a team sport. And I thank the team of PIH warriors around the world with all my heart. I am so proud to be on your team! My deep gratitude goes first to my brothers and sisters from Haiti—Fernet Léandre, Maxi Raymonville, Wesler Lambert, Charles Patrick Almazor, Jean-Gregory Jerome,

Paul Pierre, Ralph Ternier, Jonas Rigodon, Anany Prosper, Maxo Luma, Patrick Ulysse, Loune Viaud, Jack St. Fleur, Reginald Fils-Aime, Dimitri Suffrin, Darius Leopold Fenelon, Michel-Ange Desulme, Mac Lee Jean Louis, Junior Bazile, Jean Louis Romain, Daniel Dure, Christophe Milien, Marc Julmisse, Kerling Israel, Sauveur Marcel, Mackinley St. Louis, Jean Paul Joseph, Frankie Lucien, Eddy Jonas, Marie Millande Tulme, Ketty Tout-Puissant, Myrka Amazan, Father Eddy Eustache, Ermaz Pierre Louis, Tatiana Therosme, Margreth Guerrier, Father Fritz Lafontant and so many others. The revolutionary spirit of the Haitian psyche will forever mark me as one of your compatriots. Scatter my ashes at Bwa Kayiman.

My gratitude, also extends to my first home at PIH, Socios en Salud in Perú. You patiently taught me Spanish, multidrug-resistant TB, and about the Latin American solidarity movement—Jaime Bayona, Felix Alcantara, Dalia Guerra, Eda Palacios, Lorena Mestzana, Katiuska Chalco, Karim Llaro, Leo Lecca, Hilda Valdivia, and beyond. We spread so many lessons from Haiti and Peru to Rwanda, Lesotho, Malawi, Mexico, Russia, Kazakhstan, the Navjo nation, Sierra Leone, and Liberia. I cannot imagine PIH without Peter Niyigena, Jean Claude Rutayisire, Didi Farmer, Evrard Nahimana, Alice Uwingabiye, Alice Nyirimana, Emmanuel Kamanzi, Peter Drobac, Corrado Cancedda, Felix Cyaramatare, Alex Coutinho, Askar Yedilbayev, Oksana Ponomarenko, Luckson Dullie, Emily Wroe, Sam Nmojole, Noel Kalanga, Chiyembekezo Kachimanga, Cate Oswald, Bryan Eustis, Viola Karanja, Lassana Jabateh, Bailor Barrie, Amidu Barrie, Yusuf Dibba, Kerry Dierberg, Katie Baron, Abera Leta, Melino Ndayizigiye, Likhapha Ntlamelle, Seyfu Abebe Desta, Ermyas Birru, Archie Ayeh, Hugo Flores, Dan and Lindsay Palazuelos, Mercedes Aguerrebere, Jafet Arrieta, Patrick Elliot. The movement for global health equity has spread far and wide beyond the countries in which PIH works directly. For that, I sincerely thank my friends who have taken up the charge elsewhere: Deogratias Niziyonkiza, Evan Lyon, Ari Johnson, Jess Beckerman, Phuoc Van Le, Sri Shramasunder, Mike Westerhaus, Amy Finnegan, Raj Panjabi, Dan Schwartz, Ryan Schwartz, Duncan Smith-Maru, Sheela Maru, Mark Arnoldy, Neil Gupta, and Hema Magge.

I could not have written this book without my friends from PIH in Boston who bring and have brought their love, dedication, and talent to the work: Sara Stulac, Michael Rich, K. J. Seung, Sheila Davis, Regan Marsh, Daniel Orozco, Hind Satti, Milenka Jean-Baptiste, Alishya Mayfield, Michelle Morse, Annie Michaelis, Jean Claude Mugunga, Manzi Anatole, Cory McMahon, Sonya Shin, Jen Furin, Keith Joseph, Louise Ivers, Kathryn Kempton, Donna Barry, Gary Gottlieb, Rebecca Rollins, Ted Philip, Ted Constan, Ann Quandt, Megan Carbone, Eva O'Brien, Sarthak Das, Ed Cardoza, Alex Sloutsky, Bepi Raviola, Gene Bukhman, David Greenberg, Ellen Ball, Mike Seaton, David DiSimone, Christopher Hamon, Lauren Greenberg, Lauren Gallinsky, Jesse Greenspan, Jon

Lascher, John Meara, Mike Steer, Robert Riviello, and so many more. The drivers who have carried me over hill and dale, the cooks who have fed me and my picky son, the staff who have kept our white-floored hospitals clean—you are all part of the story of global health delivery and of the human dignity it requires. I also remember, nearly every day, my three good friends whose lives were lost in the long, international fight for health care as a human right—Dr. Josue Augustin, Dr. Max Raymond Jr., and Jean-Gabriel Fils. These three men touched my heart in different ways. I carry their indefatigable spirits with me.

This book would not have been possible without the vision of Global Health as an academic field, a vision supported by the faculty of Harvard Medical School and the Brigham and Women's Hospital. From the faculty, I am particularly indebted to Howard Hiatt, Byron and Mary-Jo Good, Mary Kay Smith Fawzi, Carole Mitnick, Salmaan Keshavjee, Meche Becerra, and Molly Franke. I am deeply grateful for the support of Dean David Golan and my tireless co-conspirator Christina Lively for supporting the creation of the Masters in Global Health Delivery at Harvard Medical School and to Dr. Agnes Binagwaho for her revolutionary energy and work to spread Global Health Delivery throughout the world, now via the new University of Global Health Equity in Rwanda. I am fortunate to teach students worldwide and train our residents in Global Health Equity alongside my dear friend Joe Rhatigan. Our department's tireless administrator Jen Puccetti afforded me the support of the magical Debbie Brace. Debbie was my cheerleader, crack researcher, brilliant critic, and ebullient friend—so much of the credit of the crafting of this book goes to her. In the critical eleventh hour, the dream team including Vincent Lin, Gabriela Sarriera, and Emilia Ling offered enormous support. As did the unflappable, kind, and generous Sara Autori.

It is so that everyone may enjoy their lives and their families that we fight for health as a human right. Like all of us, my family is a cornerstone of everything I am and have done. My late father, Dr. Kalinath Mukherjee, set sail from India and met my American mom in 1957. My dad passed on his work ethic, his deeply held ethical principles, his pursuit of kindness, and perhaps an epigenetic understanding of poverty and suffering to me. I am ever grateful to my mother Patricia for her adventurous spirit, unflagging hopefulness, and constant, often lovingly exaggerated, belief in my abilities. I am also connected with and indebted to my brilliant siblings Maia and Jami who in so many ways contribute to my understanding of what is beautiful and difficult in the world. We shared a bicultural and international world before it was "a thing." It is a world that shaped us all. And last, I thank my beloved son Che, who wanted me to title this book "Booky McBookface" after the boat of a similar name. Che accompanied me throughout the world for many years, forbearing 5 AM flights to Haiti, 2 AM arrivals in Rwanda, jetlag in Siberia, and a revolving door of uncles and aunts from all corners of the world. Che took his first steps in the mountains of Lesotho, learned how to say "wawa" in Chichewa before he could say "hello" in English, and was blessed by Father Lafontant in Legiz Bon Sauveur in Cange, Haiti, after his bout with cancer. It is for Che, my beautiful nephew Patrick, and the world they will inherit that we must continue this fight.

Adelante.

Introduction

Why Global Health Delivery

On December 23, 2013, a two-year-old child named Emile died of an unidentified hemorrhagic fever in Guinea.[1] Soon after, his grandmother, mother, and sister all died.[1] This was the beginning of the West African Ebola pandemic, which killed more than 11,000 people in Guinea, Liberia, and Sierra Leone by 2016.[2] This epidemic shocked the world and threw into stark relief global inequities in health care.[3] Why did thousands of West Africans get sick and die when patients treated in the United Kingdom and the United States survived? Why were simple treatments, such as the administration of intravenous fluids to combat dehydration, inaccessible? The answer to these questions is not found solely in biology or medicine, but instead in the "collective failure to ensure the availability. . . of high-quality health care services."[3] Global health in the modern era must focus on building systems to address this collective failure. To that end this book analyzes the history of health inequities and presents the principles of global health delivery needed to realize the right to health for all.

Global health inequity is inextricably tied to poverty caused by slavery, colonial and postcolonial resource extraction as well as other forms of subjugation and oppression. In the postcolonial period, even as countries gained their independence, former colonial powers and multinational corporations controlled the natural resources of the formerly colonized states. This persistent power imbalance impoverished countries in Africa, Asia, and Latin America. Leaving impoverished governments unable to provide health care for their people. Cash-strapped governments had no choice but to seek loans from the World Bank and International Monetary Fund. The loans demanded privatization of services like health and education and opposed public sector spending. These factors restricted health budgets in impoverished countries to less than 5 dollars per person per year, leaving health systems moribund and unable to provide quality health care. With little money available, 20th-century public health efforts focused solely on cheap, discreet prevention campaigns.[4]

Yet, prevention alone is insufficient. The provision of clinical care is desperately needed. In every corner of the world, illness, suffering, and death disproportionately affect the poor. Against this backdrop, acquired immune deficiency syndrome (AIDS) swept across the globe in 1980s and became a global pandemic within a decade. AIDS treatment requires long-term care, the consistent supply of drugs, well-trained health workers, and adequate health infrastructure. AIDS activists fought for access to treatment as a basic human right. This struggle successfully shifted the public health paradigm from prevention to comprehensive care.[5,6]

Beyond AIDS, health disparities between the rich and the poor are profound. A child born in the richest country will live 30 years longer than a child born in the poorest country.[7] Similar disparities exist within countries. These stark differences expose profoundly unequal access to resources and to health care. There is an ethical and moral imperative to make the fruits of science available to all. In this book, "global health" is defined as the emerging discipline of health care delivery in impoverished settings and the term "global health era" refers to the period after 2000, during which the delivery of medical care was finally considered a cornerstone of human rights and global development.

The shift from prevention-only to comprehensive care delivery is the underlying premise of this book. With this premise, the discipline of global health is based on:

1. the delivery of care to meet the burden of disease,
2. the implementation of programs to achieve health equity,
3. understanding and addressing the social determinants of health,
4. developing a rights-based approach to health care—through the public sector and with communities,
5. building local human capacity and enduring health systems to achieve Universal Health Coverage as a basic right.

This book builds on efforts to standardize and coordinate global health education. Significant international dialog went into the crafting of the 2015, list of core competencies for global health practitioners and scholars[8] stewarded by the Consortium of Universities for Global Health (CUGH) published (Figure I.1). This book is explicitly written for an undergraduate audience, at levels I and II of this framework. However, there is material in the book that may be of interest to all levels of learners. Competencies highlighted by the Consortium are central to this book including: the global burden of disease, the globalization of health and health care, social and environmental determinants of health, capacity

Level I: Global Citizen Level
Competency sets required of all post-secondary students pursuing any field with bearing on global health.

Level II: Exploratory Level
Competency sets required of students who are at an exploratory stage considering future professionals pursuits in global health or preparing for a global health field experience working with individuals from diverse cultures and/or socioeconomic groups.

Level III: Basic Operational Level
Competency sets required of students aiming to spend a moderate amount of time, but not necessarily an entire career, working in the field of global health.

Two sub-categories exist in Level III:

Practitioner-Oriented Operational Level: Competency sets required of students: 1) practicing discipline-specific skills associated with the direct application of clinical and clinically-related skills acquired in professional training in one of the traditional health disciplines; and 2) applying discipline-specific skills to global health-relevant work from fields that are outside of the traditional health disciplines (e.g., law, economics, environmental sciences, engineering, anthropology, and others).

Program-Oriented Operational Level: Competency sets required of students within the Basic Operational Level in the realm of global health program development, planning, coordination, implementation, training, evaluation, or policy.

Level IV: Advanced Level
Competency sets required of students whose engagement with global health will be significant and sustained. These competencies can be framed to be more discipline-specific or tailored to the job or capacity in which one is working. This level encompasses a range of study programs, from a masters level degree program, up to a doctoral degree with a global health-relevant concentration. Students enrolling in these programs are usually committed to a career in global health-related activites.

FIGURE 1.1 Four Proposed Levels of Global Health Competency.

Kristen Jogerst, Brian Callender, Virginia Adams, Jessica Evert, Elise Fields, Thomas Hall, Jody Olsen, Virginia Rowthorn, Sharon Rudy, Jiabin Shen, Lisa Simon, Herica Torres, Anvar Velji, Lynda L. Wilson

Identifying Interprofessional Global Health Competencies for 21st-Century Health Professionals

Annals of Global Health, Volume 81, Issue 2, 2015, 239–247

http://dx.doi.org/10.1016/j.aogh.2015.03.006

strengthening, collaboration, partnering and communication, ethics, professional practice, health equity and social justice, program management, sociocultural and political awareness, and, finally, strategic analysis.[8]

This book is divided into four sections: the history and emergence of the field of global health, the values that underpin this discipline, the technical aspects of care delivery, and the need for advocacy and governance to realize the promise of Universal Health Coverage to achieve the right to health.

Section I: History of Global Health

The first section of this book (Chapters 1–3) examines the emergence of the field of global health. Chapter 1 begins with the history of impoverishment of developing countries and the global power imbalances that cause profound health disparities. Chapter 1 also highlights important historical developments including the Universal Declaration of Human Rights, the World Bank and the IMF's structural adjustment programs, the Alma Ata conference on primary health care, and the Bamako Initiative. Chapter 2 details the rise of the AIDS pandemic and its impact on people and health systems. It documents the unprecedented movement led by people living with human immunodeficiency virus (HIV) that called for AIDS treatment for all as a matter of human rights. Chapter 3 describes the launch of the Millennium Development Goals and the utilization of HIV/AIDS funding to achieve health systems goals.

Section II: Principles of Global Health Delivery

This section (Chapters 4–6) lays out some of the common language and frameworks needed to understand the successes and challenges in global health delivery. Chapter 4 introduces the concept of the burden of disease and how it is measured. It reviews common terms used to describe the health of populations. Chapter 5 outlines social determinants of health and the biosocial nature of health. Finally, Chapter 6 introduces a value-based model of health care called the *care delivery value chain*, a tool used to analyze health systems.

Section III: Health Systems Strengthening

This section (Chapters 7–10) focuses on the WHO building blocks of health systems, the key elements needed to provide high-quality health care. Chapter 7 discusses the need to strengthen human resources for health. Chapter 8 explores the role and necessity of community health workers. Chapter 9 focuses on the evolution of drug access. Finally, Chapter 10 describes the data systems required to monitor patients and evaluate programs.

Section IV: Toward the Right to Health

The final section (Chapters 11–14) focuses attention on the geopolitical goals and forces needed to realize the right to health. Chapter 11 introduces the global goal of Universal Health Coverage. Chapter 12 describes how health care is financed.

Chapter 13 covers the levels and influence of global health governance. Finally, the book culminates with an exploration of the advocacy needed to realize the right to health for all.

Throughout the book, cases and exercises are used to illustrate the challenges of delivering care in impoverished countries. The book strives to serve as a useful guide for those seeking to understand the past challenges, present struggles, and future promises of global health.

References

1. Davis R. Ebola epidemic 2014: Timeline. *The Guardian*. Oct 15, 2014. Available from: https://www.theguardian.com/world/2014/oct/15/ebola-epidemic-2014-timeline. Accessed May 22, 2017.
2. World Health Organization (WHO). *Situation report: Ebola virus disease*. Geneva: World Health Organization; 2016.
3. Boozary AS, Farmer PE, Jha AK. The ebola outbreak, fragile health systems, and quality as a cure. *JAMA*. 2014;312(18):1859–1860.
4. Fielding JE. Public health in the 20th century. *Ann Rev Public Health*. 1999;20:xx.
5. Messac L, Prabhu K. Redefining the possible: The global AIDS response. In: Farmer P, Kim JY, Kleinman A, Basilico M, editors. *Reimagining global health, an introduction* (pp. 111–132). Berkeley/London: University of California Press; 2013.
6. Mann JM. *AIDS: A worldwide pandemic*. Current Topics in AIDS Volume 2. New York: John Wiley & Sons; 1989.
7. World Health Organization (WHO). Life expectancy increased by 5 years since 2000, but health inequalities persist. Available from: http://www.who.int/mediacentre/news/releases/2016/health-inequalities-persist/en/. Accessed Sep. 27, 2016.
8. Jogerst K, Callender B, Adams V, et al. Identifying interprofessional global health competencies for 21st-century health professionals. *Ann Global Health*. 2015;81(2):239–247.

Introduction to Global Health Delivery

Online Resources

A series of lectures by Dr. Joia S. Mukherjee and colleagues on global health can be found on the YouTube channel:
  http://bit.ly/introtoGHD

Dr. Joia S. Mukherjee is a faculty member in the Department of Global Health and Social Medicine at Harvard Medical School and is part of the Global Health Delivery Project.
Case studies on Global Health Delivery can be found at :
  http://www.globalhealthdelivery.org/case-collection/

To connect with an international community of global health delivery practitioners and scholars please visit and join:
  https://www.ghdonline.org/

PART ONE

History of Global Health

1

The Roots of Global Health Inequity

Key Points

- Weak health systems have deep historical roots.
- Colonized and exploited countries have the weakest health systems.
- The legacy of slavery and colonialism impacts health in the present day through racially based oppressive policies that result in differential risk, poor access to care, and unequal health outcomes.
- Neoliberal economic policy impaired the ability of impoverished governments to deliver health care as a basic right.
- The 1978 global conference on primary health care, held in Alma Ata in the former Soviet Union, declared that "health for all" was the future.
- *Selective primary health care* proposed in 1979, supplanted the broader aspirations of health as a human right.
- The history of impoverishment from colonialism and slavery to the neoliberal economic policies in the postcolonial period led to a near-absence of medical care in impoverished countries in the 1970s through the late 1990s.

Introduction

A child born today in Japan will live to the age of 83, whereas a child born in Sierra Leone will only live until the age of 50.[1] Similar disparities exist between rich and poor communities within countries.[2] These differences in life expectancy are not caused by genetics, biology, or culture. Health inequities are caused by poverty, racism, a lack of medical care, and other social forces that influence health. A critical analysis of the historical roots of this gross and systemic inequality is a fundamental part of the study of global health.

The slave trade and colonialism impoverished countries throughout the world. Even as the world recognized a universal set of human rights in 1948, African countries were still under the colonial yoke. Human rights were not the norm in any colonial state. Few systems were built to support the health or education of colonized people. Even after the successful African liberation struggles of the 1950s–1970s, the economic policies promoted by the World Bank indebted the very countries impoverished by the slave trade and the colonial project. There was little money for the delivery of health care. Instead, international actors proposed a set of simple, preventive interventions, called *selective primary care*, which could be delivered cheaply and without significant staff or infrastructure. These same actors imposed patient user fees to pay for drugs and supplies. The fees served as a barrier to health care for the poor, drove down utilization of services, and did not provide significant financial support for the health sector. By the end of the 20th century, the exclusive focus on prevention and the imposition of user fees crippled the delivery of health care in impoverished countries. This chapter presents the key historical events that influenced, and continue to influence, global health delivery.

Slavery and Colonialism

The world's poorest countries suffer from the consequences of slavery, colonialism, oppression, and resource extraction. Knowledge of the historical underpinnings of impoverishment is crucial to understand the disparities in health and health systems that result in the sickness and death of millions today. In this book, what are normally referred to as "resource-limited settings," "developing countries," or "low-income countries" will be referred to as "impoverished countries." This term credits the historical and ongoing processes that cause poverty.

The transatlantic slave trade began in the early 1400s, when the demand for labor-intensive commodities such as sugar, cotton, and tobacco increased.[3] European imperial powers enslaved Africans to fill the new demand for hard labor. Although forms of slavery existed since ancient times, the transatlantic slave trade was unprecedented in scale, both geographically and temporally. It spanned three continents for almost five centuries. Europeans and Americans, backed by their governments and civil institutions, committed crimes against humanity and violence of the most extreme order to enslave people. These atrocities enabled massive and continued profits for the United States and Europe, shaping the distribution of resources in the world today. By 1700, slaves had replaced gold as West Africa's most profitable export. An estimated 15 million Africans were forced into slavery. The crossing of the Atlantic alone killed at least 20 percent of those forced onto slave ships.[4] The slave trade wrought immediate suffering and fragmentation of the population as well as protracted impoverishment of countries. In contrast, the United States' economic and political hegemony was built, in large part, by slave labor. The gross domestic product (GDP) per capita in the United States today is $56,116, whereas it is only $818 in France's former slave colony of Haiti and $653 in England's former colony of Sierra Leone.[5] Between 1619 and 1865, European settlers in the United States extracted an estimated 222,505,049 hours of forced labor from African slaves, worth $97 trillion at the current US minimum wage. This amount is more than the combined GDP of all of the world's countries today.[6]

Europeans arrived in the Americas in 1492 and killed the vast majority of the indigenous people through disease, murder, slavery, and starvation. Their genocidal rule reduced the indigenous population from 50–100 million to 3.5 million by the mid-1600s.[6] European powers, using indigenous and later African slave labor, extracted 100 million kilograms of silver alone from land in what is now Latin America by the end of the 18th century. 100 million kilograms of silver invested in 1800 would be worth $165 trillion today.[6] Silver also provided "much of the capital for the industrial revolution" in Europe.[6]

White slavers and their governments undertook extreme efforts at every level to uphold slavery through the dehumanization of enslaved people. They attempted to justify their vicious inhumanity toward enslaved Africans at every opportunity and fabricated a network of lies to characterize Africans as inferior, nonhuman beings.[3]

The transatlantic slave trade devastated African societies through both the enslavement of people and the dismantling of political and economic structures. European powers and their allies forcibly removed entire populations and pitted neighboring civilizations against each other in armed conflict, producing long-lasting animosity for generations to come.[4] Slave uprisings—most notably the Haitian revolution—made the enslavement of free people a frightening proposition to colonists. The successful Haitian revolution, the many slave uprisings, and a global abolitionist movement finally ended the transatlantic slave trade in 1807. This made it illegal to enslave free people. However, slavery continued in the United States and Europe as people born into slavery were still considered private property and thus could be bought and sold.

By decimating populations and institutionalizing a narrative of white supremacy the transatlantic slave trade primed Africa for the taking by European colonial powers at the end of the 19th century. European colonialism accelerated in sub-Saharan Africa when European powers established colonial governments across the continent during the infamous *scramble for Africa* in the late 1800s. At the Berlin Conference in 1884, Britain, France, Germany, Portugal, Belgium, and others European countries divided the African continent. The Europeans concerned with maintaining their share of African resources and imposed violence on millions of Africans to do so.[7] When European powers colonized Africa, they provided land and opportunities for their own growing populations and they extracted natural resources and labor from the continent to amass wealth for individuals and empires.[8] The Congo, for example, was a private venture for Belgium's King Leopold, from which he extracted an estimated $1.1 billion worth of rubber.[9] Apart from resource extraction, the colonial rule of Africa also changed the societal structure of the continent.[8] Through brutal conditions and the justification of Africans as lesser beings, Europe "imposed its will on Africa at the point of a gun."[7] Colonial powers committed numerous human rights atrocities across the continent.[9]

The impact of slavery and colonialism on the human mind of the oppressed and the oppressor is profound and is the subject of past and present scholarship by exceptional black thinkers. Aime Césaire, a famous author from Martinique, was part of the pan-Africanist struggles of the 1950s. Césaire wrote, in his famous essay "Discourse on Colonialism" that to understand what colonialism is, is "to agree on what it is not: [it is] neither evangelization nor a philanthropic enterprise, nor a desire to push back the frontiers of ignorance, disease, and tyranny, nor a project undertaken for the greater glory of God, nor an attempt to extend the rule of law."[10] Césaire saw colonialism, simply, as plunder. Similarly, one of the greatest thinkers on black identity, Dr. Frantz Fanon, a psychiatrist from Martinique.[11] Underlined the violent mental subjugation of the colonized black psyche.[11,12] The choke-hold he described was perpetuated by the notion of white supremacy and the black inferiority it demands. In "The Wretched of the Earth," Fanon writes: "When we revolt it's not for a particular culture. We revolt simply because, for many reasons, we can no longer breathe."[11] In the United States, many voices have rejected and continue to reject the notion of white racial superiority. Prominent thinkers, from Frederick Douglass[13] to James Baldwin[14] to Ta-Nehisi Coates[15] identify race as a social construct needed to justify the oppression of a group and the creation of an underclass needed to maximize profit. Coates says: "race is the child of racism."[15] These authors and others document the powerful, race-based hatred and the notion of white supremacy that permeates Western society. Many of these beliefs undergird the global distribution of resources today. Africa is the richest continent. Yet resource extraction continues to enrich the powerful outside of Africa and impoverish the people of the continent (Figure 1.1). Descendants of the slave trade throughout the Americas and the Caribbean also continue to bear this burden of impoverishment.

This brief overview does not fully cover the complicated, long-term impacts of slavery and colonialism, nor does it cover resistance movements. It simply points out the vast injustices that have taken place throughout history that set the stage for today's profound inequality. Rooting the analysis of global health

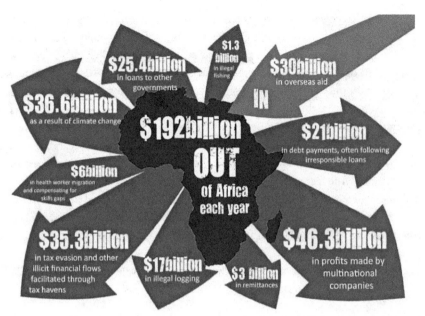

FIGURE I.I Since colonialism, the continent of Africa has been subject to massive amounts of resource extraction, both legal and illegal. This figure highlights the massive ongoing resource extraction from Africa, the world's richest continent. In comparison, only a small amount of aid is received, barely larger than the payment on debt.

Source: Sharples N, Jones T, Martin C. Honest accounts? The true story of Africa's billion dollar losses. Curtis Research. 2014.

inequalities in the ideology of white supremacy helps to elucidate why severe inequality is accepted today. Achieving justice against this backdrop will require significant transfers of wealth and, some would say, reparations. Yet, as anthropologist Dr. Jason Hickel points out, "the reparations debate is threatening because it completely upends the usual narrative of development. Talk of reparations, as opposed to charity or development assistance, suggests that poverty in the global south is not a natural phenomenon, but has been actively created. The idea of reparations casts western countries in the role not of benefactors, but of plunderers."[6]

The colonial state was unconcerned with the health of indigenous populations. Colonial medicine (the antecedent to tropical medicine and international health) was practiced largely to protect colonists against local diseases.[16,17] The narrative of protection against African diseases continues into the present day. The discourse of biosecurity is based on a fear of contagion rather the right to health or compassion for the suffering. In the 2013–2016 Ebola pandemic, disease control was promoted to protect the wealthy rather than to treat the sick. The US press, for example, focused more attention on the potential import of bush-meat into the country than on the thousands of Africans who were dying without treatment. The cover of *Newsweek* on August 29, 2014, featured a large photograph of a chimpanzee with the heading "A Back Door for Ebola, Smuggled Bushmeat Could Spark a US Epidemic."[18] The focus on bushmeat was factually incorrect. Even in Ebola-affected countries where some people hunt, sell, and consume wild animals, the epidemic was due to human-to-human transmission: there was never a verified case that the disease came from bushmeat. Furthermore, the focus on bushmeat serves a racist narrative that exoticizes Africans. For example, two Rwandan children were excluded from school in New Jersey due to fears of Ebola in Africans. Rwanda, 2,600 miles from West Africa, never had a single case of the disease.[19] The fear seen during the Ebola pandemic also represents a powerful undercurrent to the wider American discourse around global health, one in which global health interventions are regarded by leading policymakers as worth funding only to expand American influence, protect the US population against epidemic threats, or prevent violent extremism. When these are the underlying reasons for aid, the politics of fear, isolationism, and racism supercede the principle of health as a human right.

Human Rights

Prior to World War II, the conduct of a government against its own people may have seemed objectionable or deplorable but was generally considered a matter of national sovereignty.[20,21] However, upon the liberation of the Nazi concentration camps, a global sea-change occurred. The sea-change was the notion that all people, regardless of their country of origin, have an inalienable set of human rights.[22] In 1948, coinciding with the Nuremberg Trials,[23] broad support for these principles was enshrined in the Universal Declaration of Human Rights (UDHR) (Figure 1.2A–C).

Remarkably, the Declaration was unanimously supported with only two abstentions: Russia and South Africa.[24,25] The Declaration held that governments were the guarantors of the rights of their citizens, and thereby responsible for "respecting, protecting and fulfilling" those rights.[26] The population—also called "civil society"[27,28]—was charged with demanding that governments uphold their responsibilities as guarantors.[29] Of note, at the time of UDHR, the only independent countries on the African continent were South Africa, Egypt, Ethiopia, and Liberia.[30] European countries that championed human rights had little problem continuing colonialism and denying colonized people their human rights.[31]

Human rights work since the drafting of the UDHR has been two-pronged. The first prong highlights the government's responsibilities to "respect, protect, and fulfill" human rights.[26] The second prong of human rights work is to educate

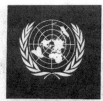

FIGURE 1.2 The Universal Declaration of Human Rights (A) English version of a poster depicting the Universal Declaration of Human Rights. The Declaration was adopted and proclaimed by United Nations General Assembly Resolution 217A III of 10 December 1948. (B) Mrs. Eleanor Roosevelt of the United States holding a Declaration of Human Rights poster in English. (C) These children of United Nations staff members are getting a closer look at the Universal Declaration of Human Rights, which is 2 years old on December 10, 1950. All nations in the world have been invited to set aside December 10 of every year as Human Rights Day.

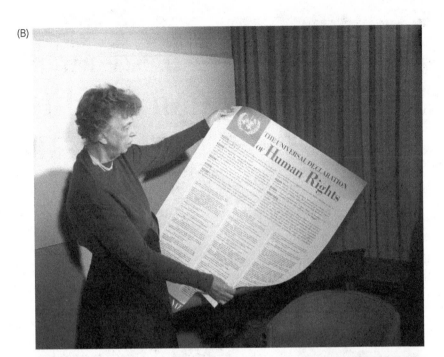

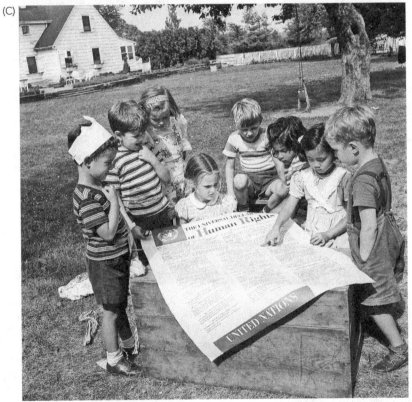

FIGURE I.2 Continued

civil society (the general populous of the country) to demand their rights.[29,32] In the UDHR, the right to health is bundled with other rights, such as food, clothing, shelter, and employment, under Article 25[26] which states:

> Everyone has the right to a standard of living adequate for the health and well-being of himself and of his family, including food, clothing, housing and medical care and necessary social services, and the right to security in the event of unemployment, sickness, disability, widowhood, old age or other lack of livelihood in circumstances beyond his control.

In the post-World War II period, the United Nations, a family of organizations, was created as a structure for international cooperation.[33] In the field of health, this responsibility fell to the World Health Organization (WHO) whose charter, drafted in 1947, contained the following statement:[34]

> The enjoyment of the highest attainable standard of health is one of the fundamental rights of every human being without distinction of race, religion, political belief, economic or social condition.

The WHO further elaborated the definition of health as "a state of complete physical, mental and social well-being and not merely the absence of disease and infirmity."[34]

Yet, as aspirational as the sentiments of the WHO or the UDHR were, such declarations and charters have no legal weight. Declarations state ideals. In contrast, treaties oblige signatories to develop a legal framework in their own country to put the language of the treaty into law.[35] Nearly two decades after the Nuremberg trial and the signing of the UDHR, there were no treaties that held signatories accountable for human rights. By the 1950s, a new conflict emerged, the Cold War. The Cold War presented a great ideological divide between economic systems and forms of governance—socialism versus capitalism and authoritarianism versus democracy. Each side accused the other of human rights violations. The US criticized the Soviet Union for denying its citizens the right to vote, to speak and associate freely, and to own property. The Soviet Union, on the other hand, pointed to the lack of guaranteed health care, housing, and job security in the United States as human rights violations.[36]

In 1966, this politicization of rights resulted in two treaties: the International Covenant on Civil and Political Rights (ICCPR) and the International Covenant on Economic, Social and Cultural Rights (ICESCR) (Table 1.1).

The ICCPR was championed by the United States. It focused on the rights associated with democratic societies, including the right to free speech, assembly,

Table 1.1 Key examples of differences in the International Covenant on Civil and Political Rights and International Covenant on Economic Social and Cultural Rights.

International Covenant on Civil and Political Rights (ICCPR)	International Covenant on Economic, Social, and Cultural Rights (ICESCR)
Article 6. The right to life, protected by law	**Article 6.** The right to gain a living by work which is freely chosen or accepted
Article 7. Freedom from cruel, inhuman, or degrading treatment or punishment	
Article 8. Freedom from slavery	**Article 9.** The right to social security, including social insurance
Article 9. The right to liberty and security	
Article 12. The right to liberty of movement	**Article 11.** The right to an adequate standard of living, including food, housing, and clothing.
Article 14. All persons are equal before court and presumed innocent until proven guilty	
Article 18. The right to freedom of thought, conscience, and religion	**Article 12.** The right to the enjoyment of the highest attainable standard of physical and mental health
Article 19. The right to freedom of expression	**Article 13.** The right to education
Article 25. The right and opportunity to vote and take part in public affairs	**Article 15.** The right to take part in a cultural life; enjoy benefits of scientific progress

voting, and access to a judiciary system. The ICESCR was backed by the Soviet Union. It focused on the rights associated with socialist societies, including the right to health, employment, shelter, and education.[37]

The right to health is not cited in the US-backed ICCPR. Rather, it appears in Article 12 of the ICESCR, which states[38]:

1. The States party to the present Covenant recognize the right of everyone to the enjoyment of the highest attainable standard of physical and mental health.
2. The steps to be taken by the States party to the present Covenant to achieve the full realization of this right shall include those necessary for:
   a) The provision for the reduction of the stillbirth-rate and of infant mortality and the health development of the child;
   b) The improvement of all aspects of environmental and industrial hygiene;

c)   The prevention, treatment and control of epidemic, endemic, occupational and other diseases;

d)   The creation of conditions which would assure to all medical service and medical attention in the event of a sickness.

Many countries, most notably the social democracies of Europe, signed and ratified both covenants,[37] thus promoting both the right to the democratic ideals of freedom of speech and electoral participation as well as the socialist ideals of protection against disease and destitution. Yet, on either side of the ideological spectrum, the anchors of the Cold War—the United States and the Soviet Union—were recalcitrant to sign the treaty championed by their adversary. Both covenants came into force in 1976—the United States ratified the ICCPR in 1992, and the Soviet Union ratified the ICESCR in 1973. To this day, neither the United States nor Russia has crossed the divide to sign the opposite covenant.[38,39]

Over the ensuing years, the United States controlled the political narrative in the West and won the Cold War.[36] Thus, the Covenant on Civil and Political Rights has primacy in human rights discussions. Human rights organizations like Amnesty International and Human Rights Watch focus their efforts on fighting governments that repress civil and political rights, such as jailing those who spoke against the government or persecuting people of religious or ethnic minorities.[32,40] Meanwhile key social and economic rights, like health care and education, became marginalized in the United States. They are often referred to as "secondary rights," "privileges," or "entitlements."[41] Even today, if one reads an article about human rights it tends to focus on a government's repression of civil or political rights,[42] whereas the lack of available health care or education is almost never framed as a violation of rights. Yet, in impoverished communities, social and economic rights are paramount. The lack of these rights results in a daily life-and-death struggle for many. When impoverished people lead human rights movements, they often focus on jobs, food, health care, and water.[43–46]

Liberation Struggles

During the Cold War period, liberation struggles were taking place on the African continent.[44,47] But newly liberated African countries, while politically free, were left impoverished by the legacy of slavery, colonialism, and resource extraction. Thus, emerging leaders did not have the resources needed to deliver on their revolutionary government's promise of human rights.[48,49] Leaders like Nkrumah of Ghana and Cabral of Guinea-Bissau wanted health care, education, and jobs for their people[50,51] but found themselves cash-strapped. Their resources were owned (and continue to be owned) by private companies held by former colonial powers and by wealthy countries like the United States.[52,53] For example, the past decade has seen an increase in mineral exploration and mining activities by multinational corporations in the African copperbelt (Zambia and southern Democratic Republic of Congo [DRC]). One of the biggest mines in the DRC is the Tenke Fungurume copper mine, responsible for about 3–4 percent of the country's GDP.[54] Until recently, the American mining company Freeport-McMoRan, owned a controlling interest, 56 percent of the mine. The DRC government, in contrast, owns only 20 percent stake in the mine. In May 2016, Freeport-McMoRan sold its shares to China Molybdenum Inc. for $2.65 billion. The Congolese government was not even aware that this deal was taking place because the large corporations hid the sale in offshore subsidiaries. The covert sale cheated the Congolese government out of tax revenue on the sale of its asset.[54] In addition to the tax revenue lost in these clandestine, multinational deals, the people of the DRC also do not profit from the extraction of natural resources from within their borders.[55] In 2011, minerals accounted for about 75 percent of all exports from the Congo, and, between 2001 and 2011, the exportation of minerals from the DRC grew from just under $1 billion to $6.5 billion.[56] Within that same time period, the GDP per capita in the DRC only grew from $150.40 to $350.30 per person.[57] Throughout the impoverished world, private economic interests are protected by the powerful armies of the former colonial states and the United States.[58] Attempts by African revolutionary governments to take control of the country's riches and nationalize resources were met with swift political and military retribution from the United States, Britain, France, and others.[59,60] The DRC gained independence from Belgium on June 30, 1960. Their first legally elected Prime Minister, Patrice Lumumba, sought to advance the ideals of national unity, economic independence, and pan-African solidarity.[61,62] At the time, Lumumba wanted to control the DRC economy and devalued American and Belgian holdings in the country. These Western capitalist countries were afraid that by losing control over the mines in the DRC (particularly the uranium mines they used to make the first atomic bombs),[61,62] the profit and the resources would fall into the hands of the Soviet Union. In 1961, the United States and Belgium combined forces to support the assassination of Lumumba and install a pro-Western government eventually led by Joseph-Désiré Mobutu (later known as Mobutu Sese Seko).[61–63] Sese Seko was one of the most corrupt and notorious dictators in the world and reigned for 32 years. During this time, he personally amassed vast sums of wealth and was abetted by the United States because of his pro-corporate stance.

Thus, even as countries gained liberation from colonial rule, economic independence remained—and continues to remain—elusive. Impoverished governments, without control of their resources, sought external financial support. At the time of African liberation, the United States and the Soviet Union were the two superpowers.[64] While the Soviet Union ideologically supported a public model for development, it had much more limited coffers than Western financial institutions. Thus, the World Bank and the International Monetary Fund [IMF] became the dominant entities in financing development.[65]

The Rise of the World Bank

In 1944, as World War II was being fought, Allied nations held an important meeting called the United Nations Monetary and Financial Conference in Bretton Woods, New Hampshire.[66] The purpose of the conference was to stabilize currency fluctuations and support the rebuilding of Europe. At the conference, the Articles of Agreement of the International Monetary Fund and the International Bank for Reconstruction and Development (IBRD, later part of the World Bank) were drafted. The IMF was created to regulate monetary policy by setting exchange rates and controlling the flow of capital. These policies aimed to prevent the hyperinflation thought to underpin the rise of fascism in Europe.[66] The IBRD was created to help rebuild Europe because all parties agreed that postwar reconstruction and development were "essential to the general economic interest" of the world.[66] Initially, the IBRD and IMF, collectively known as the international financial institutions (IFI), focused on Europe's need for large-scale development projects such as dams and roads.[67]

Several factors shaped the World Bank and IMF in the 1970s and '80s. First, when the United States implemented the Marshall Plan[68] to support the reconstruction of Europe, the World Bank shifted its attention to impoverished countries. Second, as the Cold War escalated, the World Bank, a US-led institution, promoted capitalism as a means to achieve economic development[69] and to prevent the spread of communism.[70] Third, when oil prices quadrupled in the 1970s, the consortium of oil-producing countries (known as the Organization of the Petroleum Exporting Countries or OPEC) invested heavily in the World Bank. OPEC expected a large return on investment based on the anticipated growth of the economies of impoverished countries.[71]

The World Bank and IMF rose in prominence just as liberated African countries searched for capital. The IFIs advanced capital to the impoverished countries of Africa, Asia, and Latin America in the form of loans. Between 1970 and the mid-1980s, the number of IMF programs doubled[67,72] and the external indebtedness of impoverished nations rose from $64 billion to $686 billion.[73] The United States is a major contributor to the IMF with 16 percent of vote.[74] The United States also holds the presidency of the World Bank.[67] The Soviet Union was never a member of the either of the IFIs.[75] Retrospective studies have found that IMF decisions on loan applications were highly political, and countries that aligned with capitalist ideologies were far more likely to be granted loans.[76] The IFIs initially gave loans with low interest rates; however, when commodity and oil prices fell[72] in the 1980s, economies crashed. Inflation racked the globe. In response, the IFIs drastically increased interest rates on the loans.[73] Countries in economic crisis could not keep up with the increased interest payments and sank further into debt.[73]

Neoliberal Economic Theory and Structural Adjustment Policies

During the 1970s and 1980s, neoliberal economic theory was the dominant model for development.[77] Neoliberal theory rests on the principle that economies should be controlled solely by the laws of supply and demand or what economists call the "invisible hand of the market"[78] and that government intervention decreases economic efficiency and therefore profit.[79] As the prominence and the available capital of the IFIs grew, Friedrich Hayek and Milton Friedman, the respective 1974 and 1976 Nobel Prize winners in Economics,[80] actively promoted neoliberalism. Their model not only derided the government provision of services to fulfill human rights (such as public education and health care), but conflated privatization with freedom. In his famous book, *Capitalism and Freedom*, Friedman stated that government regulations hampered the free market and made people less free to pursue their self-interests.[79]

Echoes of Hayek and Friedman continue to permeate political discourse around the world. In 2017, the U.S. Congress debated the repeal of the Affordable Care Act—a government-subsidized plan to increase health insurance coverage. U.S. Speaker of the House of Representatives Paul Ryan (Republican from Wisconsin) used Friedman's neoliberal language linking capitalism to freedom in describing why he sought to end the government subsidies for health insurance under the US Affordable Care Act (Obamacare) (Figure 1.3 (A, B)). Ryan and other neoliberals prioritize market freedom over freedom rooted in human rights that comes from having good health and not facing destitution because of health care costs. The Speaker's description of freedom was rejected by many in government and civil society.[81] His bill to repeal the Affordable Care act did not pass.

In the 1990s, U.S. President Ronald Reagan and British Prime Minister Margaret Thatcher, staunch anticommunists, believed that neoliberal principles and unfettered free-market capitalism was a critical part of their Cold War armamentarium. Reagan and Thatcher promoted neoliberalism at home and abroad.[82,83] At home, they tried to dismantle the government provision of social and economic rights, such as old-age pensions and low-income housing.[84] Abroad, Reagan and Thatcher shaped World Bank and IMF lending policies for impoverished countries throughout the 1980s and 1990s.[85]

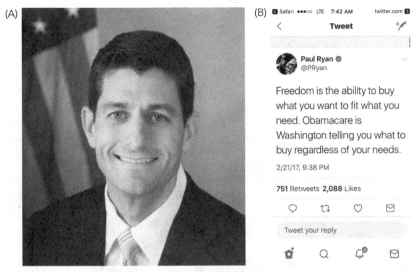

FIGURE 1.3 A, B In attempt to end the US Affordable Care Act which provides government subsidies for health insurance as a means to cover the poor and vulnerable US Speaker of the House of Representatives Paul Ryan (A) tweeted (B) "Freedom is the ability to buy what you want to fit what you need. Obamacare is Washington telling you what to buy regardless of your needs." Feb 21, 2017, 12.38 PM. Tweet by Ryan (PRyan). Ryan's tweet reiterates a common theme of neoliberalism stemming from Milton Friedman's *Capitalism as Freedom*.[79] Friedman, Ryan, and others believe that a free market without control of government intervention is freedom. This is in contrast with the human rights approach to freedom which links the fulfillment of rights to a decrease in suffering by assuring protection against harm and destitution.

A is courtesy of House.gov. Biography of Paul D. Ryan. 2017. Available from: http://paulryan. house.gov/. Accessed May 4, 2017.

World Bank loans and IMF fiscal controls were tied to conditions known as *structural adjustment programs* (SAPs).[76] The SAPs forced recipient countries to severely reduce public expenditures and favor private-sector investments by giving tax breaks to businesses, reducing protective import tariffs, or awarding private contracts for infrastructure.[86] Governments accepting SAPs were not permitted to spend government money that would create a deficit. While it may seem like sound fiscal advice not to create a deficit, the United States and Europe have relied on deficit spending for infrastructure and other government programs to build the middle class and protect citizens from destitution.[87,88] The aggregate impact of SAPs resulted in fewer civil servants (including doctors, teachers, and nurses) on the government payroll, little money for public infrastructure (hospitals, schools, and water sanitation), and no money for public goods (medicines).[89,90] The excellent film *Life and Debt* is a primer on the effect of World Bank and IMF policy in Jamaica.[91] The movie highlights the impact of SAPs on

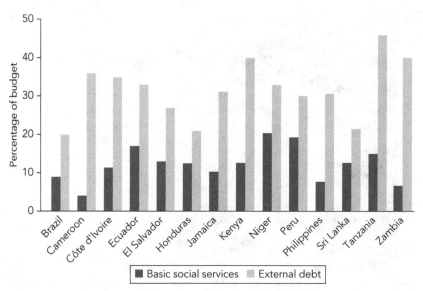

FIGURE 1.4 This figure demonstrates the overwhelming debt compared to funds dedicated to basic social services, including health care, in 1998. (UNICEF and UNDP figures, 1998).

Adapted from Vandemoortele J. *Absorbing social shocks, protecting children, and reducing poverty: The role of basic social services.* UNICEF Staff Working Paper. New York: UNICEF, January 2000, p. 26.

agriculture subsidies and the massively unequal power dynamic between the IFIs and the Jamaican government. The principles of this story were repeated throughout the world as SAPs hit health care, education, and other public services while debt repayments skyrocketed (Figure 1.4).

The restrictions on public expenditures and the prohibition on deficit spending meant that countries that were already impoverished by colonialism were left unable to deliver on social and economic rights—from health to education, job security to housing. By the late 1980s, health budgets in many African and Asian countries were less than $5 per person per year.[92]

The Alma Ata International Conference on Primary Health Care

Despite the economic constraints faced by impoverished countries, health remained an obvious and critical need. The leaders of newly liberated yet impoverished countries looked for models to provide care to large numbers of the poor and sick. In 1978, the International Conference on Primary Health Care was held in Alma Ata in the Soviet Union (currently Almaty, Kazakhstan). The Conference, also known as Alma Ata, hosted 600 representatives from the 150

WHO member states, including health ministers and experts.[93] The conference, sponsored by the WHO and United Nations International Children's Emergency Fund (UNICEF), aimed to discuss models for care delivery and develop solutions to reach the 2 billion people living without health care.

In parallel to the Cold War, socialist republics and capitalist states debated how to deliver health care in impoverished countries. The socialist republics advocated for government funds to deliver on the promise of health as a human right by building public health systems with doctors, nurses, and hospitals. Capitalist states argued that health systems could not be built until economic growth occurred. In the meantime, capitalist states reasoned, volunteers could be used to deliver health basic services in impoverished countries. The majority of delegates advocated for the public provision of health as a human right. Despite the deep ideological differences between the United States and the Soviet Union, the meeting was reported to "have ended with a strong sense of a landmark achieved."[93]

The landmark was a consensus document known as the Declaration of Alma Ata.[94] It famously proposed "Health for all by the Year 2000" (Box 1.1). The declaration advocated for health as a human right and included the need to address the social factors related to ill health, such as lack of food, water, and sanitation.[95] Alma Ata's goals for the progressive realization of the right to health were modest yet concrete: 90 percent of children should have weight for age that corresponds to reference values, every family should be within a 15-minute walk of potable water, and women should have access to medically trained attendants for childbirth.[94]

The Declaration also recognized the need for international financing to achieve "health for all"[94]:

> An acceptable level of health for all the people of the world by the year 2000 can be attained through a fuller and better use of the world's resources, a considerable part of which is now spent on armaments and military conflicts. A genuine policy of independence, peace, détente, and disarmament could and should release additional resources that could well be devoted to peaceful aims and in particular to the acceleration of social and economic development of which primary health care, as an essential part, should be allotted its proper share.[94]

The concepts that health demanded more resources than those available within an impoverished country's budget and that health should be financed through international collaboration were radical notions. The declaration placed part of the burden of the fulfillment of the right to health on the international community, not just on the nation state itself. Yet, the theory that reduced military spending would allow governments to invest in health and other social and economic rights

BOX 1.1

Declaration of Alma-Ata

I. Health is a fundamental human right and attainment of the highest possible level of health is a most important worldwide social goal.

II. The existing gross inequality in the health status of the people, particularly between developed and developing countries is politically, socially and economically unacceptable and is of common concern to all countries.

III. Economic and social development is of basic importance to the fullest attainment of health for all. The promotion and protection of the health of the people is essential to sustained economic and social development and contributes to a better quality of life and to world peace.

IV. The people have the right and duty to participate individually and collectively in the planning and implementation of their health care.

V. Governments have a responsibility for the health of their people which can be fulfilled only by the provision of adequate health and social measures. The goal is the attainment by all the peoples of the world by the year 2000 a level of health that will permit them to lead a socially and economically productive life. Primary health care is the key to attaining this target as part of development in the spirit of social justice.

VI. Primary health care is essential health care based on practical, scientifically sound and socially acceptable methods and technology made universally accessible to individuals and families in the community.

VII. Primary health care:
   A. Reflects and evolves from the economic conditions and sociocultural and political characteristics of the country and its communities
   B. Addresses the main health problems in the community, providing promotive, preventive, curative and rehabilitative services accordingly
   C. Includes at least: education concerning prevailing health problems, promotion of food supply and proper nutrition, adequate supply of safe water and basic sanitation, maternal and child health care including family planning, immunization, prevention and control of locally endemic diseases, provision of essential drugs, appropriate treatment of common diseases

D. Involves all related sectors and aspects of national and community development

E. Requires and promotes maximum community and individual self-reliance and participation in planning

F. Should be sustained by integrated, functional and mutually supportive referral systems, giving priority to the most in need

G. Relies on health workers suitably trained socially and technically to work as a health team

VIII. All governments should formulate national policies and plans of action to launch and sustain primary health care as part of a comprehensive national health system.

IX. All countries should cooperate in a spirit of partnership and service to ensure primary "health care for all people."

X. An acceptable level of health for all people by 2000 can be attained through a fuller and better use of the world's resources.

was not met with the commensurate political will to do so.[96,97] Rapidly after Alma Ata, the notion of sustainability—that is, to do only what a country can afford on its domestic health budget—became the yardstick for assessing if a country could expand access to care. And at this time, the domestic health budgets of African countries were still about $5 per person per year (Figure 1.5). The international collaboration to finance health that was proposed at Alma Ata was decades away. Programs that could be sustained on just $5 per person per year took center stage for the next 25 years.

Selective Primary Health Care: An Interim Strategy?

The year after the Alma Ata conference, Julia Walsh and Kenneth Warren published a seminal paper in the prestigious *New England Journal of Medicine* entitled, "Selective Primary Health Care: An Interim Strategy for Disease Control in Developing Countries."[98] The paper offered an alternative approach to the aspiration of "health for all." These authors argued that while the goals set at Alma Ata were laudable, their achievement was unrealistic given the impoverishment of those countries with the highest disease burden. Instead, Walsh and Warren argued that it was more realistic to target scarce resources to prevent and control

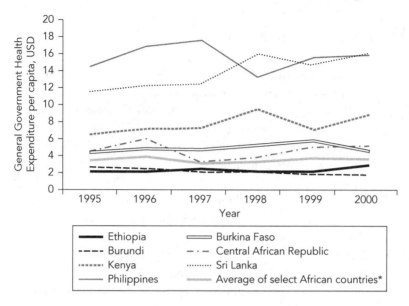

* Countries included are Burkina Faso, Burundi, Ethiopia, and Central African Republic

FIGURE 1.5 Graph of government health expenditure per capita in selected regions and countries, 1995–2000. Government health spending on health care depends on geographical location and economic development. African countries have by far the lowest government spending on health. All values in 2016 US dollars per capita.

Data adapted from WHO Global Health Expenditure Database, last updated Oct 24, 2016 http://apps.who.int/nha/database.

the spread of diseases that accounted for the highest mortality and morbidity. They called this approach *selective primary health care* (SPHC).[98]

The concept of selective primary health care was based on the notion of sustainability, rooted in the neoliberal economic paradigm. It was promoted by donors, particularly the United States, who did not support the development of publicly financed health systems. The authors and supporters of selective primary health care reasoned that simple interventions could be administered by lay, volunteer health workers and sustained on the very meager budgets of the impoverished countries. The diseases marked as priorities for this approach were those that could be easily prevented or controlled by low-cost technology (such as a vaccination). This, too, is a legacy of colonization and is often referred to as "problem choice" by historians. Colonial governments chose to fund only public health measures that protected Europeans. The legacy of "problem choice" that focused on disease control instead of treatment continued to define health priorities in African countries for generations.[16]

Estimated Annual Costs of Different Systems of Health Intervention

Intervention	Per capita cost ($)	Cost per infant and/or child death averted* ($)
Basic primary health care†		
Range	0.40–7.50	144–20,000 (I)
Median	2.00	700
Mosquito control for malaria	2.00	600 (I)
Onchocerciasis control program	0.90	Few infant & child deaths
Mollusk control for schistosomiasis	3.70	Few infant & child deaths
Community water supplies & sanitation	30–54	3600–4300 (I,C)
Narangwal nutrition supplimentation	1.75	213 (I) 3000 (C)
Selective primary health care‡	0.25	200–250 (I,C)

*I denotes infant & C child.   † Delivered by village health workers.
‡In this case, delivered by mobile units.

FIGURE 1.6   Estimated annual costs of selective primary health care interventions, 1979. *Source*: Walsh JA, Warren KS. Selective Primary Health Care an Interim Strategy for Disease Control in Developing Countries. *N Engl J Med.* 1979;301:967–974.

Selective primary care focused on the prevention not treatment of disease.[98] Of note, the cost for selective primary health care at that time was estimated at $0.25 per person per year (Figure 1.6).

UNICEF adopted selective primary health care because it focused on children under five years of age. In 1983, UNICEF, under the leadership of the charismatic American Executive Director Jim Grant, launched what Grant called the "child survival revolution."[99] In UNICEF's 1982–1983 report, "The State of the World's Children," a plan was proposed for a package of interventions, based on selective primary health care, to combat common causes of child mortality. The concept was later dubbed GOBI. [99] GOBI stands for:

- *Growth* monitoring of children (with nutritional education for mothers if the children are underweight)
- The distribution of a salt and sugar mixture called *oral* rehydration solution (ORS) to prevent death from dehydration associated with diarrheal disease
- The promotion of exclusive *breastfeeding* until age six months and continuation of breastfeeding until age two years
- *Immunization* of children

When GOBI was launched, ORS and childhood immunizations were considered scientific advancements. Oral rehydration salts (first used in 1964[100]) and measles vaccination (developed in 1960[101]) were portable and could be delivered in communities from backpacks. This strategy was appealing because it leap-frogged over inadequate health systems.[102,103] Due to its simplicity and the backing of UNICEF, GOBI was widely adopted.[99,102] For the next 25 years, impoverished countries delivered little curative health care for children or adults. However, the child survival revolution did improve under-five child mortality. In the 15 years between 1983 and 1998, under-five child mortality dropped from 107.3 to 80.6 per 1,000 live births globally.[104] This success was credited to widespread use of ORS and infant vaccinations as well as to economic development in India and China.[105,106]

Some decried GOBI because it only targeted specific diseases and ignored the need for human resources.[107] Many also recognized that GOBI did not address the underlying socioeconomic factors that led to ill health.[108] It was widely understood that GOBI did not address the need for more comprehensive health systems; but, without donor funds, these simple interventions, applied under the rubric of neoliberalism, remained ubiquitous.[107] While selective primary health care and GOBI started as an interim strategy, further plans and resources for the progressive realization of the right to health were not forthcoming.

The Bamako Initiative

Governments of impoverished countries knew that GOBI was inadequate to address the needs of their populations. However, on their meager national health budgets and restricted by SAPs, clinics and hospitals were woefully underfunded. Health care workers were infrequently paid and pharmacies lacked basic medications and supplies.[109] The sick therefore sought consultations and drugs in private clinics or pharmacies. Those who could not afford private care sought care from local healers, who also charged for services. Those who did seek care at moribund public facilities were asked for fees to cover gloves, syringes, and medicines. This fragmentation resulted in a high death rate in impoverished countries and unequal outcomes between the rich and the poor.[110]

In order to finance the public provision of care, Jim Grant of UNICEF and Dr. Halfdan Mahler, then-Director General of the WHO, held a meeting of African health ministers in Bamako, Mali, in 1987.[111] At this meeting, UNICEF suggested a plan for generating revenue to pay for health locally by charging a fee to patients.[112] This initiative was based on reportedly successful pilot projects in Benin and Ghana in communities with populations of 12,000 and 30,000 people, respectively.[112] In these pilot programs, drugs were sold at a two- to threefold markup, and the profits were deposited in a revolving fund to restock the drugs and pay health workers. The Bamako Initiative proposed scaling up these pilot programs throughout Africa as the standard model for public facilities at the primary care level. Many expressed serious concerns about the inequity that would result if this approach was used.

Critics understood that the poorest and most vulnerable people would be least able to pay the fees.[112,113] A World Bank study from that time showed that 40 percent of Kenyans could not afford the proposed fees.[111] Despite these concerns, the Bamako Initiative of 1987 promoted the idea of cost recovery through the implementation of user fees[112] and had wide support from African governments and international partners. African Ministers signed on. The Initiative received significant funding from UNICEF[112,114] for the initial supply of drugs.

The Bamako Initiative became gospel in the ensuing decades—user fees were part of the pay mix throughout most of the impoverished world.[115] A payment of about $0.50 to $1 dollar was levied for medical consultation, needed drugs, and sometimes basic laboratory services. There were two problems with user fees. First, any user fee, copay, or cost recovery is a barrier to health for poor people.[114,116] The initiative resulted in unequal access to care and drove down utilization.[114,116] Second, the money collected through user fees was not enough to adequately pay staff or stock pharmacies. Clinics financed through the meager government health budget and the Bamako Initiative's user fees were plagued by staff absenteeism, frequent stock-outs, and low utilization.[116] Despite these problems, many African governments were stuck with about $5 per capita to spend on health from federal budgets and the local, paltry inputs from user fees. Ultimately, the sum of this money was not enough to fulfill the right to health (Table 1.2).

Table 1.2 Cost of some interventions, post Bamako, 1990s.

Intervention	Cost (USD)
Measles, mumps, and rubella vaccination	$1.30 per person (1998)
Diphtheria and tetanus vaccination	$0.07 per person (1998)
Polio vaccination	$0.13 per dose, minimum 3 doses required (1998)
Standard 6 months non–multidrug resistant tuberculosis treatment (rifampicin, isoniazid, and pyrazinamide)	$55.45 per person (1999)
Permethrin impregnated rectangular bednet, cost per year (Binka, Mensah, and Mills 1997, 229–239)	$2.40 (1993/1994)
Standard 1-year HIV medication (ART)	$10,000 (1998)
Reduced osmolarity ORS per patient	$0.13 (1999)

All data from the International Drug Price Indicator Guide, unless otherwise indicated. (MSH and WHO).

ART, antiretroviral therapy.

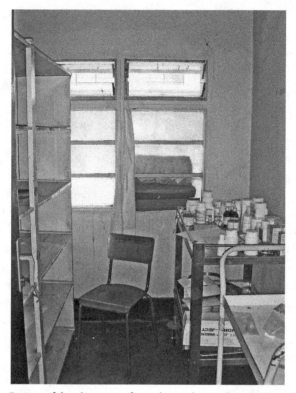

FIGURE 1.7 Picture of the pharmacy of Rwinkwavu hospital, 2005. War and decades of impoverishment leaves the public health sector destitute. At that time, the hospital was indeed open. But had few staff, almost no medications and saw just a few patients per day. Courtesy of Joia Mukherjee. Rwinkwavu, Rwanda.

Table 1.2 shows some of the costs for the commodities needed to provide health. The cost of even simple interventions (vaccines, bed nets, ORS) comes close to the $5 per capita budget. There is no room in the budget to pay health workers, operate and maintain facilities, and supply essential drugs. To this day, it is common to see only one or two staff in a clinic that serves 10,000 or 20,000 people, an empty pharmacy with only ORS sachets, a small propane fridge for vaccines (donated by UNICEF), and a building in disrepair without electricity or running water (Figure 1.7).

Conclusion

It is impossible to understand global health delivery without understanding the destructive history of slavery, colonialism, and neoliberalism that left governments impoverished and unable to fulfill the right to health. Despite the aspiration of "health for all" laid out in the Declaration of Alma Ata, selective primary health care was the sole focus of health delivery in most impoverished countries for decades. GOBI was developed to prevent some childhood illnesses and was delivered on the meager health budgets of impoverished countries with the support of UNICEF. Although the "child health revolution" succeeded in decreasing under-five mortality, it did not address the health needs of populations nor the underlying causes of ill health. Impoverished governments agreed to implement the recommendations of the Bamako Initiative to create revolving funds for essential medicines and payroll. The fees proved to be an insurmountable barrier for poor people to access health systems and did not fund needed services. By the mid-1990s, impoverished countries had huge debts, meagre health budgets, and exceptionally weak health systems.

References

1. World Health Organization (WHO). Life expectancy at birth (years) 2000–2015. Available from: http://gamapserver.who.int/gho/interactive_charts/mbd/life_expectancy/atlas.htm
2. Dickman SL, Himmelstein DU, Woolhandler S. Inequality and the health-care system in the USA. *Lancet.* 2017;389(10077):1431–1441.
3. Iliffe J. *Africans: The history of a continent.* New York: Cambridge University Press; 1995.
4. Hazard A. The Atlantic slave trade: What too few textbooks told you. Available from: http://ed.ted.com/lessons/the-atlantic-slave-trade-what-your-textbook-never-told-you-anthony-hazard. Accessed May 26, 2017.
5. World Bank. World Bank Country and Lending Groups. Available from: https://datahelpdesk.worldbank.org/knowledgebase/articles/906519-world-bank-country-and-lending-groups. Accessed March 29, 2017.
6. Hickel J. Enough of aid—let's talk reparations. *The Guardian.* Nov 27, 2015. Available from: https://www.theguardian.com/global-development-professionals-network/2015/nov/27/enough-of-aid-lets-talk-reparations. Accessed May 23, 2017.
7. Pakenham T. *The scramble for Africa. White man's conquest of the dark continent from 1876–1912.* New York: Avon Books; 1992.
8. Rodney W. *How Europe underdeveloped Africa.* Washington, DC: Howard University Press; 1982. p. 85–89.
9. Hochschild A. *King Leopold's ghost: A story of greed, terror, and heroism in colonial Africa.* Boston, MA: Mariner Books—Houghton Mifflin Harcourt; 1998.
10. Césaire A. *Discourse on colonialism.* New York: Présence Africaine; 1955.
11. Fanon F. *The wretched of the Earth.* New York: Grove Press; 1963.
12. Fanon F. *Black skin, white masks.* New York: Grove Press; 1967.

13. Douglass F. *Narrative of the life of Frederick Douglass, an American slave.* Harmondsworth, UK; New York: Penguin Books; 1982.

14. Leeming DA. *James Baldwin: A biography.* 1st ed. New York: Alfred A. Knopf Inc.; 1994.

15. Coates T. *Between the world and me.* 1st ed. New York: Spiegel & Grau; 2015.

16. Farmer P, Kim JY, Kleinman A, Basilico M. *Reimagining global health: An introduction.* Berkeley: University of California Press; 2013.

17. Greene J, Weigel J, Motgi A, Bor J, Keshavjee S. Colonial medicine and its legacies. In: Farmer P, Kim JY, Kleinman A, Basilico M, editors. *Reimagining global health* (pp. 33–73). Berkeley: University of California Press; 2013.

18. Flynn G, Scutti S. Smuggled bushmeat is Ebola's back door to America. *Newsweek.* 2014.

19. McMurry E. Elementary school throws Ebola tantrum over two kids from Rwanda. Available from: http://www.mediaite.com/tv/elementary-school-throws-ebola-tantrum-over-two-kids-from-rwanda/. Accessed May 29, 2017.

20. Axworthy L. Human security and global governance: Putting people first; *Global Governance.* 2001;7(1):19–23.

21. Dubow S. *South Africa's struggle for human rights.* Athens: Ohio University Press; 2012. Available from: http://nrs.harvard.edu/urn-3:hul.ebookbatch.PMUSE_batch:muse9780821444405. Accessed September 30, 2016.

22. Morsink J. *The Universal Declaration of Human Rights.* Philadelphia: University of Pennsylvania Press; 2000. Available from: http://muse.jhu.edu.ezp-prod1.hul.harvard.edu/book/305. Accessed September 30, 2016.

23. Taylor T. *Nuremberg Trials: War crimes and international law.* New York: Literary Licensing, LLC; 1949.

24. Glendon MA, Abrams E. Reflections on the UDHR. *First Things.* 1998;82:23–27. Available from: http://ezp-prod1.hul.harvard.edu/login?url=http://search.ebsco-host.com.ezp-prod1.hul.harvard.edu/login.aspx?direct=true&db=a6h&AN=ATLA0000991787&site=ehost-live&scope=site. Accessed September 30, 2016.

25. Glendon MA. *A world made new: Eleanor Roosevelt and the Universal Declaration of Human Rights.* 1st ed. New York: Random House; 2001.

26. United Nations GA. *Universal Declaration of Human Rights. Final authorized text.* New York: United Nations Dept. of Public Information; 1952.

27. Carothers T, Barndt W. Civil society. *Foreign Policy.* 1999(117):18–29. Available from: http://www.jstor.org/stable/1149558. Accessed October 3, 2016. doi:10.2307/1149558.

28. Hegel GWF. *The philosophy of right; the philosophy of history.* Chicago, IL: Encyclopædia Britannica; 1952.

29. Amnesty International. Amnesty International. 2017. https://www.amnesty.org/en/

30. Brittain V. The 20th century: Africa. *The Guardian.* Jan 2, 1999. Available from: https://www.theguardian.com/world/1999/jan/02/uganda.westafrica. Accessed May 3, 2017.

31. Elkins C. *Imperial reckoning: The untold story of Britain's Gulag in Kenya.* 1st ed. New York: Henry Holt and Company; 2005.

32. Human Rights Watch. Human Rights Watch. 2017. https://www.hrw.org/

33. United Nations. History of the United Nations. Available from: http://www.un.org/en/sections/history/history-united-nations/index.html. Accessed May 3, 2017.

34. World Health Organization. *Chronicle of the World Health Organization.* Geneva: World Health Organization; 1947.

35. Flowers N. A human rights glossary. University of Minnesota Human Rights Resource Center Website. Available from: http://hrlibrary.umn.edu/edumat/hreduseries/hereandnow/Part-5/6_glossary.htm. Accessed May 3, 2015.

36. Dudziak ML. *Cold War civil rights: Race and the image of American democracy.* Rev. ed. Princeton, NJ: Princeton University Press; 2011.

37. Beddard R, Hill DM. *Economic, social and cultural rights: Progress and achievement.* New York: Springer; 2016.

38. UNTC. International covenant on economic, social and cultural rights. Available from: https://treaties-un-org.ezp-prod1.hul.harvard.edu/pages/ViewDetails.aspx?src=TREATY&mtdsg_no=IV-3& chapter=4&clang=_en. Accessed October 6, 2016.

39. Carter J. US finally ratifies human rights covenant. The Carter Center. 1992. Available from: https://www.cartercenter.org/news/documents/doc1369.html.

40. Amnesty International. Campaigns. Available from: http://www.amnestyusa.org/our-work/campaigns. Accessed April 5, 2017.

41. Wolff J. *The human right to health.* 1st ed. New York: W.W. Norton & Co.; 2012.

42. The New York Times. Human rights and human rights violations. Available from: https://www.nytimes.com/topic/subject/human-rights-and-human-rights-violations. Accessed May 3, 2017.

43. Moore JT. *A search for equality: The National Urban League, 1910–1961.* University Park: Pennsylvania State University Press; 1981.

44. Sapire H, Saunders CC. *Southern African liberation struggles: New local, regional and global perspectives.* Cape Town: University of Cape Town Press; 2013.

45. Farmer P. *The uses of Haiti.* Monroe, ME: Common Courage Press; 1994.

46. Olivera O. *Cochabamba!: Water war in Bolivia.* Cambridge, MA: South End Press; 2004.

47. Gibson R. *African liberation movements: Contemporary struggles against white minority rule.* Published for the Institute of Race Relations. London/New York: Oxford University Press; 1972.

48. Fink C. *Cold War: An international history.* Boulder, CO: Westview Press; 2014.

49. Patman RG. *The Soviet Union in the Horn of Africa: The diplomacy of intervention and disengagement.* New York: Cambridge University Press; 1990.

50. Birmingham D. *Kwame Nkrumah: The father of African nationalism.* Rev. ed. Athens: Ohio University Press; 1998.

51. Chabal P. *Amílcar Cabral: Revolutionary leadership and people's war.* Cambridge: Cambridge University Press; 1983.

52. Dearden N. Africa is not poor, we are stealing its wealth. Al Jazeera. May 24, 2017. Available from: http://www.aljazeera.com/indepth/opinion/2017/05/africa-poor-stealing-wealth-170524063731884.html. Accessed May 29, 2017.

53. Rodney W. How Europe underdeveloped Africa. In: How Europe Undeveloped Africa. Washington, DC: Howard University Press; 1982. p. 173.

54. Brophy K. DRC's largest mine was just sold. And DRC got nothing. Oxfam. Available from: https://politicsofpoverty.oxfamamerica.org/2016/08/drcs-largest-mine-was-just-sold-and-drc-got-nothing/. Accessed May 23, 2017.

55. Konadu-Agyemang K, Panford MK. *Africa's development in the twenty-first century: Pertinent socio-economic and development issues.* Aldershot, UK/Burlington, VT: Ashgate; 2006.

56. OPM. The impact of mining in the Democratic Republic of Congo: Performance to date and future challenges. *Oxford Policy Management, Synergy.* 2013. http://www.opml.co.uk/sites/default/files/DRC%20mining%20report%20-%20OPM%20-%20Final%20Eng.pdf

57. World Bank. World development indicators. Available from: http://databank.worldbank.org/data/reports.aspx?source=world-development-indicators. Accessed March 29, 2017.

58. Southall R, Melber H, eds. *A new scramble for Africa?: Imperialism, investment and development.* Scottsville, SA: University of KwaZulu-Natal Press; 2009.

59. Zeilig L. *Lumumba: Africa's lost leader.* London: Haus; 2008.

60. Botchway FN. *Natural resource investment and Africa's development.* Cheltenham, UK/Northampton, MA: Edward Elgar; 2011.

61. Nzongola-Ntalaja G. Patrice Lumumba: The most important assassination of the 20th century. *The Guardian.* Jan 17, 2011. Available from: https://www.theguardian.com/global-development/poverty-matters/2011/jan/17/patrice-lumumba-50th-anniversary-assassination. Accessed May 23, 2017.

62. De Witte Ld. *The assassination of Lumumba.* London/New York: Verso; 2001.

63. Ramsdell M. *When elephants fight.* 2015.

64. Tarp F, Hjertholm P. *Foreign aid and development: Lessons learnt and directions for the future.* London/New York: Routledge; 2000.

65. Donaldson RH. *The Soviet Union in the Third World: Successes and failures.* Boulder, CO/London: Westview Press/Croom Helm; 1981.

66. US Department of State. *Proceedings and documents of the United Nations Financial and Monetary Conference.* Washington, DC: United States Government Printing Office; 1948.

67. Lateef KS. *The evolving role of the World Bank: Helping meet the challenge of development.* Washington, DC: World Bank; 1995.

68. US Department of State. Marshall Plan, 1948. Office of the Historian Website. Available from: https://history.state.gov/milestones/1945-1952/marshall-plan. Accessed April 13, 2017.

69. Hickel J. The World Bank and the development delusion. Aljazeera. Sept 27, 2012. Available from: http://www.aljazeera.com/indepth/opinion/2012/09/201292673233720461.html. Accessed May 3, 2017.

70. Sargent D. The Cold War and the international political economy in the 1970s. *Cold War History*. 2013;13(3):393–425.

71. Decoodt P. The debt crisis of the third world: Some aspects of causes and solutions. *Columbia J World Bus*. 1986;21(3):3.

72. Reinhart C, Trebesch C. The international monetary fund: 70 years of reinvention. Faculty Research Working Paper Series. Boston: Harvard Kennedy School. 2015.

73. Walton J, Ragin C. Global and national sources of political protest: Third World responses to the debt crisis. *Am Soc Rev*. 1990;55(6):876–890.

74. IMF. IMF members' quotas and voting power, and IMF board of governors. International Monetary Fund Website. Available from: https://www.imf.org/external/np/sec/memdir/members.aspx. Accessed May 23, 2017.

75. Bradsher K. Toward the summit; Soviet bid to join I.M.F. still a puzzle. *The New York Times*. July 29, 1991. Available from: http://www.nytimes.com/1991/07/29/world/toward-the-summit-soviet-bid-to-join-imf-still-a-puzzle.html. Accessed May 23, 2017.

76. Thacker SC. The high politics of IMF lending. *World Politics*. 1999;52(1):38–75.

77. Owusu F. Pragmatism and the gradual shift from dependency to neoliberalism: The World Bank, African leaders and development policy in Africa. *World Dev*. 2003;31(10):1655–1672.

78. Smith A. *An inquiry into the nature and causes of the wealth of nations*. Edwin Cannan, ed. London: Methuen & Co., Ltd. 1904. Library of Economics and Liberty. Available from: http://www.econlib.org/library/Smith/smWN.html.

79. Friedman M. *Capitalism and freedom*. 40th anniversary edition ed. Chicago, IL: University of Chicago Press; 2002.

80. Nobelprize.org. The Sveriges Riksbank Prize in Economic Sciences in Memory of Alfred Nobel. Available from: http://www.nobelprize.org/nobel_prizes/economic-sciences/laureates/1975/. Accessed April 13, 2017.

81. Pear R, Kaplan T, Haberman M. In major defeat for Trump, push to repeal health law fails. *The New York Times*. March 24, 2017. Available from: https://www.nytimes.com/2017/03/24/us/politics/health-care-affordable-care-act.html. Accessed May 3, 2017.

82. Kim JY, Millen JV, Irwin A. *Dying for growth: Global inequality and the health of the poor*. Monroe, ME: Common Courage Press; 2000.

83. Navarro V. Neoliberalism, "globalization," unemployment, inequalities, and the welfare state. *Intl J Health Serv*. 1998;28(4):607–682.

84. Pierson P. *Dismantling the welfare state?: Reagan, Thatcher, and the politics of retrenchment*. Cambridge/New York: Cambridge University Press; 1994.

85. Dreher A. A public choice perspective of IMF and World Bank lending and conditionality. *Public Choice*. 2004;119(3):445–464.

86. Babb S. The social consequences of structural adjustment: Recent evidence and current debates. *Annu Rev Sociol.* 2005;31:199–222.

87. Swain M. Pat Harrison and the Social Security Act of 1935. In: Chambers DB, Watson K, Prenshaw PW, editors. *The past is not dead.* Jackson: University Press of Mississippi; 2012. doi:10.14325/mississippi/9781617033032.003.0006.

88. Kennedy DM. What the New Deal did. *Pol Sci Q.* 2009;124(2):251–268.

89. Laurell A. Three decades of neoliberalism in Mexico: The destruction of society. *Intl J Health Serv.* 2015;45(2):246–264.

90. Lustig N. *Mexico, the remaking of an economy.* Washington, DC: The Brookings Institution; 1992.

91. Black S, Kincaid J, Fisher S, et al. *Life and debt.* New York: New Yorker Films/Axiom Films; 2003.

92. World Health Organization (WHO). NHA indicators. World Health Organization—Global Health Expenditure Database Website. Available from: http://apps.who.int/nha/database/ViewData/Indicators/en. Accessed March 29, 2017.

93. High hopes at Alma-Ata. *Lancet.* 1978;312(8091):666. http://www.thelancet.com/journals/lancet/article/PIIS0140-6736(78)92768-X/abstract

94. World Health Organization (WHO). Declaration of Alma-Ata International Conference on Primary Health Care, Alma–Ata, USSR, 6-12 September 1978. *Development.* 1978 Sept;47(2):159–161.

95. Bryant JH, Richmond JB. Alma-Ata and primary health care: An evolving story. In: Heggenhougan K, editor. *International encyclopedia of public health.* Oxford: Elsevier; 2008. p. 152–174.

96. Marshall A. What happened to the peace dividend?: The end of the Cold War cost thousands of jobs. Andrew Marshall looks at how the world squandered an opportunity. *Independent.* Jan 3, 1993. Available from: http://www.independent.co.uk/news/world/what-happened-to-the-peace-dividend-the-end-of-the-cold-war-cost-thousands-of-jobs-andrew-marshall-1476221.html. Accessed April 18, 2017.

97. Knight M, Loayza N, Villanueva D. The peace dividend: Military spending cuts and economic growth. *Staff Papers—International Monetary Fund.* 1996;43(1):1.

98. Walsh J, Warren K. Selective primary health care: An interim strategy for disease control in developing countries. *Soc Sci Med.* 1980;14c(2):145–163.

99. Grant JP. *The state of the world's children 1982–1983.* Geneva: United Nations Children's Fund (UNICEF); 1982.

100. Cash RA. A history of the development of oral rehydration therapy (ORT). *J Diarrhoeal Dis Res.* 1987;5(4):256–261.

101. Enders JF, Katz SL, Milovanovic MV, Holloway A. Studies on an attenuated measles-virus vaccine: Development and preparation of the vaccine: Technics for assay of effects of vaccination. *N Engl J Med.* 1960;263(4):153–159.

102. Claeson M, Waldman R. The evolution of child health programmes in developing countries: From targeting diseases to targeting people. *Bull World Health Org.* 2000;78(10):1234–1245.

103. Warren KS. The evolution of selective primary health care. *Soc Sci Med.* 1988;26(9):891–898.

104. UNICEF. Under-five mortality rate (trend data including uncertainty ranges). *UNICEF Data: Monitoring the Situation of Children and Women.* New York: UNICEF; 2015.

105. Claeson M, Bos E, Mawji T, Pathmanathan I. Reducing child mortality in India in the new millennium. *Bull World Health Org.* 2000;78(10):1192–1199.

106. UNICEF. *The State of the World's Children 2008: Child Survival.* New York: UNICEF; 2008.

107. Wisner B. GOBI versus PHC? Some dangers of selective primary health care. *Soc Sci Med.* 1988;26(9):963–969.

108. Victora CG, Wagstaff A, Schellenberg JA, Gwatkin D, Claeson M, Habicht J. Applying an equity lens to child health and mortality: More of the same is not enough. *Lancet.* 2003;362(9379):233–241.

109. Riddell J. Things fall apart again: Structural adjustment programmes in Sub-Saharan Africa. *J Mod Afr Studies.* 1992;30:53–68.

110. Loewenson R. Structural adjustment and health policy in Africa. *Intl J Health Serv.* 1993;23(4):717–730.

111. Chabot J. The Bamako Initiative. *Lancet.* 1988;332(8621):1177–1178. Available from: http://www.sciencedirect.com.ezp-prod1.hul.harvard.edu/science/article/pii/S0140673688902413. doi: //dx.doi.org.ezp-prod1.hul.harvard.edu/10.1016/S0140-6736(88)90241-3.

112. Kanji N. Charging for drugs in Africa: UNICEF's "Bamako Initiative." *Health Policy Plan.* 1989;4:110–120.

113. Ridde V. Fees-for-services, cost recovery, and equity in a district of Burkina Faso operating the Bamako Initiative. *Bull World Health Org.* 2003;81(7):532.

114. Carol Bellamy. The Bamako Initiative. UNICEF. March 1999. Available from: http://www.unicef.org/media/media_11991.html. Accessed October 6, 2016.

115. Gilson L, Russell S, Buse K. The political economy of user fees with targeting: Developing equitable health financing policy. *J Intl Dev.* 1995;7(3):369–401.

116. Lagarde M, Palmer N. The impact of user fees on health service utilization in low- and middle-income countries: How strong is the evidence? [Impact de la participation dont s'acquittent les utilisateurs des services de sante dans les pays a revenu faible ou moyen: Les donnees sont-elles solides? Impacto del cobro de honorarios a los usuarios en el uso de los servicios de salud en los paises de ingresos bajos y medios: Grado de evidencia.] *Bull World Health Org.* 2008;86(11):839.

2

Reversing the Tide

LESSONS FROM THE MOVEMENT FOR AIDS
TREATMENT ACCESS

Key Points

- AIDS was a new disease identified in the 1980s.
- People living with AIDS fought against discrimination and linked AIDS to human rights.
- Activists pushed for research, which led to the discovery of new drugs.
- On the African continent, the global AIDS pandemic caused significant decreases in life expectancy and increases in child mortality.
- A global movement of people living with AIDS in wealthy and impoverished countries worked in solidarity to increase access to treatment.
- Activism for AIDS treatment generated new money for the delivery of care.
- The success of this movement launched an era of global health focused on the delivery of care, treatment, and the strengthening of health systems.

Introduction

The selective primary health care approach in impoverished countries continued throughout the 1980s and into the late 1990s. Prevention efforts increased child survival but paid little attention to the provision of treatment or the development of health systems.[1] By the end of the 1990s, impoverished countries had oral rehydration solutions (ORS), vaccines, and educational materials but virtually no access to drugs, diagnostics, or functioning health facilities. In the early 1980s, against this backdrop, AIDS emerged.

This chapter reviews the AIDS epidemic chronologically from the discovery of a new disease to the movement for access to antiretroviral therapy. The chapter emphasizes the importance of AIDS activists in the fight for treatment access and the explicit connection between the AIDS pandemic and the right to health. AIDS changed many things in global health, from patient-led activism to drug discovery to the long-term provision of care.

A New Disease

In 1981, sporadic cases of two rare diseases—Kaposi's sarcoma (KS; a type of cancer) and *Pneumocystis carinii* pneumonia (PCP; a rare parasitic infection)—were reported among men who have sex with men (MSM) in New York and San Francisco.[2-4] The US Centers for Disease Control (CDC) published a paper in its journal, *Morbidity and Mortality Weekly Report*, entitled "Kaposi's Sarcoma and Pneumocystis carinii Pneumonia Among Homosexual Men— New York and California."[4] Within a few weeks, another report was published in the *New England Journal of Medicine* describing four men sick with PCP and yeast infections who appeared to have what was termed "a new acquired cellular immunodeficiency."[5]

Immune deficiency describes a state in which the body's normal defenses against infection or cancer are weakened. When researchers started investigating these cases of PCP and KS, the underlying immune deficiency had no apparent cause. The only common factor among these patients was that they were all identified as MSM. Within the next two years, the condition that led to KS and PCP became known by the pejorative term, the "gay plague."[6] It was later called acquired immune deficiency syndrome (AIDS).

In 1983, a landmark paper reported that the first 1,000 documented cases of KS and PCP came from two-thirds of all American states. The authors concluded that "AIDS appears to be a new illness of rapidly increasing incidence."[7] This paper identified that 93 percent of the patients were homosexual or bisexual men, intravenous drug users, Haitians, or hemophiliacs (those with a blood disorder requiring frequent blood transfusions). Another publication documented that the average lifespan of AIDS patients was six months.[8] As AIDS claimed the lives of several hundred men, it led to widespread panic and stigma.[8,9] The risk groups identified by these early papers became known as the "4-H club" (a disparaging reference to homosexuals, Haitians, heroin-users, and hemophiliacs).[9] The distinction of being a member of the 4-H club became synonymous with carrying the disease. Thus began an epidemic of discrimination.[10] Members of all four groups were banned from giving blood[11]; some were denied housing[12] and employment.[13] In the 1980s, people with AIDS or from a risk group for AIDS were also victims of violence and discrimination.[14,15] In Haiti, the stigma of AIDS as a Haitian disease caused the entire tourist economy to come to a grinding halt.[16]

In 1983, a letter to the editor was published in the British medical journal, *Lancet*, entitled "Acquired Immune Deficiency Syndrome in Black Africans."[17] The authors noted that there had yet to be a case of AIDS in previously healthy Africans. Yet that same year, there was a brief report about a white Danish surgeon who traveled to Africa in 1976 and died of an immunodeficiency syndrome upon her return to Denmark.[18] Around the same time several African patients from Zaire (now the Democratic Republic of Congo) were treated in Europe for a fungal infection known as cryptococcosis, also primarily a disease affecting people with weakened immune systems.[19] In retrospect, these patients likely had AIDS. By the mid 1980s, there were reports of people with AIDS in countries throughout Africa—from South Africa to Rwanda to Zaire to Uganda.[20-24] These cases suggested that the origins of the AIDS epidemic may have been in Africa, where it appeared a decade before it was recognized in the United States. The idea of a "Black African"[17] origin of AIDS led to further stigma along racial lines and promoted racist narratives of sexuality.[25]

Fear of AIDS promoted not only homophobia and racial bias, but class-based gender bias as well. This first paper about women with HIV was published in 1983 and was titled "Acquired Immunodeficiency . . . in Infants Born to Promiscuous and Drug-Addicted Mothers."[26] The very title of the paper cast blame on mothers for failing their innocent children. Blame pervaded the epidemic.

From Disease to Pandemic

In 1984, Drs. Françoise Barré-Sinoussi, Luc Montagnier, and their team at the Pasteur Institute in France connected the disease of AIDS with the presence of a virus.[27,28] The virus became known as the human immunodeficiency virus, or HIV.[29] In 1985, an antibody test for HIV was developed and used to screen the blood supply to prevent HIV transmission through transfusions. However, widespread clinical testing was unavailable and even controversial without a treatment for AIDS.[30] Scientists began to investigate how HIV was transmitted. They identified male-to-male, male-to-female, and female-to-male transmission of HIV. Transmission through blood products, needles, and other instruments containing infected fluids was also documented.[31,32] Finally, transmission was documented from mother to child, through the exchange of body fluids in utero, during the birthing process, and through breastfeeding.[33]

The new availability of a diagnostic test made it possible to document the spread of HIV around the world. The World Health Assembly created an AIDS program within the World Health Organization (WHO), called the Special Programme on AIDS, to track the spread of the disease.[34] By late 1986, there were about 34,000 cases of AIDS worldwide, which almost doubled to about 60,000 in 1987 (Figure 2.1).[34]

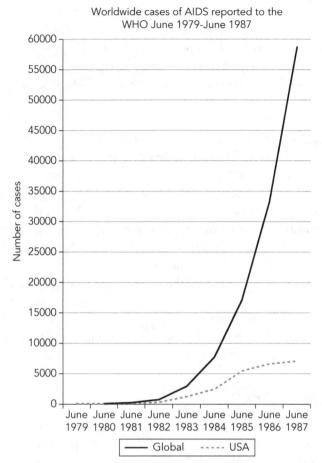

Worldwide cases of AIDS reported to the
WHO June 1979-June 1987

FIGURE 2.1 The graph depicts the rise in AIDS cases reported to the World Health Organization (WHO) in the United States and globally between 1979–1987.

Data adapted from Mann JM. The World Health Organization's global strategy for the prevention and control of AIDS. *West J Med.* 1987;147(6):732.

That year, the US government instituted a travel ban forbidding the entry of anyone with HIV into the country. The ban was active for 22 years and was officially lifted in 2009.[35]

The Global Pandemic

The Special Program on AIDS later became the United Nations AIDS Program (UNAIDS).[36] The goal of UNAIDS was to raise awareness and money for prevention efforts. UNAIDS also helped countries develop national plans to combat the disease.[37] The great AIDS crusader, Dr. Jonathan Mann, the inaugural director of the Special Program, wrote that "global AIDS control requires global leadership and coordination."[38] He believed that there were three important things that would help to control the disease: "the concept and infrastructure of primary health care" that would allow people to access needed services, "modern behavioral science" that would use public health information to craft prevention messages, and the "emergence of a global conscience" that would inspire the international community to work together and finance the response in coordination with the WHO.[38] Mann advocated for money, political will, and cheaper and more available HIV testing in impoverished countries.[39] Yet the call for resource mobilization went unanswered, and international coordination remained weak. The epidemic continued to spread, and the death toll mounted.[37]

AIDS Activism and Its Role in the Right to Health

As the global AIDS pandemic expanded at a terrifying pace, people living with AIDS (PLWA) were dying. In the United States and Europe, PLWA were dying of rare conditions (so-called opportunistic infections, which attack those with weakened immune systems). PLWA in impoverished countries were dying even more rapidly.[40,41] In Africa, tuberculosis (TB) became the number one cause of death for PLWA.[42,43] As TB cases increased, the disease spread to both HIV-positive and HIV-negative people.[43,44] The noxious synergy of AIDS and TB overwhelmed health systems already weakened by neoliberal economic policies and structural adjustment programs (SAPs).[45,46]

Around the world, PLWA and their loved ones banned together to combat hopelessness, fear, and discrimination. In 1987, Dr. Noerine Kaleeba (whose husband had AIDS) and others formed the AIDS Support Organization (TASO) in Uganda.[47] TASO began to provide community-based support, promote positive living, and encourage community acceptance.[48] As one of the first African AIDS organizations, TASO became an important peer support organization in the country, region, and, eventually, the world.

A fight was raging against AIDS-related discrimination in the United States as well, as the award-winning film, *How to Survive a Plague,* beautifully documents.[49] The community that had been fighting for gay rights for decades now found its ranks decimated by AIDS. AIDS increased the stigma and marginalization that they already faced. AIDS activist Larry Kramer remembers New York at the height of the epidemic: "[you couldn't] walk down the street without running into somebody who said: 'Have you heard about so and so? He just died.' Sometimes you could learn about three or four people just walking the dog. I started making a list of how many people I knew, and it was hundreds.

People don't comprehend that. People really were dying like flies."[50] Rather than retreat from the epidemic, the gay community and its allies organized a movement. The Gay Men's Health Crisis (GMHC) was founded in 1982 by Kramer and other activists to educate the public about AIDS, provide support for PLWA, and advocate for policies to protect PLWA.[51] As politicians continued to willfully dismiss the epidemic, activists grew angrier. In 1987, Kramer and others founded a more militant group—the AIDS Coalition to Unleash Power (ACT UP).[52] ACT UP's strategy relied on direct action to call attention to AIDS and to the silence of policymakers. ACT UP fought to end discrimination and accelerate research for an AIDS cure. Their now-famous logo is a pink triangle—the symbol used to identify suspected homosexual men who were sent to Nazi death camps—over the phrase SILENCE = DEATH (Figure 2.2).

In 1987, ACT UP held its first protest on Wall Street, calling for investors in pharmaceutical companies to accelerate the release of their AIDS drugs.[53] ACT UP demanded that AIDS drugs be reasonably priced and widely accessible[54] (Figure 2.3A, B).

ACT UP directly targeted the US Food and Drug Administration (FDA) and policymakers including conservative Senator Jesse Helms and President Ronald Reagan.[55] The American government not only dismissed PLWA, it legislated policies that increased stigma and homophobia associated with AIDS. Senator Jesse Helms, a Republican from North Carolina, became particularly outspoken against PLWA. He introduced an amendment to the 1988 appropriations bill for the Departments of Labor, Health and Human Services, and Education to prevent the US Centers for Disease Control (CDC) from funding AIDS programs

designed by the silence=death project for act up

FIGURE 2.2 Logo used first used by US-based AIDS activist group ACT UP in the 1980s. Silence=death was a rebuke of the neglect of the epidemic by policy makers, the pink triangle a reminder of the Nazi's persecution of presumably homosexual men. Courtesy of ACT UP New York.

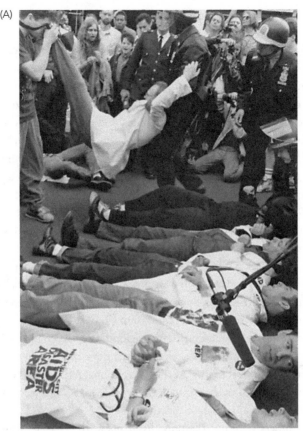

(A)

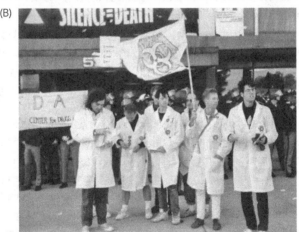

(B)

FIGURE 2.3 (A) Members of activist group ACT UP are arrested during protest, 1989. (B) Members of activist group ACT UP protest outside the US Food and Drug Administration (FDA) headquarters, October 1988.

Photo A courtesy of Manuscripts and Archives Division, The New York Public Library. "ACT UP. [Police arrest prone protesters. "AIDS DISASTER AREA" sign.]" New York Public Library Digital Collections. Accessed Dec 9, 2016. Available from: http://digitalcollections.nypl.org/items/5e9c3290-c178-0130-1b4b-58d385a7b928. Photographer: Rowell Douglass. Photo B courtesy of Mark Harrington.

that "promote, encourage or condone homosexual activities."[56] In referring to gay men in his introduction, he stated "We have got to call a spade a spade and a perverted human being a perverted human being."[56] He blamed GMHC for perpetuating the epidemic.[56] Activist Peter Staley of ACT UP orchestrated a response to Jesse Helms's homophobic policies. Staley and other members of ACT UP placed an enormous condom over Jesse Helms's home in Arlington, Virginia. On the side of the condom, they wrote, "A condom to stop unsafe politics. Helms is deadlier than a virus."[57] President Reagan, while less outspoken against those affected by AIDS, was certainly no less destructive: Reagan's presidency from 1981 to 1989 corresponded with the beginning of the AIDS epidemic. Reagan made no public mention of AIDS in his first five years in office and waited seven years before making a speech on the health crisis.[58]

Within ACT UP, some members recognized the need to understand the science and policies that underpinned drug development. In 1992, Mark Harrington, Gregg Gonsalves, Peter Staley, Spencer Cox, and more than a dozen other AIDS activists formed the Treatment Action Group (TAG), a nonprofit organization that pushed for increased funding for pharmaceutical research for AIDS, particularly drug trials. TAG members challenged the devastatingly slow pace of drug development and clinical trials.[59] At the International AIDS Society (IAS) meeting in Amsterdam in 1992, the group presented a 66-page critique of the National Institutes of Health's approach to clinical trials.[60,61]

TAG members were not the only dissidents at the 1992 IAS meeting. The theme of the conference was "A World United Against AIDS" and was originally supposed to be held in the United States. However, due to the US travel ban against PLWA,[35] the conference was moved to Amsterdam. Eight-thousand people attended, and many attendees were dying of AIDS. At this conference, PLWA from wealthy countries came into direct contact with PLWA from impoverished countries. Some of the participants from Africa were so ill that they were taken to hospitals in Holland. Other African attendees received medicines from American and European participants who were moved to solidarity with their brothers and sisters from impoverished countries.[62] The connections that grew between organizations and people from wealthy and impoverished countries strengthened global alliances between groups like ACT UP and TASO. The groups shared an agenda to value the dignity and worth of all human beings, to fight stigma and discrimination, and to expand access to AIDS treatment and health care. By 1993, there were more than 18 million people infected with HIV around the world (16 million in Africa).[63] At the Ninth International AIDS conference in Berlin, Germany, WHO Special Programme on AIDS Director Mann decried the insufficient political will, dwindling resources, and lack of treatment or prevention options.[64] The AIDS pandemic was causing a decrease in life expectancy across Africa (Figure 2.4).

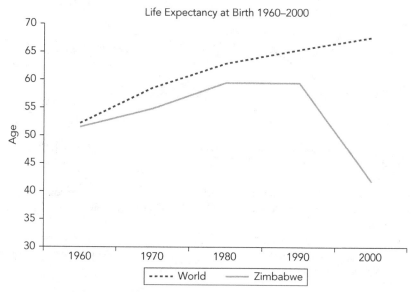

FIGURE 2.4 Life expectancy at birth in selected African countries, 1960–2000. Shown is the abrupt drop in life expectancy in the late 1980s and early 1990s due to the growing HIV/AIDS epidemic.

Data adapted from World Bank. World development indicators. The World Bank Databank Web site. 2017. Available from: http://databank.worldbank.org/data/reports.aspx?source=world-development-indicators. Accessed Mar 29, 2017.

African children were dying at an alarming rate. Preceding the AIDS pandemic, selective primary health care programs, while narrowly focused on prevention, did improve child survival.[65] These gains, however, were reversed as the pandemic spread. Although only about 10 percent of PLWA were children, child survival plummeted as parents developed AIDS and could not care for their families.[65] By 1996, the "AIDS orphan crisis" generated attention. It was predicted then that there would be 40 million orphans by 2010.[66] Orphans and vulnerable children (OVCs) became an important group that highlighted the dire nature of the unremitting pandemic. Providers and patients alike were losing hope as AIDS claimed nearly 8,000 lives per day.[67]

The Lazarus Effect

The work of the AIDS activists to break down political, regulatory, and scientific barriers to accelerate the development of AIDS medicines bore remarkable fruit. Activists worked with Dr. Emilio Emini of the Merck corporation and together discovered a remarkable treatment.[68] In 1995, a third and novel drug (indinivir) used

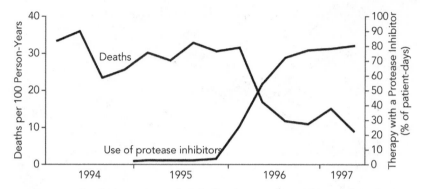

FIGURE 2.5 Graph shows the marked decline in mortality as the use of combination antiretroviral therapy including a protease inhibitor increased among people living with AIDS.

Source: Palella FJ, Delaney KM, Moorman AC, et al. Declining morbidity and mortality among patients with advanced human immunodeficiency virus infection. *N Engl J Med*. 1998;338(13):853–860.

in combination with two existing HIV drugs suddenly turned AIDS from a fatal illness into a manageable, chronic condition.[69] This cocktail of drugs, originally known as *highly active antiretroviral therapy* (HAART, later ART) resulted in a 90 percent reduction of mortality for AIDS patients with access to the drugs.[70] The reversal of AIDS symptoms was nothing short of miraculous (Figure 2.5). Many likened the effect of the drugs to the Biblical resurrection of Lazarus, as bedridden AIDS patients recovered from the edge of death.[71,72]

Despite the success of ART, access to these life-saving drugs mirrored the economically stratified population affected by the global AIDS pandemic. The cost of the drug cocktail, priced at more than $10,000 per patient per year,[74,75] excluded millions of PLWA from treatment in both the United States and around the world. In the United States, patients judged as high risk for nonadherence, such as those who used intravenous drugs, those who were homeless, or those who were involved in commercial sex work, were not offered ART.[73] Despite the fact that 95 percent of the epidemic was in Africa, there was no movement to bring ART to the then 16 million African PLWA.[74]

Yet, despite the large global inequity in access, fueled by the heady optimism of ART's success, the International AIDS Society meeting was held in Vancouver in 1996 with the slogan, "One World, One Hope."[76] Eric Sawyer, one of the founders of ACT UP who was by then receiving ART, addressed the opening session of the conference. However, rather than basking in the victory of ART, Sawyer painted a grim picture of the lack of treatment access in impoverished countries. Sawyer said:

The headlines that PLWA want you to write from this conference would read: "Human Rights Violations and Genocide continue to kill millions of impoverished people with AIDS." That is the truth about AIDS in 1996. The truth is, genocide continues against poor people with AIDS, especially those from developing countries, by AIDS Profiteers who are more concerned about maximizing profits than saving lives. Drug Companies are killing people by charging excessive prices. This limits access to treatments. The greed of AIDS Profiteers is killing impoverished people with AIDS. The truth is, the governments of the world are killing people with AIDS, because they think public health is isolating their rich often white populations from the diseases of the poor by instituting immigration barriers instead of providing healthcare to the sick. [Rich] Governments are killing poor people in developing countries because they are providing only a tiny amount of AIDS funding which is limited to prevention efforts and does not pay for AIDS care.

The truth is, hatred of the poor and of the disenfranchised communities continues to allow discrimination, stigmatization, violence and even the murder of people living with AIDS to remain unchecked. People with AIDS do not have any protection against Human Rights Violations.[77]

Sawyer ended his fiery speech with the statement "Greed Kills, Access for All," which was then chanted by participants. It was a powerful connection between access to medicines and human rights. Sawyer's speech captured the mood of the conference, one of solidarity between PLWA from rich and impoverished countries. Leaders of the AIDS movement, most of whom were living with the disease, placed the right to health and access to medicines at center stage.

But equitable access to treatment was far away. In 1996, most impoverished countries burdened with debt, constricted by structural adjustment, and without control of their natural resources, continued to have less than $5 per capita per year for health. This left only meager funding for AIDS prevention and none for treatment.[78] Even as more than 8,000 people died each day of what was then a treatable disease, there was no access to ART in impoverished countries.[79–82] After the Vancouver meeting, activists argued a human rights–based approach was needed. Instead of focusing exclusively on prevention, they reasoned that treatment should be available for all. Global activism for ART access grew in force and, for the first time, challenged the neoliberal notion of doing only what could be sustained on impoverished countries' budgets.[80]

Zackie Achmat, a gay man, antiapartheid activist, and PLWA in South Africa, founded the Treatment Action Campaign (TAC) in 1998 (Figure 2.6).

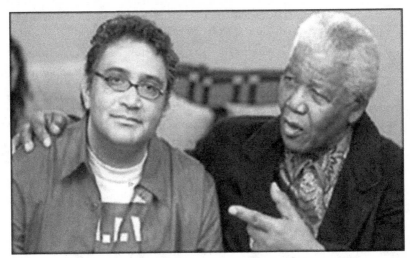

FIGURE 2.6 South African AIDS activist and founder of the Treatment Action Campaign Zackie Achmat with Nelson Mandela (2003). Although highly active antiretroviral therapy (HAART) was available to wealthy South Africans by that time, Mr. Achmat famously refused treatment until the South African government changed its policies and provided ART to all. His actions—personal and through the Treatment Action Campaign (TAC)—were equated with those of Nelson Mandela and other human rights leaders.
Photo courtesy of Mark Harrington.

TAC members worked to educate people living with AIDS about ARTs through treatment literacy campaigns. They also organized communities of PLWA to demand access to ART from the South African government. The members bravely wore T-shirts that proclaimed themselves "HIV POSITIVE" even as PLWA in South Africa were murdered for being HIV positive.[83] TAC members also took action against the AIDS denialism of South African President Thabo Mbeki[84] and his Minister of Health Dr. Tshabalala.[85] Mbeki claimed that HIV did not cause AIDS and that ART was not needed.[86] It is estimated that Mbeki's denial of AIDS and the efficacy of ART resulted in the premature deaths of about 330,000 South Africans.[86,87] The 16,000 members of TAC organized to hold the government accountable for the right to AIDS treatment through protests, media, meetings with officials, and legal battles. Since the right to health was enshrined in the post-apartheid South African constitution, these actions took on important significance.[88]

Yet despite the efforts of activists, in 2000, four years after Eric Sawyer's proclamation that the lack of access to ART was tantamount to genocide against the poor, there was still no movement for treatment access in impoverished countries. That year, the IAS conference was held in Durban, South Africa. The slogan of the conference was "Break the Silence."[89] It was the first time that the AIDS

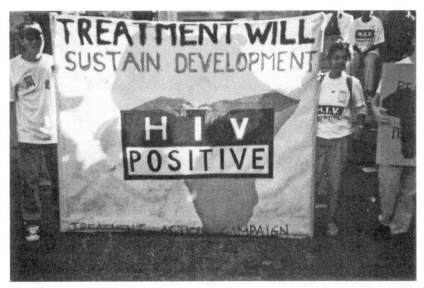

FIGURE 2.7 Treatment Action Campaign (TAC) protest at the 2000 International AIDS Society conference in Durban.

Photo courtesy of Mark Harrington.

meeting was held in an impoverished or high-prevalence country. The result was transformative. Massive protests were staged by TAC and other activist groups including ACT UP, TAG, and TASO. The global solidarity, disciplined, non-violent protests, and consistent messaging received significant media coverage. Activism raised the awareness of millions of people to the magnitude of the crisis in impoverished countries[89] (Figure 2.7).

The Durban protests spurred Nelson Mandela to speak about decreasing the price of ART and even to wear an "HIV POSITIVE" shirt.[90] The conference and civil action crystallized a consensus that AIDS must be treated even in countries without the financial means to procure the drugs or the systems to deliver them.

HIV Drug Pricing

The drugs contained in ART were developed by private, for-profit American pharmaceutical companies that protected their discoveries through patents or intellectual property (IP) laws. Patents protect a company's exclusive right to produce a medicine. Under patent, the price of a medicine can be set at whatever the company believes the market can bear without fear of competition. Pharmaceutical companies justified a very high price of ART, more than $10,000 dollars per patient per year,[75] stating they needed to recuperate the costs of research and development. ART was extremely profitable and the price of drugs remained the major barrier to their use in impoverished countries. Patents and IP laws ensure that the profit associated with a new discovery goes to the person or institution that led the research. Patents are generally issued in wealthy countries where companies seek a large paying market.[91] In the era of market globalization, the World Trade Organization (WTO) was launched in 1995 to assure global adherence IP laws.[92] Countries that signed on to the WTO agreement received favorable terms of trade, such as lower tariffs, in exchange for respecting patent protections.[92] In the late 1990s, when ART came to the market with the patent-protected drugs priced at $10,000 per patient per year, WTO signatories were obliged to respect patents and were not allowed to purchase less-expensive generic drugs from India.[93] Activists demanded generic access. They disrupted shareholder meetings at the ART-producing pharmaceutical companies. They also protested WTO meetings on trade to demand access to generic ART.[94,95] The activists' fight for access to generic ART continued in the streets and in courts around the world.[96]

In 2000, ART-producing corporations finally agreed to give concessional prices to the South African government, reducing the price of branded ART by up to 90 percent.[96,97] However, TAC activists knew that these concessional prices were simply a move to block entry of cheaper generic drugs into the market.[97] TAC activists searched for potential legal solutions to import generic ART into the country despite the fact that South Africa was a WTO signatory. Activists targeted a clause within the WTO treaty, known as the *trade-related aspects of intellectual property* (TRIPS).[98] TRIPS states that, in the case of a national emergency, a government may seek a generic option for a patented product in one of two ways. The first option is known as *parallel importing*. It allows a WTO member country to import generic products to address the national emergency. In the case of AIDS, most impoverished countries utilized this clause to import generic ART from India. The second option of TRIPS is *compulsory licensing*. In a national emergency, a WTO signatory may seek to purchase the license to manufacture a product for their own citizens. Thailand and Brazil used this strategy because they had the manufacturing capabilities.[99,100]

TAC and Médicins Sans Frontieres (MSF, or Doctors Without Borders) supported the use of TRIPS clauses. They knew that negotiations with private companies would make countries beholden to the free market instead of to needs their citizens.[101] Their concerns about concessional prices from private pharmaceutical companies proved prescient. In 1997, the South African government passed the "The Medicines and Related Substances Act."[102] The purpose of the law was to improve access to ART for the 4.2 million South Africans living with HIV through compulsory licensing, parallel importing, and transparent pricing.[102,103] The law gave the Minister of Health the power to circumvent patent laws.[103] Thirty-nine drug companies sued the South African government.[102] The pharmaceutical companies argued that this law was in direct violation of the WTO treaty.[104] However, under enormous civil society pressure, the companies withdrew their suit two months later.[104] Meanwhile, TAC continued to pressure the South African government for increased treatment access. In 2001, TAC filed a lawsuit in South Africa's Constitutional Court on behalf of pregnant HIV-positive women who did not have access to ART to prevent transmission of the virus to their children.[96] TAC won the lawsuit when the court held that the government was responsible, under the constitution, to guarantee access to health care. The Court ordered the government to take a series of steps to ensure access to comprehensive services to prevent mother-to-child HIV transmission including the public provision of ART.[105]

On the other side of the world, the government of Brazil took a very progressive approach to HIV from the earliest days of the epidemic.[106] With an active civil society, a new democracy, and a constitution that guaranteed the right to health, the country decided that all people living with HIV would receive treatment through the public sector.[107] Beginning in 1993, Brazil implemented a state-supported program to manufacture AIDS drugs domestically, enabled by compulsory licensing. Brazil was able to bring the price from $10,000 per patient per year down to $3,000.[108] This price was beyond the scope of impoverished countries but was affordable for a middle-income country like Brazil.[108,109] While Brazil's program was a major success story, it was not without critics. The most notable critic was then-President Bill Clinton, who threatened Brazil with sanctions for violating patent laws.[110] Despite the threat, Brazil continued with its national HIV program. The program achieved 30 percent coverage of ART by 2005 (compared with 2 percent in South Africa, a country of similar income).[111] The Brazilian National AIDS program was also credited by the World Bank for halving the rate of new infections.[109]

Feasibility of ART in Impoverished Settings

In impoverished countries, local production of ART was not an option because these countries lacked manufacturing capabilities. Yet countries feared retaliation from the US if they violated the WTO policies by importing generic drugs. Furthermore, prominent US policymakers thought people from impoverished countries would not be able to adhere to a life-long course of drugs even if it was available.[112] In 1998, Partners in Health (PIH), a nonprofit organization founded by Dr. Paul Farmer in Haiti, began to treat a handful of patients with ART. The organization received donations of unexpired drugs from a group of American

PLWA who had switched their therapies. The medicines were collected by PIH's staff and supporters. One supporter, an undergraduate student and former PIH intern named Sanjay Basu, was criticized by the *Wall Street Journal* for sending ART to Haiti citing concerns over patents.[113] Yet the donation program continued, and patients in rural Haiti began to take ART. The program, called the HIV Equity Initiative, was a success.[114] Not surprisingly, the rural poor in Haiti also experienced the Lazarus effect. Because the organization did not have enough drugs to cover the whole population of PLWAs, the team led by Dr. Farmer and Dr. Fernet Léandre chose the sickest patients to receive the limited supply of ART. PLWA who did not start ART were counselled, educated on preventing transmission, and treated for other opportunistic infections—most commonly TB. The team's experience with community-based TB therapy was instructive. Community health workers assured adherence to ART, provided social support, and accompanied patients to clinics. The team published the results of the HIV Equity Initiative—just 60 patients—in *Lancet* in 2001. The paper documented that all patients on ART gained weight and resumed work.[115] Partners in Health's team published a second paper that year in the WHO's *Bulletin* as a round table discussion, which invited critique.[114] Public health scholars argued that the study was not scientific and impossible to replicate.[116] One of the chief critics was Sir Richard Feachem, a doctor who had a long career with the World Bank.[112] Feachem argued that impoverished countries with underfunded health systems did not have the capability to provide ART to PLWA. Instead, Feachem said that efforts should be focused on regions with strong and reliable systems so as not to waste ART. Feachem wrote, "an international effort focused on establishing and sustaining a number of islands of learning and good practice is likely to make a greater contribution to the reduction of suffering and unnecessary death than spreading limited resources thinly across the low-income countries."[112]

Feachem was not alone in his criticism. Despite the work of the Brazilian government, PIH in Haiti, MSF in South Africa,[117] and the tireless of work of activists, many believed that HIV treatment simply could not be done in impoverished countries. Andrew Natsios, the former head of the US Agency for International Development (USAID), was quoted in the *New York Times* as saying;

[Africans] don't know what Western time is. You have to take these (AIDS) drugs a certain number of hours apart each day, or they don't work. Many people in Africa have never seen a clock or a watch in their entire lives. And if you say one o'clock in the afternoon, they do not know what you are talking about. They know morning, they know noon, they know evening, they know the darkness at night.[118]

The claims of ignorance and the backwardness of Africans by highly placed officials echoed the colonial mindset and enraged activists. These views pervaded the discourse on the provision of ART in impoverished countries, to the detriment of many people waiting for treatment.

The Fight for Financing

Activists continued to rally in support of global treatment access. PLWA in impoverished countries were the strongest voices. In February 2000, MSF and TAC collaborated to open an AIDS treatment center in Khayelitsha, on the outskirts of Cape Town. The success of this program and the stories of the recovering patients prompted the opening of more clinics in South Africa and Zimbabwe.[117] In Cange, Haiti, PLWA receiving treatment through the HIV Equity Initiative knew that their own Lazarus stories shattered conventional wisdom. In 2001, the patients, then numbering more than 150, penned the "Declaration of Cange."[119] In the Declaration, the PLWA defied the claim that they could not take medicines[119]:

> We have a message for you who suffer from the same sickness as we do. We would like to tell you not to get discouraged because you do not have medications. We pledge to remain steadfast in this fight and never to tire of fighting for the right of everyone to have necessary medications and adequate treatment.
>
> We also have a message for the big shots—for those from other countries as well as from Haiti, and from big organizations like the World Bank and USAID. We ask you to take consciousness of all that we continually endure. We too are human beings, we too are people. We entreat you to put aside your egotism and selfishness, and to stop wasting critical funds by buying big cars, constructing big buildings, and amassing huge salaries.
>
> Please also stop lying about the poor. It has been alleged that we don't know how to tell time and that is the reason we are ineligible or unworthy of medications that have to be taken at scheduled intervals. Stop accusing us unjustly and propagating erroneous assumptions about our right to health and our unconditional right to life. We are indeed poor, but just because we are poor does not automatically mean we are also stupid!
>
> It is our ardent wish that this message not be put aside or relegated to the files as just another paper document. As Haitian popular wisdom asserts, "As long as the head is not cut off, the hope of wearing a hat remains."

The combination of these programs and activist pressure forced the reduction of ART prices from private pharmaceutical companies from $10,000 to $600–800 per patient per year by 2003.[120,121] However, even at the reduced price, impoverished countries could not afford large-scale HIV treatment. The remaining challenge to assure access to ART as a human right was financing. By the year 2000, more than 30 million people were living with HIV and dying without medicines.[122] During the late 1990s, the pandemic had massive effects on health and development. It became abundantly clear that the neoliberal policies enforced by the IMF and World Bank were inextricably linked to the AIDS crisis. Peter Piot, then the director of UNAIDS, stated that "structural adjustment raises particular concern for governments because most of the factors which fuel the AIDS pandemic are also those factors that seem to come into play in structural adjustment programmes."[123] Piot meant that impoverished countries were being crushed by their debts and that the health systems, stripped bare by SAPs, could not respond to the crisis. In 2001, Tanzania was home to around 1.4 million PLWA and more than half a million children orphaned by the epidemic.[111] That year, the country's payment on its World Bank debt was three times higher than its health budget.[124,125]

The Creation of the Global Fund

At the 2000 IAS conference in Durban, Jeffrey Sachs, a development economist and chairman of the WHO's Commission on Macroeconomics and Health, proposed the idea of a donor-supported fund for AIDS treatment.[126] Sachs visited Haiti to estimate the cost of the HIV Equity Initiative. In 2001, Sachs led a meeting at Harvard that produced the Consensus Statement on the Use of Antiretroviral Therapy. The Statement was based on the work in Haiti, the costing done by Sachs, and inputs from faculty members who had been doing research in South Africa, Botswana, and elsewhere.[127] The authors proclaimed their support for massive and rapid expansion of access to ART in impoverished countries. The Statement contained a figure that showed the escalating death toll in Africa as compared to the trajectory of the epidemic in the United States[127] (Figure 2.8).

All of this work led to high-level discussions at the G8 summit in Okinawa, Japan, in 2000, and at the African Union summit in Apr 2001. That year, under the crushing weight of 32.5 million HIV infections, UN Secretary-General Kofi Annan called a UN General Assembly Special Session on AIDS (UNGASS). Annan called for the creation of a fund that would support the large-scale treatment of AIDS.[128] This fund was endorsed by the G8 in July 2001. A Transitional Working Group was established to determine the principles and working modalities of the new organization, and the Global Fund to fight AIDS, TB, and Malaria came into being in January 2002.[129]

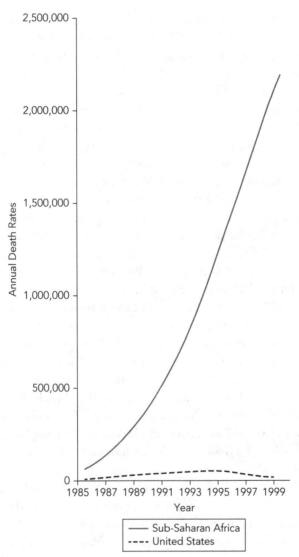

FIGURE 2.8 This graph shows the trend in age-adjusted AIDS death rates (1985–1999) for sub-Saharan Africa (*solid line*) and the United States (*dashed line*). In the United States, highly active antiretroviral therapy (HAART) was introduced in 1995, accounting for the visible decline in deaths. Almost no treatment was available in Sub-Saharan Africa until 2003. During this period, it is estimated that 8000 people died per day.

Source: Individual Members of the Faculty of Harvard University. Consensus statement on antiretroviral treatment for AIDS in poor countries. *Top HIV Med.* 2001;9(2):14–26.

The Global Fund, as it became known, first called for proposals in 2002 and rapidly became the world's largest financing institution for health. Sir Richard Feachem, once a critic of the HIV Equity Initiative in Haiti, was selected as the first Executive Director of the Global Fund.[129,130] It was and continues to be managed as an independent fund that accepts country proposals to finance AIDS, TB, and malaria programs and disperses money based on the success of the programs.[129,130] At the country level, proposal writing and oversight are done through a country coordinating mechanism (CCM), which brings together government and civil society partners—always including PLWA. The CCM serves a three-fold function: coordination for more efficient use of grants, capacity-building of weaker sectors through collaborative grant writing and administrative processes, and improved reach of service delivery to all populations.[131] In 2003, the first round of the Global Fund disbursed more than $600 million to 30 countries across the globe. Large-scale AIDS treatment began. In 2003, President George W. Bush announced the creation of the President's Emergency Plan for AIDS Relief (PEPFAR), which promised an additional $15 billion over five years to prevent and treat HIV.[132] In the first wave of PEPFAR funding, bilateral agreements were made between the United States and 14 high-burden countries.

Finally, 22 years after the first cases of HIV were reported and 8 years after the miracle of ART was seen in rich countries, the realization of the right to AIDS treatment was possible for the world's poor. In 2003, as the first checks from the Global Fund were cut and PEPFAR planning was under way, Farmer's group Partners In Health in Cange, Haiti, along with Dr. Jean William Pape's Group Haitien pour l'Etude de le Sarcome Kaposi et Infeciones Opportunistiques (GHESKIO) held an international conference in Haiti called "Models to Implementation," where experts from around the world came to the rural village of Cange to see first-hand the delivery of HIV care in a setting of great poverty. In 2003, Dr. Jim Kim, a founder of Partners in Health, left the organization to promote HIV treatment access at the WHO. Kim became the Director of the WHO's AIDS program and launched the 3 × 5 initiative with a goal of treating 3 million people by 2005.[133] On the cover of the WHO's brochure was a before-and-after picture of Joseph Jeune, a PLWA from rural Haiti who lived more than 13 years after his initial presentation, thanks to ART (Figure 2.9A, B).

Joseph Jeune passed away on January 21, 2015, at the age of 37. He will always be remembered as an international icon and advocate for treatment access. His story can be found on the PIH website, in a blog post entitled "Remembering Ti Joseph: Patient, Friend, and HIV Advocate."[134] By 2016, 18.2 million people were on ART. This massive achievement could not have happened without activism. Yet there is still work to do.

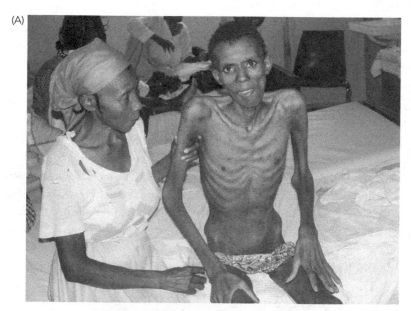

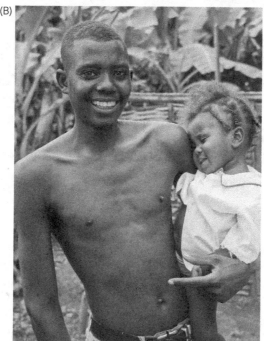

FIGURE 2.9 (A,B) Joseph Jeune, a Haitian person living with AIDS (PLWA) before and after receiving HIV treatment at Partners in Health facility; March 2003, shortly after his diagnosis, and with his niece in September 2003, after starting treatment for AIDS and completing treatment for tuberculosis.

Source: Partners in Health, 2003; photos courtesy of David Walton.

AIDS Today

In 2011, US Secretary of State Hillary Clinton announced the bold goal of an "AIDS free generation."[135] Yet despite scientific advancements, activism, and funding, AIDS is still a major threat to human life today. The opportunity to realize the "beginning of an end of AIDS" is not being met with the necessary political will or resources.[136,137] While the 2016 UNAIDS report documented that 18.2 million people are on ART, that is only half of the 36.7 million people living with AIDS. In 2015, there were roughly 1.1 million AIDS-related deaths, or about 3,000 per day.[138] Under new guidelines, all PLWA should be on treatment to save lives and prevent transmission. Disparities in access to treatment still occur today. In Europe and North America, there were 22,000 AIDS-related deaths in 2015, while there were about 800,000 in sub-Saharan Africa. In both regions, the poor and marginalize suffer significantly worse outcomes.[138] These deaths come despite the fact that studies have shown a near-normal life expectancy for people on ART, in both the United States and impoverished countries.[139,140] Therefore, to achieve the goal of an AIDS-free generation, it is imperative to call for "bold leadership and stronger investment."[141]

Recently, UNAIDS announced their 90-90-90 campaign. This campaign targets treatment as a means to end the AIDS epidemic and calls for 90 percent of all people living with HIV knowing their status, 90 percent of all people with a positive diagnosis of HIV receiving sustained ART, and 90 percent of all people receiving ART achieving viral suppression by 2020.[142] In a 2016 press statement, UNAIDS Executive Director Michel Sidibé estimated that, to reach these targets, global investment will need to increase by about one-third to reach $26.6 billion. Sidibé said, "Lack of investment now will result in the epidemic being prolonged indefinitely. . . . AIDS is not over yet but it can be."[141]

Conclusion

AIDS hit the world by storm in the 1980s and 1990s. The emergence of this deadly infection, for which no treatment or cure was known, created an environment of fear, stigma, and discrimination. The exponential spread of the virus, compounded with its propensity to unequally affect already vulnerable populations, led many countries, particularly those in the sub-Saharan Africa, into a state of national emergency. Under pressure from activists, ART was discovered. Despite this successful development, life-saving treatment was not accessible to all. However, thanks to the tireless work of many, the movement for AIDS treatment access created the field of global health delivery. By 2016, the Global Fund and PEPFAR dispersed $102 billion.[130,132] The success of this movement is profound. Most of the 18 million people on ART receive the treatment free of charge in public facilities.[143] After years of pitting prevention versus treatment, in 2011, studies documented that with large scale treatment, new infections were averted.[144] Yet the long-awaited money for HIV laid bare the ravages of decades of willful neglect of public infrastructure and human resources for health. To treat AIDS human capacity laboratory and clinic infrastructure, drug supply chains, and monitoring systems must be built. The delivery of health as a human right began with laying the building blocks for AIDS treatment.

References

1. Claeson M, Bos E, Mawji T, Pathmanathan I. Reducing child mortality in India in the new millennium. *Bull World Health Org.* 2000;78(10):1192–1199.
2. Altman LA. Rare cancer seen in homosexuals. *New York Times.* 1981;2016. http://www.nytimes.com/1981/07/03/us/rare-cancer-seen-in-41-homosexuals.html
3. Gottlieb GJ, Ragaz A, Vogel JV, et al. A preliminary communication on extensively disseminated Kaposi's sarcoma in young homosexual men. *Am J Dermatopathol.* 1981;3(2):111–114.
4. US Centers for Disease Control. Kaposi's sarcoma and Pneumocystis pneumonia among homosexual men—New York City and California. *Morb Mort Wkly Rep.* 1981;30(25):305–308.
5. Gottlieb MS, Schroff R, Schanker HM, et al. Pneumocystis carinii pneumonia and mucosal candidiasis in previously healthy homosexual men. *N Engl J Med.* 1981;305(24):1425–1431.
6. VerMeulen M. The gay plague. *New York Magazine.* 1982:52.
7. Jaffe HW, Bregman DJ, Selik RM. Acquired immune deficiency syndrome in the United States: The first 1,000 cases. *J Infect Dis.* 1983;148(2):339–345.
8. Conant MA. The AIDS epidemic. *J Am Acad Dermatol.* 1994;31(3):S50.
9. Vicira J, Franck E, Spiria, T J et al. Acquired immune deficiency in Haitians. *N Engl J Med.* 1983;308:125–129.
10. Farmer P. *AIDS and accusation: Haiti and the geography of blame.* Berkeley: University of California Press; 2006.
11. Wainberg MA, Shuldiner T, Dahl K, Gilmore N. Reconsidering the lifetime deferral of blood donation by men who have sex with men. *CMAJ.* 2010;182(12):1321.
12. Howe M. For people with AIDS, housing is hard to find. *New York Times.* 1984:B4. https://partners.nytimes.com/library/national/science/aids/062584sci-aids.html
13. Leonard AS. Employment discrimination against persons with AIDS. *Clearinghouse Rev.* 1986;19(11):1292–1302.
14. Malcolm A, Aggleton P, Bronfman M, Galvão J, Mane P, Verrall J. HIV-related stigmatization and discrimination: Its forms and contexts. *Crit Public Health.* 1998;8(4):347–370.
15. Blendon R, Donelan K. Discrimination against people with AIDS: The public's perspective. *N Engl J Med.* 1988;319(15):1022–1026.

16. Simons M. For Haiti's tourism, the stigma of AIDS is fatal. *New York Times*. Nov 29, 1983: A2.

17. Clumeck N, Mascart-Lemone F, De Maubeuge J, Brenez D, Marcelis L. Originally published as volume 1, issue 8325 Acquired Immune Deficiency Syndrome in black Africans. *Lancet*. 1983;321(8325):642. doi://dx.doi.org.ezp-prod1.hul.harvard.edu/10.1016/S0140-6736(83)91808-1.

18. Bygbjerg IC. Originally published as volume 1, issue 8330 AIDS in a Danish Surgeon (ZAIRE, 1976). *Lancet*. 1983;321(8330):925. doi://dx.doi.org.ezp-prod1.hul.harvard.edu/10.1016/S0140-6736(83)91348-X.

19. Vandepitte J, Verwilghen R, Zachee P. Originally published as volume 1, issue 8330 AIDS and Cryptococcosis (Zaire, 1977). *Lancet*. 1983;321(8330):925–926. doi://dx.doi.org.ezp-prod1.hul.harvard.edu/10.1016/S0140-6736(83)91349-1.

20. Biggar R. The AIDS problem in Africa. *Lancet*. 1986;327(8472):79–83.

21. Van De Perre P, Lepage P, Kestelyn P, et al. Acquired immunodeficiency syndrome in Rwanda. *Lancet*. 1984;324(8394):62–65.

22. Piot P, Taelman H, Bila Minlangu K, et al. Acquired immunodeficiency syndrome in a heterosexual population in Zaire. *Lancet*. 1984;2(8394):65–69.

23. Ras GJ, Simson IW, Anderson R, Prozesky OW, Hamersma T. Acquired immunodeficiency syndrome. A report of 2 South African cases. *S Afr Med J*. 1983;64(4):140–142.

24. Lyons SF, Schoub BD, Mcgillivray GM, Sher R, Dos Santos L. Lack of evidence of HTLV- III Endemicity in Southern Africa. *N Engl J Med*. 1985;312(19):1257.

25. Yeboah IEA. HIV/AIDS and the construction of sub-Saharan Africa: Heuristic lessons from the social sciences for policy. *Soc Sci Med*. 2007;64(5):1128–1150.

26. Rubinstein A, Sicklick M, Gupta A, et al. Acquired immunodeficiency with reversed T4/T8 ratios in infants born to promiscuous and drug-addicted mothers. *JAMA*. 1983;249(17):2350–2356.

27. Papaevangelou G, Economidou J, Kallinikos J, et al. Lymphadenopathy associated virus in AIDS, lymphadenopathy associated syndrome, and classic Kaposi patients in Greece. *Lancet*. 1984;324(8403):642. doi://dx.doi.org.ezp-prod1.hul.harvard.edu/10.1016/S0140-6736(84)90635-4.

28. Laurence J, Brun-Vezinet F, Schutzer SE, et al. Lymphadenopathy-associated viral antibody in AIDS. *N Engl J Med*. 1984;311(20):1269–1273.

29. Coffin J, Haase A, Levy JA, et al. Human immunodeficiency viruses. *Science*. 1986;232((4751)):697.

30. Acheson ED. AIDS: A challenge for the public health. *Lancet*. 1986;327(8482):662–666. doi://dx.doi.org.ezp-prod1.hul.harvard.edu/10.1016/S0140-6736(86)91736-8.

31. Royce RA, Seña A, Cates W, Cohen MS. Sexual transmission of HIV. *N Engl J Med*. 1997;336(15):1072–1078.

32. Curran JW. The epidemiology and prevention of the acquired immunodeficiency syndrome. *Ann Intern Med*. 1985;103:662.

33. Curran JW, Morgan WM, Hardy AM, Jaffe HW, Darrow WW, Dowdle WR. The epidemiology of AIDS: Status and future prospects. *Science.* 1985;229(4720):1352–1357.

34. World Health Assembly. Resolutions of the thirty-ninth world health assembly of interest to the executive committee. Jun 1986. http://apps.who.int/iris/bitstream/10665/162252/1/WHA39_1986-REC-1_eng.pdf

35. Preston J. Obama lifts a 22-year ban on entry into U.S. by H.I.V.- positive people. *New York Times (1923-Current file).* 2009:A9. http://www.nytimes.com/2009/10/31/us/politics/31travel.html

36. Piot P, Russell S, Larson H. Good politics, bad politics: The experience of AIDS. *Am J Public Health.* 2007:1934–1936. http://ajph.aphapublications.org/doi/10.2105/AJPH.2007.121418

37. Mann JM, ed. *AIDS: A worldwide pandemic.* Current Topics in AIDS, vol. 2, 2nd ed. New York: Wiley; 1989.

38. Mann JM. The World Health Organization's global strategy for the prevention and control of AIDS. *West J Med.* 1987;147(6):732–734.

39. Mann J, Francis H, Mwandagalirwa K, et al. Elisa readers and HIV antibody testing in developing countries. *Lancet.* 1986;327(8496):1504. doi://dx.doi.org.ezp-prod1.hul.harvard.edu/10.1016/S0140-6736(86)91541-2.

40. Black RE, Morris SS, Bryce J. Where and why are 10 million children dying every year? *Lancet.* 2003;361(9376):2226–2234.

41. Cegielski JP, Mcmurray D. The relationship between malnutrition and tuberculosis: Evidence from studies in humans and experimental animals. *Int J Tuberc Lung Dis.* 2004;8(3):286–298.

42. Grant AD, Djomand G, De Cock KM. Natural history and spectrum of disease in adults with HIV/AIDS in Africa. *AIDS.* 1997;11 Suppl B:S43.

43. Raviglione M, Nunn PP, Kochi A, O'Brien RJ. The pandemic of HIV-associated tuberculosis. In: Mann J, Tarantola D, editors. *AIDS in the world II.* New York: Oxford University Press; 1996. p. 87–96.

44. Corbett EL, Watt CJ, Walker N, et al. The growing burden of tuberculosis: Global trends and interactions with the HIV epidemic. *Arch Intern Med.* 2003;163(9):1009–1021.

45. Raviola G, Machoki M, Mwaikambo E, Good M. HIV, disease plague, demoralization and burnout: Resident experience of the medical profession in Nairobi, Kenya. *Cult Med Psychiatry.* 2002;26(1):55–86.

46. World Health Organization (WHO). *Taking stock: Health worker shortages and the response to AIDS.* Geneva: World Health Organization; 2006.

47. TASO. The AIDS support organization (TASO). Available from: https://www.tasouganda.org/index.php/about-taso. Accessed Nov 15, 2016.

48. Kalibala S, Kaleeba N. AIDS and community-based care in Uganda: The AIDS support organization, TASO. *AIDS Care.* 1989;1(2):173–175.

49. France D, Richman TW, Walk TH, et al. *How to survive a plague.* New York: Sundance Selects, MPI Media Group; 2013.

50. Leland J. Twilight of a difficult man: Larry Kramer and the birth of AIDS activism. May 19, 2017. Available from: https://www.nytimes.com/2017/05/19/nyregion/larry-kramer-and-the-birth-of-aids-activism.html.

51. New York Public Library. Gay Men's Health Crisis records. Available from: http://archives.nypl.org/mss/1126. Accessed Jun 28, 2016.

52. ACT Up. ACT UP capsule history. Available from: http://www.actupny.org/documents/cron-87.html. Accessed Jun 28, 2016.

53. Sotomayor J. Homosexuals arrested at AIDS drug protest. Available from: http://www.nytimes.com/1987/03/25/nyregion/homosexuals-arrested-at-aids-drug-protest.html. Updated 1987. Accessed Jun 28, 2016.

54. ACT UP. Flyer of the first ACT UP Action Mar 24, 1987, Wall Street, New York City. Available from: http://www.actupny.org/documents/1stFlyer.html. Accessed Jun 28, 2016.

55. Shepard BH, Hayduk R. *From ACT UP to the WTO: Urban protest and community building in the era of globalization.* London/New York: Verso; 2002.

56. Koch EI. Senator Helm's callousness toward AIDS victims. *New York Times.* Nov 7, 1987. Available from: http://www.nytimes.com/1987/11/07/opinion/senator-helms-s-callousness-toward-aids-victims.html. Accessed May 23, 2017.

57. Strub S. Condomizing Jesse Helm's House. 2011. The Blog. http://www.huffingtonpost.com/sean-strub/condomizing-jesse-helms-h_b_113329.html

58. La Ganga ML. The First Lady who looked away: Nancy and the Reagans' troubling AIDS Legacy. *The Guardian.* Mar 11, 2016. Available from: https://www.theguardian.com/us-news/2016/mar/11/nancy-ronald-reagan-aids-crisis-first-lady-legacy. Accessed May 23, 2017.

59. TAG. News: Treatment action group. Treatment Action Group Web site. Available from: www.treatmentactiongroup.org. Accessed Nov 16, 2016.

60. IAS. *VIII International Conference on AIDS/III STD World Congress, Amsterdam, The Netherlands 19–24 Jul 1992.* Amsterdam: Congrex Holland B. V.; 1992.

61. Gonsalves G, Harrington M, editors. *AIDS research at the NIH: A critical review.* New York: Treatment Action Group; 1992.

62. Davidson K, Kos P. *Bending the arc.* USA:2017.

63. Mann J. Acquired immunodeficiency syndrome in the 1990s: A global analysis. *Am J Infect Control.* 1993;21(6):317–321. doi://dx.doi.org.ezp-prod1.hul.harvard.edu/10.1016/0196-6553(93)90389-L.

64. Mann JM. We are all Berliners: Notes from the ninth international conference on AIDS. *Am J Public Health.* 1993;83(10):1378–9.

65. Preble EA. Impact of HIV/AIDS on African children. *Soc Sci Med.* 1990;31(6):671–680.

66. Foster C, Williamson J. A review of current literature on the impact of HIV/AIDS on children in sub-Saharan Africa. *AIDS.* 2000;14:S284.

67. Jong-Wook L. WHO/UNAIDS/GFAT media pack for the global launch of the "3by5" initiative and World AIDS Day, 2003. Geneva: WHO, UNAIDS, GFATM; 2003.

68. France D. *How to survive a plague: The inside story of how citizens and science tamed AIDS.* First edition. New York: Knopf; 2016.

69. Hammer SM, Squires KE, Hughes MD, et al. A controlled trial of two nucleoside analogues plus indinavir in persons with human immunodeficiency virus infection and CD4 cell counts of 200 per cubic millimeter or less. *N Engl J Med.* 1997;337(11):725–733.

70. Palella FJ, Delaney KM, Moorman AC, et al. Declining morbidity and mortality among patients with advanced human immunodeficiency virus infection. *N Engl J Med.* 1998;338(13):853–860.

71. Voelker R. Protease inhibitors bring new social, clinical uncertainties to HIV care. *JAMA.* 1997;277(15):1182–1184.

72. Leland J. The end of AIDS? *Newsweek.* 1996;128(23):64.

73. Bangsberg D, Tulsky JP, Hecht FM, Moss AR. Protease inhibitors in the homeless. *JAMA.* 1997;278(1):63–65.

74. Quinn TC. Global burden of the HIV pandemic. *Lancet.* 1996;348(9020):99–106.

75. Deeks SG, Smith M, Holodniy M, Kahn JO. HIV-1 protease inhibitors: A review for clinicians. *JAMA.* 1997;277(2):145–153.

76. International AIDS Society. One world. One hope. Proceedings of the XI International Conference on AIDS. Vancouver, Canada, 7–12 Jul 1996. *AIDS.* 1996;10 Suppl 3:S1.

77. Sawyer E. Remarks at the opening ceremony. Available from: www.actupny.org/Vancouver/sawyerspeech.html. Accessed Nov 17, 2016.

78. Ravishankar N, Gubbins P, Cooley RJ, et al. Financing of global health: Tracking development assistance for health from 1990 to 2007. *Lancet.* 2009;373(9681):2113–2124.

79. Cohen B, Trussell J. *Preventing and mitigating AIDS in Sub-Saharan Africa: Research and data priorities for the social and behavioral sciences.* Washington, DC: National Academy Press; 1996.

80. Messac L, Prabhu K. Redefining the possible: The global AIDS response. In: Farmer P, Kim JY, Kleinman A, Basilico M, editors. *Reimagining global health, an introduction.* Berkeley: University of California Press; 2013.

81. Marseille E, Hofmann PB, Kahn JG. HIV Prevention before HAART in Sub-Saharan Africa. *Lancet.* 2002;359(9320):1851–1856.

82. Creese A, Floyd K, Alban A, Guinness L. Cost-effectiveness of HIV/AIDS interventions in Africa: A systematic review of the evidence. *Lancet.* 2002;359(9318):1635–1642.

83. Robins S. "Long live Zackie, long live": AIDS activism, science and citizenship after apartheid. *J S Afr Studies.* 2004;30(3):651–672.

84. Malan M. Exposing AIDS: Media's impact in South Africa. *Georgetown J Intl Affairs.* 2006;7(1):41–49.

85. Boseley S. Discredited doctor's cure: For AIDS ignites life-and-death struggle in South Africa. *The Guardian.* May 14, 2005. Available from: https://www.theguardian.com/world/2005/may/14/southafrica.internationalaidanddevelopment. Accessed Apr 18, 2017.

86. Nattrass N. *Mortal combat: AIDS denialism and the struggle for antiretrovirals in South Africa.* Scottsville, SA: University of KwaZulu-Natal Press; 2007.

87. Chigwedere P, Seage GR, Gruskin S, Lee T, Essex M. Estimating the lost benefits of antiretroviral drug use in South Africa. *J Acquir Immune Defic Syndr.* 2008;49(4):410.

88. Republic of South Africa Constitutional Court. The Constitution of the Republic of South Africa. 1996. http://www.gov.za/sites/www.gov.za/files/images/a108-96.pdf

89. International AIDS Society. History of the IAS—Episode 4, 2000: AIDS denialism and treatment equity at the Durban Conference. International AIDS Society—At the Durban XIII International AIDS conference.

90. Denny C. Mandela hits out at AIDS drug firms. *The Guardian.* Apr 16, 2001. Available from: https://www.theguardian.com/business/2001/apr/16/aids. Accessed Apr 18, 2017.

91. Chirac P, Von Schoen-Angerer T, Kasper T, Ford N. AIDS: Patent rights versus patient's rights. *Lancet.* 2000;356(9228):502.

92. WTO. Understanding the WTO. 2015. https://www.wto.org/english/thewto_e/whatis_e/tif_e/tif_e.htm

93. Chaudhuri S. *The WTO and India's pharmaceuticals industry: Patent protection, TRIPS, and developing countries.* New Delhi/New York: Oxford University Press; 2005.

94. Treatment Action Campaign. 1998–2010 fighting for our lives: The history of the treatment action campaign. 2010. http://www.tac.org.za/files/10yearbook/files/tac%2010%20year%20draft5.pdf

95. ACT UP. ACT UP accomplishments and partial chronology. Available from: http://actupny.com/actions/index.php/the-community. Accessed Nov 21, 2016.

96. Schneider H, Fassin D. Denial and defiance: A socio-political analysis of AIDS in South Africa. *AIDS.* 2002;16:S51.

97. Baleta A. Cautious welcome for antiretroviral cost reduction in South Africa. *Lancet.* 2000;355(9217):1799.

98. World Trade Organization. Understanding the WTO: The Agreements Intellectual Property: Protection and enforcement. Available from: https://www.wto.org/english/thewto_e/whatis_e/tif_e/agrm7_e.htm. Accessed Jul 1, 2016.

99. Ford N, Wilson D, Cawthorne P, et al. Challenge and co-operation: Civil society activism for access to HIV treatment in Thailand. [Défi et coopération: Activisme de société civile pour l'accès au traitement du VIH en Thaïlande. point de vue; retos y cooperación: Activismo de la sociedad civil para el acceso al tratamiento de VIH en Tailandia. Punto de vista.] *Trop Med Intl Health.* 2009;14(3):258–266.

100. Ford N, Wilson D, Chaves G, Lotrowska M, Kijtiwatchakul K. Sustaining access to antiretroviral therapy in the less- developed world: Lessons from Brazil and Thailand. *AIDS*. 2007;21:S29.

101. Medecins Sans Frontieres. Access campaign. Available from: https://www.msfaccess.org/. Updated 2017. Accessed May 4, 2017.

102. Sidley P. Drug companies sue South African government over generics. *BMJ*. 2001;322(7284):447.

103. Bombach KM. Can South Africa fight AIDS? Reconciling the South African medicines and related substances act with TRIPS agreement (agreement on trade- related aspects of intellectual property rights). *Boston U Intl L J*. 2001;19(2):273–306.

104. Sidley P. Drug companies withdraw law suit against South Africa. *BMJ*. 2001;322. (7293):1011.

105. Kapczynski A, Berger JM. The story of the TAC case: The potential and limits of socio-economic rights litigation in South Africa. In: Hurwitz DR, Satterthwaite ML, Ford D, editors. *Human rights advocacy stories*. New York: Thomson Reuters/ Foundation Press; 2009.

106. Francisco I, Pinkusfeld BM, Nunn A, Hacker MA, Malta M, Szwarcwald CL. AIDS in brazil: The challenge In: Celentano David, Beyrer Chris, editors. *Public health aspects of HIV/AIDS in low and middle income countries*. New York: Springer-Verlag; 2009:629–654.

107. Nunn AS, Fonseca EM, Bastos FI, Gruskin S, Salomon JA. Evolution of antiretroviral drug costs in Brazil in the context of free and universal access to AIDS treatment. *PloS Med*. 2007;4(11):1804.

108. Levi GC, Vitória MA, A. Fighting against AIDS: The Brazilian experience. *AIDS*. 2002;16(18):2373.

109. Rosenberg T. Look at Brazil. *New York Times (1923-Current file)*. New York Times Magazine; 2001:SM26.

110. Ashraf H. USA and Brazil end dispute over essential drugs. *Lancet*. 2001;357(9274):2112.

111. World Bank. Health nutrition and population statistics. 2017. http://data.worldbank.org/data-catalog/health-nutrition-and-population-statistics

112. Feachem R. HAART: The need for strategically focused investments. *Bull World Health Org*. 2001;79(12):1152.

113. Zimmerman R. Sending AIDS drugs to Haitians in need is MIT Student's Project. Available from: http://www.wsj.com/articles/SB1016061549375397320. Accessed Jun 30, 2016.

114. Farmer P, Léandre F, Mukherjee J, Gupta R, Tarter L, Kim JY. Community-based treatment of advanced HIV disease: Introducing DOT-HAART (directly observed therapy with highly active antiretroviral therapy). *Bull World Health Org*. 2001;79(12):1145–1151.

115. Farmer P, Léandre F, Mukherjee JS, et al. Community-based approaches to HIV treatment in resource-poor settings. *Lancet*. 2001;358(9279):404–409.

116. Gilks C, AbouZahr C, Turmen T. HAART in Haiti: Evidence needed. *Bull World Health Org.* 2001;79(12):1154.

117. Neuman M. South Africa. MSF, an African NGO? Available from: http://www.msf-crash.org/livres/en/south-africa-msf-an-african-ngo. Accessed Apr 18, 2017.

118. Herbert B. Americans refusing to save Africans. *New York Times.* Jun 11 2001. Available from: http://www.nytimes.com/2001/06/11/opinion/in-america-refusing-to-save-africans.html.

119. PIH. Cange declaration: PIH's first HIV patients advocate for equal access to treatment. Available from: http://www.pih.org/blog/cange-declaration-pihs-first-hiv-patients-advocate-for-equity-in-access-to. Accessed Nov 21, 2016.

120. Katzenstein D, Laga M, Moatti JP. The evaluation of the HIV/IDS drug access initiatives in cote D'Ivoire, Senegal and Uganda: How access to antiretroviral treatment can become feasible in Africa. *AIDS.* 2003;17:S4.

121. Mcneil DG. Companies to cut cost of AIDS drugs for poor nations. *The New York Times on the Web.* 2000:4. https://partners.nytimes.com/library/world/africa/051200africa-aids.html

122. UNAIDS. *Report on the global HIV/AIDS epidemic June 2000.* Geneva: Joint United Nations Programme on HIV/AIDS; 2000.

123. Piot P. United Nations University Address. Aug 8, 2001. http://archive.unu.edu/media/archives/2001/pre28.01.html

124. Colgan AL. *Africa's debt.* Africa Action position paper. 2001:4. https://www.globalpolicy.org/component/content/article/210/44717.html

125. Poku NK. Poverty, debt and African's HIV/AIDS crisis. *Intl Affairs.* 2002;78(3):531–546.

126. Attaran A, Sachs J. Defining and refining international donor support for combating the AIDS pandemic. *Lancet.* 2001;357(9249):57–61.

127. Individual Members of the Faculty of Harvard University. Consensus statement on antiretroviral treatment for AIDS in poor countries. *Topics HIV Med.* 2001;9(2):14–26.

128. United Nations. Declaration of commitment on HIV/AIDS: United Nations General Assembly Special Session on HIV/AIDS 25–27 June 2001. New York: United Nations; 2001.

129. Tan DHS, Upshur REG, Ford N. Global plagues and the global fund: Challenges in the fight against HIV, TB and malaria. *BMC Intl Health Human Rights.* 2003;3:2.

130. The Global Fund. Global fund overview. Available from: http://www.theglobalfund.org/en/overview/. Accessed Nov 21, 2016.

131. Brugha R, Donoghue M, Starling M, et al. The global fund: Managing great expectations. *Lancet.* 2004;364(9428):95–100.

132. Dybul M. Lessons learned from PEPFAR. *JAIDS.* 2009;52:S13.

133. World Health Organization (WHO). The 3 by 5 initiative. Available from: http://www.who.int/3by5/about/initiative/en/. Accessed Apr 18, 2017.

134. Partners in Health. Remembering Ti Joseph: Patient, friend, and HIV advocate. Available from: http://www.pih.org/blog/remembering-ti-joseph-patient-friend-and-hiv-advocate. Accessed Apr 10, 2017.

135. Editorial. The beginning of the end of AIDS? *Lancet.* 2012;380(9858):1967. Available from: http://www.thelancet.com/journals/lancet/article/PIIS0140-6736(12)62137-0/fulltext?rss=yes.

136. Havlir D, Beyrer C. The beginning of the end of AIDS? *N Engl J Med.* 2012;367(8):685–687.

137. McMahon JH, Medland N. 90-90-90: How do we get there? *Lancet HIV.* 2014;1(1):e11.

138. UNAIDS. *AIDS data.* Geneva: Joint United Nations Programme on HIV/AIDS; 2016.

139. Trickey A, May MT, Vehreschild J, et al. Survival of HIV- positive patients starting antiretroviral therapy between 1996 and 2013: A collaborative analysis of cohort studies. *Lancet HIV.* 2017;4(8):e349–e356. https://www-clinicalkey-com.ezp-prod1.hul.harvard.edu/#!/content/playContent/1-s2.0-S2352301817300668?returnurl=null&referrer=null

140. Mills EJ, Bakanda C, Birungi J, et al. Life expectancy of persons receiving combination antiretroviral therapy in low-income countries: A cohort analysis from Uganda. *Ann Intern Med.* 2011;155(4):209.

141. Sidibe M. Calling on innovators, implementers, investors, activists and leaders to fast-track ending the AIDS epidemic by 2030. UNAIDS Web site. Available from: http://www.unaids.org/en/resources/presscentre/pressreleaseandstatementarchive/2016/june/20160603_EXD_HLM_message. Accessed May 23, 2017.

142. UNAIDS. *90-90-90: An ambitious treatment target to help end the AIDS epidemic.* Geneva: Joint United Nations Programme on HIV/AIDS; 2017.

143. UNAIDS. Fact sheet November 2016. Available from: http://www.unaids.org/en/resources/fact-sheet. Updated 2016. Accessed Nov 21, 2016.

144. Cohen MS, Chen YQ, McCauley M, et al. Prevention of HIV-1 infection with early antiretroviral therapy. *N Engl J Med* 2011;365:493–505.

3

The Millennium Development Goals and Sustainable Development Goals

Key Points

- In 2000, the international community agreed on a set of goals for development. These were called the Millennium Development Goals (MDGs).
- Three of the eight MDGs would measure concrete progress on child health, women's health, and access to infectious disease treatment by 2015.
- To achieve the MDGs, health systems needed to be strengthened.
- Only MDG 6—the treatment of AIDS, tuberculosis (TB), and malaria—received dedicated funding.
- MDG 6 was the most successful MDG.
- The international community launched the Sustainable Development Goals (SDGs) at the end of the MDG period in 2015. The SDGs set new targets for 2030 including Universal Health Coverage.

Introduction

In 2001, all 189 United Nations member states signed onto the Millennium Development Goals (MDGs). The MDGs were a set of eight goals with time-bound targets to improve the health and development of impoverished nations by 2015.[1] The three health-related MDGs focused on children, women, and infectious diseases. The other MDGs addressed social factors related to health: hunger, gender equality, education, and environmental sustainability. MDG 8 called for a global partnership for development and encouraged international coordination, cooperation, and financing to achieve the agreed upon targets.[1] The turn of the millennium renewed the sense of urgency for political and economic commitments to achieve health as a human right.

Given the history of selective primary health care, achieving the MDGs was impeded by significant health system weaknesses. Health systems strengthening requires attention to multiple components including human resources, infrastructure, and supply chain. Money is required to implement these components. However, the MDGs did not provide any money for impoverished countries to achieve these goals. The Global Fund and the President's Emergency Plan for AIDS Relief (PEPFAR) are the notable exceptions. Unsurprisingly, AIDS treatment was the most successful component of the MDGs. Finally, this chapter discusses the shift from the MDGs to the Sustainable Development Goals (SDGs). This chapter addresses the creation of the MDGs and the use of AIDS-specific funding to improve entire health systems.

The Millennium Development Goals

The MDGs were developed with the shared purpose of improving the health and development of the world's poor. Yet the health care delivery needed to achieve the MDGs was in stark contrast with the reality of how little health care was being delivered in impoverished countries.[2] For example, at that time, the cornerstone of selective primary health care was childhood vaccinations campaigns. Yet even these simple programs faced enormous challenges. Data from the World Bank show that childhood immunizations in the 1990s for polio; measles; and diphtheria, pertussis, and tetanus (DPT) in sub-Saharan Africa never reached more than 55 percent coverage.[3] In 2000, the average health budgets of impoverished governments ranged from $5 to $10 per capita per year.[4] Health systems suffered from a small, poorly trained, and erratically paid health workforce, lack of drugs, and insufficient health infrastructure.[4] According to the World Development Report of 2000,[5] poverty in most regions, particularly in sub-Saharan Africa, was increasing. More people were dying (Figure 3.1A, B).

By the late 1990s, it was clear that the health of the world's poor had received insufficient attention.[5] The structural adjustment policies of the World Bank and the International Monetary Fund (IMF) were increasingly criticized for hampering the ability of governments to deliver comprehensive health care.[2] A series of development meetings held by the UN, the Organization for Economic Cooperation and Development (OECD), the World Bank, and the IMF in the 1990s focused on reducing global inequality.[6] These meetings concluded that the debt burdens in impoverished countries and low levels of overseas development assistance (ODA) from wealthy countries limited economic development.

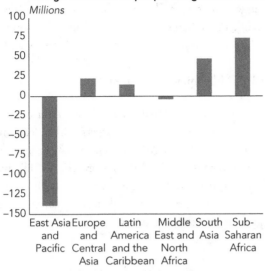

(A) **Where poverty has fallen, and where it has not**

Change in number of people living on less than $1 a day, 1987–98

(B) **Infant mortality rates vary widely across the world**

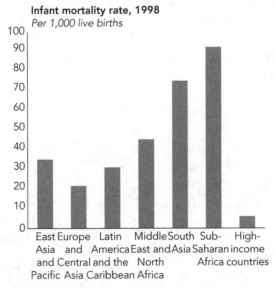

Infant mortality rate, 1998

FIGURE 3.1 (A) Number of people living on less than $1 per day increased in South Asia and sub-Saharan Africa 1987–1996. This increase in poverty mirrors the worsening infant mortality rates (B).

Source: World Bank. 2001. World Development Report 2000/2001: Attacking poverty. License: Creative Commons Attribution (CC BY 3.0 IGO).

The OECD's Development Assistance Committee (DAC) penned its ambitious International Development Goals (IDGs) in 1996. The IDGs included global targets for reducing hunger, illiteracy, and ill health.[7] In 2000, the IDGs were formalized at the UN Millennium Summit.[8] At this summit, 189 member states drafted the MDGs to address poverty, health, environmental threats, and human rights violations.[9]

Leaders signing the UN Millennium Declaration were:

> Committing their nations to a new global partnership to reduce extreme poverty and setting out a series of time-bound targets, with a deadline of 2015, that have become known as the Millennium Development Goals. The Millennium Development Goals (MDGs) are the world's time-bound and quantified targets for addressing extreme poverty in its many dimensions-income poverty, hunger, disease, lack of adequate shelter, and exclusion—while promoting gender equality, education, and environmental sustainability.[10]

The creation of the MDGs was criticized for the lack of civil society engagement in the process, the difficulty of measuring progress toward the goals, and the belief that countries had insufficient funds to achieve the targets.[11,12] Despite these criticisms, the MDGs were widely endorsed and addressed hunger (MDG 1), education (MDG 2), gender equality (MDG 3), child health (MDG 4), women's health (MDG 5), infectious disease (MDG 6), and environmental sustainability (MDG 7)[13] (Figure 3.2).

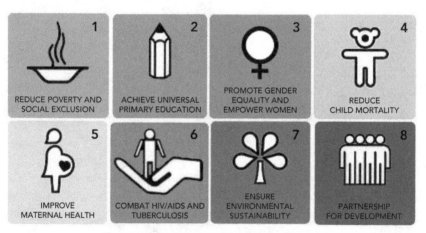

FIGURE 3.2 The Millennium Development Goals (MDGs). The MDGs were launched in 2000. They comprise of a set of eight goals for development. The three health-related goals are MDG 4, 5, and 6.

Icons developed by and courtesy of UNDP Brazil.

Health Systems Coordination

Achieving the three health-related MDGs required that impoverished governments deliver comprehensive health care. To achieve MDG 4, a reduction of under-five child mortality by two thirds, countries had to address diarrheal disease, respiratory infection, malaria, and malnutrition.[14] Countries would have to train clinicians to diagnose and treat these ailments and build laboratories to support these efforts.[15] Countries needed to provide an even more complex set of interventions to achieve MDG 5, the reduction of maternal mortality by three-quarters. The majority of maternal deaths are due to five things—bleeding, infection, uncontrolled high blood pressure (eclampsia), obstructed labor, or incomplete or unsafe abortion (Figure 3.3).[16] To avert deaths of this type, health systems need well-trained staff to deal with the complications of childbirth and prevent women from dying in pregnancy and childbirth. Hospitals must be equipped to provide the surgery, blood, antibiotics, and anticonvulsants necessary to save women's lives.[17] For MDG 6, expanding treatment for AIDS, tuberculosis (TB), and malaria, clinicians need to manage longitudinal treatments. A robust supply chain is needed to avoid drug stock-outs, and laboratories are needed to diagnose disease and monitor response to treatment.

Due to the complex and interdependent nature of the elements needed to deliver health care, achieving the MDGs required moving from vertical campaigns, like programs for child growth monitoring, oral rehydration, breastfeeding, and immunization (GOBI),[18] to broad-based health systems strengthening.[19] The term "vertical program" is used to describe disease-specific efforts.[20] AIDS treatment activism succeeded in generating massive funding for MDG 6 (Figure 3.4). Countries, however, were concerned that AIDS funding would be vertical and used only for the treatment of AIDS rather than to also strengthen health systems.[21–23] Impoverished governments worried that nongovernmental organization (NGO)-run, vertical AIDS programs would weaken government health systems. International actors recognized the need for coordination of new AIDS funding and held multiple meetings to address these concerns. At the International Conference on AIDS and Sexually Transmitted Infections (STIs) (ICASA) in Nairobi, Kenya, in September 2003,[24–26] African ministers, donors, leaders of NGOs, and representatives of the private sector met to discuss the coordination of money for AIDS. They outlined a consensus that became known as the "three ones."[27] Participants agreed that countries should have:

- one national AIDS plan (HIV/AIDS Action Framework) to coordinate the work of all partners,
- one national coordinating authority (with multisectoral participation; e.g., beyond health),
- one country-level monitoring and evaluation system.

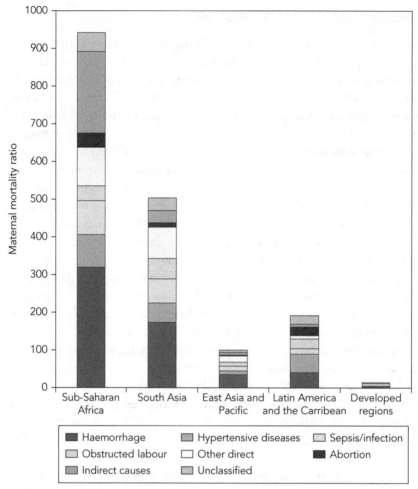

FIGURE 3.3 Maternal mortality by cause and region (2000).

Source: Ronsmans C, Graham WJ. Maternal mortality: Who, when, where, and why. *Lancet.* 2006;368(9542):1189–1200.

This consensus of a coordinated approach was novel because it explicitly stated that the "three ones" ought to shift power to governments from NGOs and donors.[27]

Government coordination of new AIDS funding to meet the MDGs began a new era in the public provision of health care.[19] Because time-bound targets required care delivery and shifted the focus from prevention programs to the delivery of health care, the World Health Organization (WHO) defined a discrete set of building blocks for a functioning health system.[28,29] These building blocks included service delivery, health workforce, information systems, medical products, vaccines, financing, and governance

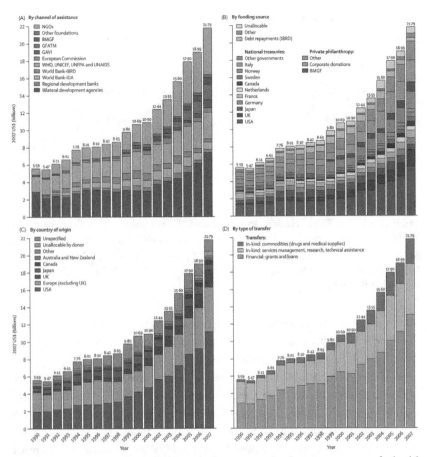

FIGURE 3.4 These graphs show the marked increase in development assistance for health by channel of assistance (1990–2007). Much of this change was driven by AIDS activism.

Source: Ravishankar N, Gubbins P, Cooley RJ, et al. Financing of global health: Tracking development assistance for health from 1990 to 2007. *Lancet*. 2009;373(9681):2113–2124.

(Figure 3.5). These six building blocks served as a framework for health system strengthening.[30] The WHO proposed that health systems would be evaluated by health outcomes, system responsiveness, social and financial risk protection, and improved efficiency.[29,31]

Leveraging Vertical Programs

Funding was needed to achieve MDG targets and strengthen health systems. AIDS activism brought forth new funding, though the lion's share of this money was earmarked for AIDS, TB, and malaria programs.[32] Although some claimed

THE WHO HEALTH SYSTEM FRAMEWORK

SYSTEM BUILDING BLOCKS   OVERALL GOALS/OUTCOMES

| SERVICE DELIVERY |
| HEALTH WORKFORCE |
| INFORMATION |
| MEDICAL PRODUCTS, VACCINES & TECHNOLOGIES |
| FINANCING |
| LEADERSHIP/GOVERNANCE |

ACCESS
COVERAGE

QUALITY
SAFETY

| IMPROVED HEALTH (LEVEL AND EQUITY) |
| RESPONSIVENESS |
| SOCIAL AND FINANCIAL RISK PROTECTION |
| IMPROVED EFFICIENCY |

FIGURE 3.5 The World Health Organization (WHO) Health System Framework. The WHO health system building blocks serve as a framework for health systems strengthening. *Source*: World Health Organization. Everybody's business: Strengthening health systems to improve health outcomes: WHO's framework for action. 2007. Available from: http://www.who.int/iris/handle/10665/43918.

there was too much money for AIDS, in actuality there was insufficient funding for all other health needs.[33] In fact, impoverished countries aimed to use new AIDS-specific funding to strengthen their health systems.[33,34]

Unfortunately, many AIDS interventions did start as vertical programs, focusing human resources, drugs, and diagnostics solely on AIDS.[35] NGOs managed most of these vertical programs, which did not strengthen government delivery of comprehensive health care. Vertical programs offered HIV testing, known as voluntary counseling and testing (VCT), in HIV clinics isolated from other services.[36] Vertical VCT programs educated populations about HIV risk factors, AIDS symptoms, and the new availability of antiretroviral treatment (ART). VCT programs were created with the hope that education would promote HIV testing. However, because VCT centers were built separately from general health care facilities, few people went to these isolated centers, and the approach largely failed.[37,38] Different claims were made for the low usage of VCT centers: some blamed a population-wide lack of education about HIV,[39] while others blamed community stigma against those who attended known HIV clinics.[40] People did not come forward for HIV testing alone, they come for care when they are sick.

PIH Efforts: HIV Monies and Health Systems Strengthening

Partners in Health and its Haitian counterpart, Zamni Lasante (ZL), supported the government of Haiti in its national plan to scale-up HIV treatment in public clinics. ZL received one of the first Global Fund grants in 2003 and used the funds to partner with the Haitian government to revitalize primary care in public facilities. The public–private partnership inaugurated its first revitalized clinic in the town of Lascahobas (with a population of 55,000 people) in 2003. Before the partnership was launched, that public facility cared for just 5 to 10 patients per day. The clinic was plagued by a lack of drugs and an irregularly paid and often absent government staff.[41] ZL knew that to find HIV cases, the clinic itself needed to be utilized and that people would come to a clinic if they were sick and if care was available. ZL reasoned that the first step in scaling up HIV testing and treatment was to deliver primary health care. Patients seeking care for general complaints would then be offered an HIV test. This strategy became known as *provider-initiated testing*.[42,43] Provider-initiated testing was different from VCT because it shifted the burden of asking for an HIV test from patients to providers. It also linked HIV testing to the provision of general medical care. ZL used funding for AIDS to support public clinics in four major ways: (1) paying the public sector staff and adding additional staff; (2) procuring essential medications (such as antimalarials and other antibiotics); (3) minimizing the financial barriers to care (reducing or exempting user fees and providing cash transfers to the vulnerable for clinic attendance); and (4) hiring, paying, and supervising community health workers who would find the sick, encourage them to come to health centers for care, and provide long-term follow-up of patients in their homes.

This strategy of buttressing health care delivery with AIDS money resulted in a 30- to 60-fold increase in utilization. The Lascahobas clinic went from seeing 5–10 patients a day to more than 300 (Figure 3.6). Attendance at other ZL-supported public clinics followed similar trajectories (Table 3.1). High levels of HIV testing took place when public clinics provided quality health services. Provider-initiated testing for HIV was offered to four groups[44]: (1) people presenting to outpatient clinics with symptoms of or risk factors for HIV, (2) people with a diagnosis or symptoms of TB (a common infection among those with HIV), (3) pregnant women presenting for prenatal care, and (4) people presenting with symptoms of other sexually transmitted diseases or STIs.

In one VCT clinic without linkage to general clinical care in Hinche, Haiti, only 306 HIV tests were done in one year.[45] In 2004, one year after ZL leveraged HIV funds to launch primary care and provider-initiated testing, more than 3,107 people were tested. By July 2006, 11,974 people had been tested and 350 were on ART.[45] Importantly, everyone screened was given condoms and preventative education. The provision of basic health services improved HIV case-finding, treated thousands of people for common conditions, provided prenatal care to many hundreds of women, and addressed the concomitant burden of TB.[44]

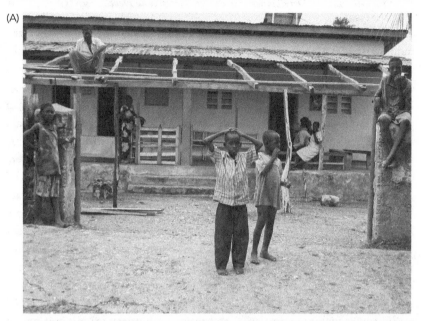

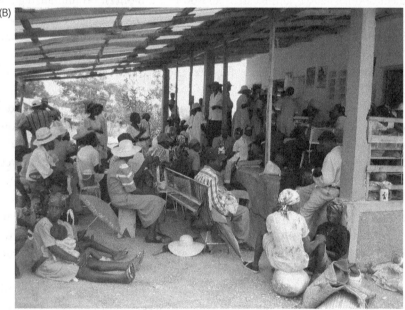

FIGURE 3.6A,B (A) A public clinic in Haiti after many decades of underinvestment. Few patients utilize the clinic. They know there are no drugs and only occasional staff. (B) The same clinic after 3 months of support for primary health care including staffing, drugs, the reduction of user fees and support from community health workers. The strategy of providing primary health care and strengthening the public system was supported by the Global Fund. But achieve far more than just HIV case finding and treatment as thousands received ongoing care in a public facility.

Courtesy of Joia Mukherjee.

Table 3.1 Use of services after the HIV–primary health care integrated model of care was implemented.

Public Clinic	July 2002, Before MSPP—Zanmi Lasante Community Partnership Average No. Ambulatory Visits per Day	December 2003, After Initiation of MSPP—Zanmi Lasante Community Partnership Average No. Ambulatory Visits per Day
Lascahobas	20	400
Belledere	10	150
Thomonde	10	250
Boucan Carre	10	250

HIV, human immunodeficiency virus; *MSPP*, Ministère de la Santé Publique et de la Population.

Utilization of health care increased dramatically in Haiti after Partners in Health and Zanmi-Lasante leveraged vertical AIDS money for the delivery of primary care.

Source: Mukherjee J, Ivers L, Leandre F, Farmer P, Behforouz H. Antiretroviral therapy in resource-poor settings: Decreasing barriers to access and promoting adherence. *JAIDS*. 2006;43:S126.

Similarly, visionaries throughout the world sought to leverage AIDS funding to improve the public provision of health care. Dr. Agnes Binagwaho, Executive Secretary of the National AIDS program in Rwanda from 2003 to 2008, Permanent Secretary of the Rwandan Ministry of Health from 2008 to 2011, and Minister of Health of Rwanda from 2009 to 2015, explained the country's approach in a 2008 interview: "we used AIDS money to assure we had a functioning system. Each district received an ambulance. Primary care clinics were built that could also provide HIV testing. Staff were trained to treat HIV but also to deliver primary care protocols."[46] Dr. Julio Frenk, the former Minister of Health of Mexico, calls the leverage of vertical funding the "diagonal approach."[47] Frenk advocated for this approach to bridge the dichotomy between vertical interventions generally supported by donors and the cross cutting needs of the health system. Mexico used a diagonal approach with child health funding to set the Mexican health system on an upward trajectory.[47]

Dr. Jim Kim, Director of the WHO's HIV/AIDS program, also understood that achieving HIV targets alone would insufficiently address the health needs of populations. At the WHO, Kim initiated a project called "Maximizing Positive Synergies" (MPS).[48] MPS was an international consortium of ministries, civil society, and academic organizations. This project researched how disease-specific funding was used by the health system. It demonstrated that Global Health Initiatives (GHIs), such as PEPFAR and the Global Fund, increased the uptake of both targeted services (such as HIV testing) and nontargeted services (such as blood pressure screening).[49] The MPS project also showed that standardized guidelines promoted by GHIs resulted in higher quality treatment. However, the project also exposed weaknesses in governance and coordination of health aid. It highlighted the potential for the distortion of government priorities toward areas of funding rather than toward the burden of disease. In summary, the project showed that when programs were designed to leverage vertical money for system strengthening they had a positive impact on the general delivery of health care. In contrast, systems designed as vertical, stand-alone programs had a negative impact on health systems, even if they achieved disease-specific targets. With this in mind, over the next several years, GHIs recognized the need to add health systems strengthening funding and metrics to vertical programs. The Global Fund continuously increased its commitments to health system strengthening over its first 15 years.[50] Researchers in Rwanda found that the diagonal implementation of HIV services increased utilization of antenatal care, screening for STIs, and the utilization of family planning.[51] Rwanda achieved remarkable success in the MDGs by using this diagonal approach (Figure 3.7).

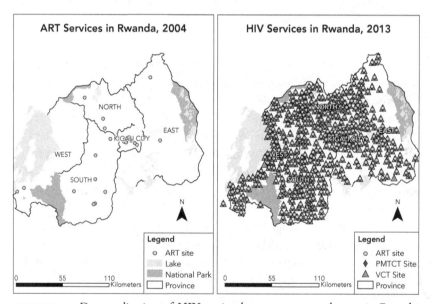

FIGURE 3.7 Decentralization of HIV testing between 2004 and 2014 in Rwanda. Because the plan for HIV testing, called VCT integré, was to integrate HIV testing within a strengthened set of primary care interventions, the expansion of HIV testing was also an expansion of access to primary care.

Source: Nsanzimana S, Prabhu K, McDermott H, Karita E, Forrest JI, Drobac P, Farmer P, Mills EJ, Binagwaho A. Improving health outcomes through concurrent HIV program scale-up and health system development in Rwanda: 20 years of experience. BMC Med. 2015 Sep 9;13:216.

Toward the Sustainable Development Goals

Despite the health system challenges, significant progress was made during the MDG era. The greatest successes were made on MDG 6.[52] In 2003, fewer than 1 million people were receiving HIV treatment; by the end of 2014, there were more than 13.6 million people on treatment.[52] ART reduced new infections by almost 40 percent between 2000 and 2013.[53,54] This finding ended years of debate that pitted AIDS prevention against treatment. Widespread ART not only saved lives but also prevented new infections. Through the distribution of 1 billion insecticide-treated nets and easy, widespread access to modern antimalarial medications,[55] more than 6.2 million malaria deaths were averted between 2000 and 2015.[52]

Despite these overall gains, progress on the health-related MDGs was uneven both between and within countries.[56] Improvements in malaria treatment profoundly impacted child survival, and under-five child deaths around the world dropped by 50 percent between 1990 and 2015.[52] The increased coverage of the treatment of pneumonia, diarrhea, and malnutrition, as well as improved childhood vaccination rates also contributed to this decrease in the deaths of children under 5 years of age.[52,57] However, less progress was made in reducing the deaths of children during the neonatal period (aged 0–28 days).[58] Saving newborns requires more sophisticated health care than does saving older children: sick newborns require intravenous medicines, breathing support, and incubators for temperature stabilization. Complications during the birthing process often cause newborns to fall ill and die.[59] The vulnerable mother–baby pair need higher level health care: a delivery room, access to emergency care, trained staff to resuscitate babies, and intravenous antibiotics for infection.[60] Without funding for women's health, MDG 5 lagged furthest behind targets.[52]

Analysis of MDG successes and failures provides several important lessons. First, goals that had dedicated funding had better outcomes. Second, goals that required higher level care were more difficult to achieve. Third, leveraging AIDS money supported primary care delivery but was insufficient to provide hospital care.

Of note, the cumulative effects of these and other development efforts did reduce extreme poverty. Countries made significant strides on MDG 1—the eradication of extreme poverty.[61] The UN MDGs report noted that the proportion of those living in extreme poverty dropped by about 50 percent from 1.9 billion in 1990 to fewer than 1 billion in 2015.[52] Most of the global drop in poverty was related to achievements in China and India, particularly due to agricultural-led economic growth for rural communities and government employment plans.[52]

To capture the interdependence of antipoverty issues, development, and the need for universal health care, the international community ended the first 15 years of the new millennium with the creation of the Sustainable Development Goals (SDGs).[62] The SDGs are a set of 17 goals which focus on diverse aspects of development. They are geared toward decreasing human suffering and reversing the dangerous trajectory of climate change by 2030. Important social movements, especially the movement to halt climate change, influenced the expansion of the SDGs.[63] The 17 SDGs are:

1. End poverty in all its forms everywhere.
2. End hunger, achieve food security and improved nutrition, and promote sustainable agriculture.
3. Ensure healthy lives and promote well-being for all at all ages.
4. Ensure inclusive and equitable quality education and promote life-long learning opportunities for all.
5. Achieve gender equality and empower all women and girls.
6. Ensure availability and sustainable management of water and sanitation for all.
7. Ensure access to affordable, reliable, sustainable modern energy for all.
8. Promote sustained, inclusive, and sustainable economic growth, full and productive employment, and decent work for all.
9. Build resilient infrastructure, promote inclusive and sustainable industrialization, and foster innovation.
10. Reduce inequality within and among countries.
11. Make cities and human settlements inclusive, safe, resilient, and sustainable.
12. Ensure sustainable consumption and production patterns.
13. Take urgent action to combat climate change and its impacts.
14. Conserve and sustainably use the oceans, seas, and marine resources for sustainable development.
15. Protect, restore, and promote sustainable use of terrestrial ecosystems, sustainably manage forests, combat desertification, halt and reverse land degradation, and halt biodiversity loss.
16. Promote peaceful and inclusive societies for sustainable development, provide access to justice for all, and build effective, accountable, and inclusive institutions at all levels.
17. Strengthen the means of implementation and revitalize the Global Partnership for Sustainable Development.

SDG 3 pertains to health. SDG 3 aims to "ensure healthy lives and promote well-being for all at all ages" (Box 3.1).[62] It builds on the successes of

---

BOX 3.1

Summary of Sustainable Development Goal 3

"Ensure healthy lives and promote well-being for all at all ages," targets for 2030:

- Reduce global maternal mortality rate to less than 70/100,000 live births.
- End preventable deaths of newborns and children under five:
  - reduce neonatal mortality to 12/1,000 live births
  - reduce under-five mortality to 25/1,000 live births
- End epidemics of AIDS, tuberculosis (TB), malaria, and neglected tropical diseases; combat hepatitis, water-borne diseases, and other communicable diseases.
- Reduce premature mortality from noncommunicable diseases by a third.
- Strengthen the prevention and treatment of substance abuse.
- By 2020, halve global deaths and injuries from road traffic accidents.
- Ensure universal access to sexual and reproductive health care services.
- Achieve universal health coverage, including financial risk protection and access to quality essential health care services.
- Substantially reduce deaths and illnesses from hazardous chemicals and air, water, and soil pollution and contamination.
- Strengthen the implementation of the World Health Organization Framework Convention on tobacco control in all countries.
- Support research and development of vaccines and medicines for the communicable and noncommunicable diseases primarily affecting developing countries and provide access to affordable medicines for all.
- Substantially increase financing, recruitment, development, training, and retention of the health workforce in developing countries.
- Strengthen the capacity of all countries for early warning, risk reduction, and management of national and global health risks.

---

health-related MDGs and significantly broadens the scope of preventive and curative interventions. It includes the diagnosis and long-term care of chronic, noncommunicable conditions and calls for Universal Health Coverage (UHC) to deliver the full-range of health services needed everywhere. UHC is defined as access to high-quality care for the diseases and conditions faced by populations without causing financial hardship for individuals and families. SDG 3 also recognizes the importance of disease surveillance and epidemic preparedness. It also recognizes the need for equitable access to scientific advancements.

Conclusion

This chapter documents the evolution in thinking about health systems through the first 15 years of the new millennium. To achieve the MDGs, countries needed to begin the task of building health systems. Progress toward the MDGs was most significant when vertical monies were leveraged to support broad health care delivery. Absent dedicated funding for health, the achievement of MDGs was uneven. In 2015, the SDGs were launched. SDG 3—to ensure healthy lives and promote well-being for all at all ages—is the only health-specific goal, but it has a broad array of targets and includes the aim of providing Universal Health Coverage.

References

1. United Nations. *United Nations Millennium Declaration*. New York: United Nations, General Assembly; 2000.
2. Kim JY, Millen JV, Irwin A. *Dying for growth: Global inequality and the health of the poor*. Monroe, ME: Common Courage Press; 2000.
3. World Bank. Health nutrition and population statistics. 2017. http://data.world-bank.org/data-catalog/health-nutrition-and-population-statistics
4. Wolff J. *The human right to health*. 1st ed. New York: Norton; 2012.
5. The World Bank. *World Development Report 2000–2001: Attacking poverty*. New York: Oxford University Press; 2000. https://openknowledge.worldbank.org/handle/10986/11856
6. United Nations. World conferences. Available from: http://www.un.org/geninfo/bp/intro.html. Accessed Apr 5, 2017.
7. OECD. *Shaping the 21st century: The contribution of development cooperation*. Paris: Organisation for Economic Co-operation and Development; 1996.
8. United Nations. Millennium Summit. Conferences, meetings and events website. Available from: http://www.un.org/en/events/pastevents/millennium_summit.shtml. Accessed Oct 11, 2016.
9. United Nations. *United Nations Millennium Declaration*. New York: United Nations Dept. of Public Information; 2000.
10. United Nations. UN Millennium Project. Available from: http://www.unmillen-niumproject.org/goals/. Accessed October 11, 2016.
11. Attaran A. An immeasurable crisis? A criticism of the Millennium Development Goals and why they cannot be measured (policy forum). *PLoS Med.* 2005;2(10):e318.
12. Fehling M, Nelson BD, Venkatapuram S. Limitations of the Millennium Development Goals: A literature review. *Global Public Health.* 2013;8(10):1109–1122.
13. United Nations. UN Millennium Project: Goals, targets and indicators. Available from: http://www.unmillenniumproject.org/goals/gti.htm.
14. Lopez AD, Mathers CD, Ezzati M, Jamison DT, Murray CJ. Global and regional burden of disease and risk factors, 2001: Systematic analysis of population health data. *Lancet.* 2006;367(9524):1747–1757.

15. World Health Organizaation. Integrated management of childhood illness (IMCI). Available from: http://www.who.int/maternal_child_adolescent/topics/child/imci/en/. Accessed Oct 12, 2016.

16. Khan KS, Wojdyla D, Say L, Gülmezoglu AM, Van Look P,F.A. WHO analysis of causes of maternal death: A systematic review. *Lancet.* 2006;367(9516):1066–1074.

17. Campbell OM, Graham WJ. Strategies for reducing maternal mortality: Getting on with what works. *Lancet.* 2006;368(9543):1284–1299.

18. UNICEF. The state of the world's children. State world's child. New York: Oxford Universtiy Press; 1983. https://www.unicef.org/about/history/files/sowc_1982-83.pdf

19. Travis P, Bennett S, Haines A, et al. Overcoming health-systems constraints to achieve the Millennium Development Goals. *Lancet.* 2004;364(9437):900–906.

20. Cairncross S, Peries H, Cutts F. Vertical health programmes. *Lancet.* 1997;349:S21.

21. Garrett L. The challenge of global health. *Foreign Affairs.* 2007;86(1):14–17.

22. Shiffman J. HIV/AIDS and the rest of the global health agenda. *B World Health Organ.* 2006;84(12):923.

23. England R. Are we spending too much on HIV? *BMJ.* 2007;334(7589):344.

24. World Health Organization. *The 13th international conference on AIDS & STIs in Africa (ICASA).* Geneva: World Health Organization; 2003.

25. Nattrass N. Millennium Development Goal 6: AIDS and the international health agenda. *J Hum Dev Capabilities.* 2014;15(2–3):232–246.

26. Bongaarts J, Over M. Global HIV/AIDS policy in transition. *Science.* 2010;328(5984):1359.

27. UNAIDS. Three ones, key principles. Available from: http://data.unaids.org/UNA-docs/Three-Ones_KeyPrinciples_en.pdf. Accessed Jul 7, 2016.

28. World Health Organization. *Health systems: Improving performance. The World Health Report 2000.* Geneva: World Health Organization; 2000.

29. World Health Organization. *Everybody's business: Strengthening health systems to improve health outcomes: WHO's Framework for Action.* Geneva: World Health Organization; 2007.

30. Navarro V. The new conventional wisdom: An evaluation of the WHO report health systems: Improving performance. *Intl J Health Serv.* 2001;31(1):23–33.

31. Murray CJ, Frenk J. A framework for assessing the performance of health systems. *Bull World Health Org.* 2000;78(6):717–731.

32. Shiffman J. Has donor prioritization of HIV/AIDS displaced aid for other health issues? *Health Policy Planning.* 2007;23(2):95–100.

33. Yu D, Souteyrand Y, Banda MA, Perriëns JH, Kaufman JA. Investment in HIV/AIDS programs: Does it help strengthen health systems in developing countries? *Globalization Health.* 2008;4:8.

34. Levine R, Oomman N. Global HIV/AIDS funding and health systems: Searching for the win-win. *JAIDS.* 2009;52:S5.

35. Commonwealth Regional Health Community Secretariat for East, Central and Southern Africa. HIV/AIDS voluntary counselling and testing: Review of policies, programmes and guidelines in East, Central and Southern Africa. Geneva: World

Health Organization, Commonwealth Regional Health Community Secretariat for East, Central and Southern Africa, USAID/REDSO; 2002.

36. Oberzaucher N. *HIV voluntary counselling and testing: A gateway to prevention and care: Five case studies related to prevention of mother-to-child transmission of HIV, tuberculosis, young people, and reaching general population groups.* Geneva: UNAIDS; 2002.

37. Obermeyer CM, Osborn M. The utilization of testing and counseling for HIV: A review of the social and behavioral evidence. *Am J Public Health.* 2007;97(10):1762–1774.

38. Hutchinson PL, Mahlalela X. Utilization of voluntary counseling and testing services in the Eastern Cape, South Africa. *AIDS Care.* 2006;18(5):446–455.

39. Mall S, Middelkoop K, Mark D, Wood R, Bekker L. Changing patterns in HIV/AIDS stigma and uptake of voluntary counselling and testing services: The results of two consecutive community surveys conducted in the Western Cape, South Africa. *AIDS Care.* 2013;25(2):194–201.

40. Kalichman SC, Simbayi LC. HIV testing attitudes, AIDS stigma, and voluntary HIV counselling and testing in a black township in Cape Town, South Africa. *Sex Transm Infect.* 2003;79(6):442.

41. Pabo E, Rhatigan J, Ellner A, Lyon E, Jain S. HIV voluntary counseling and testing in Hinche, Haiti. The Global Health Delivery Project: Harvard University; 2008. http://www.globalhealthdelivery.org/case-collection/case-studies/latin-america-and-caribbean/hiv-voluntary-counseling-and-testing-in-hinche-haiti

42. Ivers LC, Freedberg KA, Mukherjee JS. Provider-initiated HIV testing in rural Haiti: Low rate of missed opportunities for diagnosis of HIV in a primary care clinic. BioMed Central: AIDS Research and Therapy; 2007.

43. UNAIDS. *Guidance on provider-initiated HIV testing and counselling in health facilities.* Geneva: World Health Organization, UNAIDS; 2007.

44. Walton D, Farmer P, Lambert W, Leandre F, Koenig S, Mukherjee J. Integrated HIV prevention and care strengthens primary health care: Lessons from rural Haiti. *J Public Health Policy.* 2004;25(2):137–158.

45. Pabo E, Ellner A, Rhatigan J, Lyon E. *Two years in Hinche.* Global Health Delivery Project. Cambridge, MA: Harvard University Press; 2011.

46. Ivers LC, Jerome JG, Sullivan E, et al. Maximizing positive synergies between global health initiatives and the health system. In: *Interactions between global health initiatives and health systems: Evidence from countries.* Geneva: World Health Organization; 2009.

47. Frenk J. Bridging the divide: Global lessons from evidence-based health policy in Mexico. *Lancet.* 2006;368(9539):954–961.

48. World Health Organization. Maximizing positive synergies between health systems and global health initiatives. Available from: http://www.who.int/healthsystems/GHIsynergies/en/. Accessed Oct 13, 2016.

49. World Health Organization. *Initial summary conclusions: Maximizing positive synergies between health systems and global health initiatives.* Geneva: World Health Organization; 2009.

50. Warren AE, Wyss K, Shakarishvili G, Atun R, de Savigny D. Global health initiative investments and health systems strengthening: A content analysis of global fund investments. *Globalization Health.* 2013;9(30).

51. Price JE, Leslie JA, Welsh M, Binagwaho A. Integrating HIV clinical services into primary health care in Rwanda: A measure of quantitative effects. *AIDS Care.* 2009;21(5):608–614.

52. United Nations. Millennium Development Goal Report, 2015. Available from: http://www.un.org/millenniumgoals/2015_MDG_Report/pdf/MDG%20 2015%20rev%20(July%201).pdf. Accessed Jul 11, 2016.

53. Steinbrook R. Controlling HIV/AIDS: The obstacles and opportunities ahead. *JAMA Intern Med.* 2013;173(1):11–12.

54. UNAIDS. *GAP report.* New York: United Nations; 2014.

55. Klayman DL. Qinghaosu (artemisinin): An antimalarial drug from China. *Science.* 1985(4703):1049–1055.

56. United Nations Development Programme. *The Millennium Development Goals Report 2015.* New York: UNDP; 2015.

57. Kuruvilla S, Schweitzer J, Bishai D, et al. Success factors for reducing maternal and child mortality. [Facteurs de reussite pour la reduction de la mortalite maternelle et infantile/factores de exito para reducir la mortalidad materna e infantile.] *Bull World Health Org.* 2014;92(7):533.

58. Liu L, Oza S, Hogan D, et al. Global, regional, and national causes of child mortality in 2000–13, with projections to inform post-2015 priorities: An updated systematic analysis. *Lancet.* 2015;385(9966):430–440.

59. Lawn J, Cousens S, Zupan J. Neonatal survival 1–4 million neonatal deaths: When? where? why? *Lancet.* 2005;365(9462):891–900.

60. Requejo JH, Bryce J, Barros AJD, et al. Countdown to 2015 and beyond: Fulfilling the health agenda for women and children. *Lancet.* 2015;385(9966):466–476.

61. United Nations. We can end poverty: Millennium Development Goals and beyond 2015. New York: United Nations; 2013.

62. United Nations. Sustainable development goals. Available from: http://www. un.org/sustainabledevelopment/sustainable-development-goals/. Accessed Jul 11, 2016.

63. Sachs J. *The age of sustainable development.* New York: Columbia University Press; 2015.

PART TWO

Principles of Global Health Delivery

4

Global Health and the Global Burden of Disease

Key Points

- Terms such as incidence, prevalence, morbidity, and mortality describe the extent to which diseases occur in a population and cause suffering and death.
- The "burden of disease" is a term that relates to the quantity and impact of diseases in a population.
- The Global Burden of Disease Project, launched in 1990, quantifies the impact of diseases worldwide on a regular basis.
- The term "epidemiological transition" describes the change in the types of illnesses in a given population based on the economic status of the country or region.
- Care delivery systems must move from a disease control framework to address the entirety of the burden of disease.

Introduction

As the previous chapter discussed, the Millennium Development Goals (MDGs) and new funding sources renewed the promise of expanding health care delivery. The largely vertical, preventative health programs that dominated health in impoverished countries in the twentieth century proved insufficient to address the AIDS pandemic or the many other causes of illness and death.[1] It is necessary to understand the global burden of disease to build the systems of care that may achieve the targets in the newer Sustainable Development Goals (SDGs). The *global burden of disease* refers to the quantity of diseases and conditions and their impact on a population. To understand the global burden of disease, it is important to become familiar with the terms used to describe the health of populations.

This chapter focuses on common terms used to describe the health of populations. It does not explain the statistical methods for calculating population health; rather, the chapter explains the common lexicon of public health and global health. The concept of epidemiological transition is also explained; an important early framework that used disease burden to help countries of differing economic strata to assign health priorities. This chapter introduces two important ongoing projects the Global Burden of Disease (GBD) project, which quantifies the state of health in every country and the Disease Control Priorities (DCP) project which uses cost-effectiveness analyses to help policymakers set priorities in national health systems.

Describing the Health of Populations

It is important to understand what diseases or conditions need to be effectively covered in a given population. One of the building blocks in the World Health Organization's (WHO) framework[2] is health system responsiveness. That means that the health of a population must be measured and understood if the health system is to appropriately respond. Descriptive statistics quantify the existence, frequency, and outcomes of conditions in a population. Health professionals use this common language to compare health within and across countries. The quantity of disease in a given population is expressed as a fraction, percentage, or ratio that represents the number of cases of a disease in the reference population. The reference population may be the total population or only those at risk for a particular condition.

For example, the Minister of Health in Malawi may want to know the number of new tuberculosis (TB) cases detected in all Malawians in a year. For TB, the whole population is considered to be at risk because the disease is airborne and anyone can contract it. The Malawian Minister learns that there are 260 new cases of TB per 100,000 people per year. The total population of the country is 15.5 million. Therefore she would want to plan for 40,300 people to be diagnosed and treated to achieve universal coverage of TB treatment for new cases of the disease.

There are many reasons to quantify the burden of a disease including planning, policymaking, design of delivery systems, and program evaluation. To continue the preceding example, the Malawian Minister needs to know not only how many TB drugs to buy for the year, but also how many nurses will be needed to provide treatment, how TB is distributed within the country, and what populations are at highest risk. By comparing the burden between two different years, the Minister may also gather evidence about the effectiveness of the TB program.

The standard denominator for describing the disease burden may be the whole population, as in the Malawi example, or it may be only a segment of the population exposed to a particular risk. For example, to represent the number of women who die in childbirth, the appropriate denominator is only women who are in the various stages associated with childbirth—pregnancy, labor, delivery, and the postpartum period. The *maternal mortality ratio* is the statistic used to describe death related to childbirth. It is calculated as the number of women who die while pregnant, during labor, or in the 42 days after pregnancy per 100,000 women who deliver a live child.

Table 4.1 outlines the common terms used to describe the health of populations. These descriptive statistics will be used in cases and examples throughout this text as well as in the majority of journal articles and texts about global health.

These ratios are used to compare populations and to analyze the association between a risk factor and the occurrence of disease. For example, the incidence of lung cancer among cigarette smokers is higher than the incidence of lung cancer in the general population. Assessing the association between a condition and a risk factor is part of the field of epidemiology, which is beyond the scope of this book. However, understanding of the descriptive terms used to elucidate the disease burden is foundational to understanding the field.

The Global Burden of Disease

The "burden of disease" refers to two things. "Disease" refers to conditions, illnesses, and injuries. "Burden" refers to the impact of diseases on a population.[3] Understanding the burden of disease requires the measurement of conditions, a process known as *disease surveillance*.[4,5] Such measurement is not a simple task, particularly in countries with weak health systems. Many people get sick and die at home without ever reaching medical care.[6] Those who reach medical care may find themselves in facilities without adequate diagnostic capabilities, and the causes of their illnesses may remain unknown. In addition, personnel trained to keep records and track patients are often in short supply. As a result, there was, historically, insufficient data with which to estimate the burden of disease.

In the 1992, the World Bank commissioned the WHO to quantify the global burden of disease.[7] The preliminary results of this work were published by the WHO in 1994[8] and in a series of papers in *The Lancet*.[9] The data needed to inform this work were, indeed, scarce. The group estimated that less than 30 percent of the data on disease and death came from medically certified records. As a result, the Global Burden of Disease (GBD) team, led by Dr. Chris Murray,

Table 4.1 Common terms related to the impact of disease on a population.

Term	Description	Example of Use	Equation
Life expectancy	The average number of years from birth that a person can be expected to live. Usually calculated for a given country based on the observed average age of death in the population.	Life expectancy in the United States in 2016 is 78.8 years: 81 years for women, 76 years for men.	N/A
Incidence	The number of new cases of a disease divided by the total population at risk for disease.	Every year, there are X newly diagnosed cases of tuberculosis (TB) in Lesotho, a country of population Y. The reported incidence of TB is #new cases/100,000 people.	
Prevalence	The total number of active cases of a particular disease, in the population at risk for the disease.	The prevalence of HIV in Haiti is 1.2% among the 15- to 49-year-old population. That is the age at which people are assumed to be at risk for acquiring HIV.	
Morbidity	Sickness	A common morbidity among diabetics is a nonhealing infection that results in lower limb amputation.	N/A
Mortality	Death	Heart attack is a major cause of mortality in the United States.	N/A
Mortality rate	The number of deaths of a specific cause divided the whole population (or exposed population) in one year. The denominator is scaled to 100,000.	There were 10 deaths from lung cancer in Smith, Wyoming, population 20,000. That means the mortality rate from lung cancer was 50 per 100,000 residents.	

Under-5 child mortality rate	The number of children who die before their fifth birthday for every 1,000 live births.	Because many children die of dehydration when they have diarrhea, the large-scale distribution of packets of salt and sugar that can be easily mixed with water to make an oral rehydration solution (ORS) for children helped to reduce the under-five child mortality rate worldwide from 107.3 per 1,000 in 1983 to 87.3 per 1,000 in 1993.
Infant mortality rate	The number of infants who die in the first year of life for every 1,000 live births (subset of under-five child mortality).	If children survive the newborn period (first 28 days of life), malaria and pneumonia are common causes of infant mortality.
Neonatal mortality rate	The number of babies who die before they are 28 days old for every 1,000 live births (a subset of both the child and infant mortality rates).	Even in countries where under-five child mortality has improved, neonatal mortality remains a difficult challenge due to complications that may arise for newborns when they are born.
Maternal mortality rate	The number of women who die while pregnant, in labor, delivering a baby, or in the immediate postpartum period per 100,000 live births.	Lack of access to services to address complications in labor and delivery is a common cause of maternal mortality.
Fertility rate	The number of births per woman.	The average number of children a woman has varies around the world according to a number of health, economic, and cultural conditions. In 2010, Portugal, the United States, and Somalia had respective fertility rates of 1.4, 1.9, and 6.9.

used data from a variety of sources including sample-registration data (from India and China) and smaller population study data. The team used a variety of analytic techniques to estimate the disease burden (both death and disability) for 107 conditions and more than 400 sequelae (secondary consequences). The conditions included in this study were categorized in three groups: (1) infections and perinatal and maternal conditions, (2) noncommunicable diseases, and (3) injuries and accidents.

Estimates were then also grouped into eight global regions: what the group called *established market economies* (high-income countries such as the United States and Western European countries), the formerly socialist economies of Europe, India, China, Asia, sub-Saharan Africa, Latin America/the Caribbean, and the Middle East.[10]

The GBD project set out to develop a consistent way to estimate the incidence, prevalence, and mortality of the selected diseases. The group also sought to characterize *sequelae,* or consequences of diseases. The GBD evaluated the average age of onset and the duration of both diseases and their sequelae. To do this, the group introduced a new metric called the disability-adjusted life year (DALY). The DALY, developed in 1994,[11] is calculated based on "years of life lost from premature death and years of life lived in less than full health."[3] DALYs are an important measure of chronic conditions such as mental illness, diabetes, or disability from injury. Prolonged illness and disability have significant impact on the opportunity of individuals to reach their full potential. Data for 107 conditions and 483 disabling sequela were used to project the burden of disease from 1990 to 2020.[8] Table 4.2 shows the distribution of DALYs for specific causes in 1990.

The study confirmed a high burden of disease and premature mortality in impoverished regions and enormous health disparities between the established market economies and the most impoverished countries. Impoverished countries suffered 98 percent of all deaths among children younger than 15 years of age and 83 percent of deaths among those aged 15–59 (Figure 4.1). While infectious diseases were a critical component of the disease burden in impoverished countries, noncommunicable diseases and injuries also played a significant role[10] (Table 4.3). These conditions were not addressed by the selective primary health care strategies promoted in the 1980s and 1990s. When the investigators considered disability, the burden was quite different. For example, in the 2010 GBD, chronic conditions—notably mental illness—become a ranking cause of DALYs lost,[12] as shown in Table 4.4.

The GBD study was updated by WHO for the years 2000–2002 and included a more extensive analysis of the burden of disease relating diseases to 26 risk factors including malnutrition (being underweight and having deficiencies in nutrients such as vitamin A, zinc, and iron), high cholesterol, lack of contraception,

Table 4.2 Distribution % of disability-adjusted life years (DALYs) for specific causes, 1990; distribution of DALYS, as a percent of total burden in developed and developing countries, 1990.

	Distribution % of DALYs for Specific Causes, 1990	
	Developed	Developing
Group 1		
Total group 1	7.8	48.7
Infectious and parasitic diseases	2.7	25.6
Respiratory infections	1.6	9.4
Maternal disorders	0.6	2.4
Perinatal disorders	1.9	7.3
Nutritional deficiencies	0.9	4.1
Group 2		
Total group 2	77.7	36.1
Malignant neoplasms	13.7	4.0
Other neoplasms	0.8	0.2
Diabetes mellitus	1.9	0.7
Endocrine disorders	0.9	0.4
Neuropsychiatric disorders	22.0	9.0
Sense organ disorders	0.1	0.8
Cardiovascular disorders	20.4	8.3
Respiratory disorders	4.8	4.3
Digestive disorders	4.4	3.3
Genitourinary disorders	1.3	1.1
Skin disorders	0.1	0.1
Musculoskeletal disorders	4.3	1.0
Congenital anomalies	2.2	2.4
Oral disorders	0.8	0.5
Group 3		
Total group 3	14.5	15.2
Unintentional injuries	10.3	11.1
Intentional injuries	4.2	4.1

Source: Adapted from Murray CJL, Lopez AD. Global mortality, disability, and the contribution of risk factors: Global burden of disease study. *Lancet.* 1997;349(9063):1436–1442.

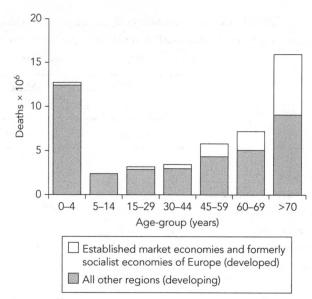

FIGURE 4.1 Distribution of deaths worldwide by age and region.
Source: Murray CJL, Lopez AD. Mortality by cause for eight regions of the world: Global burden of disease study. *Lancet*. 1997;349(9061):1269–1276.

smoking, drug and alcohol use, unsafe water, sanitation and hygiene, and climate change.[13] The GBD project continues to be carried out on a regular basis to analyze trends in disease burden with time.[14]

Epidemiological Transition

In 1971, Abdel Omran put forth a concept called the *epidemiological transition*. This concept describes the observed shift in the types of diseases that affect populations as economic conditions improve. For example, malnutrition and infectious diseases become less frequent as a population gains food security, clean water, and sanitation. Some noncommunicable diseases increase as a country develops economically, such as diseases related to obesity and smoking.[15] Omran describes four stages of population health (Figure 4.2):

1. Age of pestilence and famine: Populations in this stage suffer from high mortality due to infectious diseases and starvation. Populations have low life expectancies.
2. Age of receding pandemics: This stage is marked by reductions in mortality, especially among infants and children. Life expectancy increases as access to food, clean water, and infrastructure improves.

Table 4.3 Leading causes of death, wealthy and impoverished countries 2015.

Wealthy			Impoverished	
Rank	Cause	Number of Deaths	Cause	Number of Deaths
1	Cardiovascular diseases	3,160,979.145	Noncommunicable diseases	2,071,864.659
2	Neoplasms	2,594,167.856	Diarrhea, lower respiratory, and other common infectious diseases	1,053,437.999
3	Ischemic heart disease	1,648,890.723	Cardiovascular diseases	864,523.3653
4	Neurological disorders	1,020,527.817	HIV/AIDS and tuberculosis	581,510.3775
5	Alzheimer disease and other dementias	879,758.0549	Injuries	492,558.7511
6	Cerebrovascular disease	842,735.0826	Lower respiratory infections	479,308.3076
7	Communicable, maternal, neonatal, and nutritional diseases	605,780.6729	Neonatal disorders	460,975.1959
8	Diabetes, urogenital, blood, and endocrine diseases	595,768.1065	Neoplasms	382,606.0798
9	Tracheal, bronchus, and lung cancer	572,268.0679	HIV/AIDS	376,555.6821
10	Injuries	551,218.9598	Neglected tropical diseases and malaria	363,442.5609

Top ten causes of mortality in wealthy and impoverished countries, 2015.

Source: Data adapted from IHME. GBD results tool. IHME Data GHDx Website. http://ghdx. healthdata.org/gbd-results-tool. Accessed May 31, 2017.

Table 4.4 Disease-specific burden of death vs. disability-adjusted life years (DALYs), 2010; disease-specific burden of disease, measured as DALYs and mortality.

All Ages DALYs in 2010 × 1,000 (UI 95%)		All Ages Deaths × 1,000 (UI 95%)	
1	Cardiovascular diseases	295,036 (273,061–309,562)	Cardiovascular and circulatory diseases	15,616 (14,512.2–16,315.1)
2	Diarrhea, lower respiratory, and other common infections	282,982 (254,312–317,466)	Neoplasms	7,978 (7,337.1–8,403.8)
3	Neonatal disorders	201,959 (182,138–221,901)	Diarrhea, lower respiratory infections, meningitis, and other common infectious diseases	5,277 (4,742.2–5,790.4)
4	Neoplasms	188,487 (174,452.199037)	Chronic respiratory diseases	3,776 (3,648.2–3,934.1)
5	Mental and substance use disorders	185,190 (154,647–218,496)	HIV/AIDS and TB	2,661 (2,358.1–2,895.7)
6	HIV/AIDS and tuberculosis (TB)	130,944 (119,310–141,121)	Neonatal disorders	2,236 (2,014.6–2,470.1)
7	Neglected tropical diseases and malaria	108,739 (87,846–137,588)	Neglected tropical diseases and malaria	1,322 (1,055.6–1,677.6)
8	Nutritional deficiencies	85,341 (68,823–106,945)	Other	721 (626.8–830.4)
9	Other	4,1957 (36,061–4,9095)	Nutritional deficiencies	684 (546.0–790.1)
10	Maternal disorders	16,104 (12,972–18,912)	Maternal disorders	255 (203.8–303.3)

Data adapted from: Lozano R, Naghavi M, Foreman K, et al. Global and regional mortality from 235 causes of death for 20 age groups in 1990 and 2010: A systematic analysis for the global burden of disease study 2010. *Lancet*. 2012;380(9859):2095–2128; and Murray CJL, Vos T, Lozano R, et al. Disability-adjusted life years (DALYs) for 291 diseases and injuries in 21 regions, 1990–2010: A systematic analysis for the global burden of disease study 2010. *Lancet*. 2012;380(9859):2197–2223.

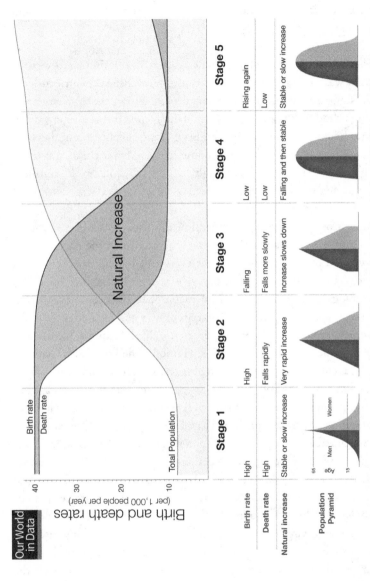

The author Max Roser licensed this visualisation under a CC BY-SA license. You find more information at the source: http://**www.OurWorldInData.org**/world-population-growth

FIGURE 4.2 Schematic shows the five stages of the epidemiological transition described in 1971. The framework specifically focuses on the linkage between decrease in fertility as children survive and the economy improves. It also links specific conditions with stages of economic development This framework has been influential in setting disease priorities throughout the world.

Source: Ortiz-Ospina E, Roser M. World population growth. 2016. Available from: https://ourworldindata.org/world-population-growth/.

3. Age of degenerative and manmade diseases: The total fertility rate declines as infant mortality continues to fall. Major causes of death are noncommunicable diseases (e.g., cancer and diabetes).

4. Age of delayed chronic diseases: Reductions occur in mortality in old age and primary prevention of chronic diseases (e.g., promotion of exercise and healthy diets).

Omran believed the age of delayed chronic diseases was beginning in wealthy countries as he was writing.[15] In contrast, because impoverished countries disproportionately suffer from infectious diseases and malnutrition, the child death rate is high. A high child death rate is one of the major factors that results in women having many children (also called high fertility).[16] Large population studies have shown that a woman more commonly chooses to have fewer children if she is educated, has greater economic opportunity, and if her children do not die.[16] Based on this observation, programs focused on child survival were considered important investments to decrease fertility.[17]

The concept of epidemiological transition was used by neoliberal policymakers to support stepwise priority-setting that promoted the cheapest and easiest preventive interventions as the first priority in impoverished countries. Unfortunately, diseases do not occur in a stepwise fashion. In reality, the epidemiological transition paints an incomplete picture of population health. The disease burden is diverse in every country and includes infectious, noncommunicable, acute, and chronic diseases.[18] Noncommunicable diseases occur across the spectrum of countries from impoverished to wealthy nations. For example, mental illness is one of the biggest causes of suffering in both impoverished and wealthy countries.[19] Conversely, infectious diseases are not present only in impoverished countries. TB is among the leading causes of death among incarcerated people in Eastern Europe,[20] and HIV prevalence is higher in South Africa, where the per capita income is $5,692, than in Chad, where the per capita income is $776.[21] Furthermore, injuries like broken bones occur in all societies and, without treatment, may cause severe morbidity and even mortality.[22] Health systems that treat a range of problems are needed not only to provide care but to respond to shocks from epidemics like Ebola to natural disasters like earthquakes.[23] In addition, treatment in many cases is a potent form of prevention.[24] This is obvious with infectious diseases like TB, in which treatment of an infected person will kill the bacteria and stop the transmission of infection.[25] But it is also true of noncommunicable diseases such as high blood pressure, in which treatment prevents the long-term consequences of heart disease, kidney disease, and stroke.[26]

Cost-Effectiveness

In 1977, Milton Weinstein and William Stason proposed the use of a formula that became known as cost-effectiveness as a way to make choices between different medical interventions. They posited that for an intervention to be cost-effective, its cost should be no more than three times the per capita health costs. In the US, this meant that an intervention could be considered cost-effective if it was several thousand dollars because the per capita health expenditure of the American health system is high.[27] In impoverished countries however, as neoliberal policymakers constricted government health budgets to about $5 per capita per year as part of structural adjustment programs very few interventions were cheap enough to be considered cost-effective. Impoverished countries, therefore, were encouraged to set priorities with only the hand full of interventions that cost under $5-15 dollars per patient per year.[28–32]

There are three major limitations of cost-effectiveness as the sole tool for priority setting. First, narrowly costed interventions do not address the true burden of disease, the social factors that underpin health, or the costs incurred to the patient. Second, the use of cost-effectiveness is problematic when fixed cost-effectiveness models are used to create 5- to 10-year strategic health plans. Fixed models assume there will be no change in the cost or effectiveness of interventions with time. Yet both cost of an intervention and the effectiveness of therapy do change with time, advocacy, and scientific advancement.[33] For example, the price of drugs may decrease as much as 100-fold over time, as was seen when AIDS activists fought for generic drugs. Similarly, effectiveness may change with time. New technologies can alter the cost of diagnosing a disease by reducing staff time or laboratory complexities.[34] Third, the provision of health care that addresses the entirety of the burden of disease is a moral issue, not something that should be related to cost-effectiveness alone. A person suffering from end-stage cancer has a right to drugs that will treat the pain. This intervention may be costly and is not always effective but it is the morally just approach. Few health interventions meet the criteria of being cost-effective in impoverished settings because the health budget is simply too low. Much more money is needed to fulfill the right to health.[35]

Priority Setting: The Disease Control Priorities Project

Simultaneous with the GBD project, economists began to understand that the significant burden of disease in impoverished countries impeded economic development.[36-38] To address this link, the World Bank's Population, Health, and Nutrition Division commissioned Drs. Dean Jamison and Henry Mosley to prioritize those interventions that would have the greatest impact on the burden of disease in impoverished countries. Drs. Jamison and Mosley published their framework for disease control priorities (DCP) in 1991.[30] The prioritization was based on three dependent inputs: (1) an understanding of the types of diseases and overall burden within a country; (2) the design of the health system to respond to the needs of the population; and (3) the ability of governments to set priorities, based on their abilities to use "the instruments that are at their disposal in the areas of persuasion, taxation, regulation and the provision of services."[30]

The work led by the DCP investigated two dozen acute and chronic diseases of adults and children. These studies were published in the book *Disease Control Priorities in Developing Countries* in 1993.[39] The work was done to help impoverished governments choose interventions that could be supported within the confines of their health budgets. The first DCP broadened the focus of interventions from child health alone. The authors of the DCP found that there were several adult interventions that were as cost-effective as the standard child health package of growth monitoring, oral rehydration, breastfeeding, and immunization (GOBI). These adult interventions included antismoking campaigns and the treatment of TB.[39]

The DCP also promoted using the data about the disease burden as a major pillar in health planning. Yet they did not propose treatment to address the disease burden. Rather, the DCP promoted disease control or prevention rather than treatment due to the constrained health budgets of impoverished countries. Additionally, the DCP advocated cost-effectiveness as a cornerstone for governments to set health priorities. The authors discouraged the treatment of many chronic diseases as too costly for impoverished countries to afford.[39,40] Low health budgets so severely constrained models of cost-effectiveness that many effective interventions were simply not considered feasible for the millions of people living in impoverished countries. In the global health era, rather than starting the analysis of what should be done from the inadequate budget of the impoverished country, AIDS activism and novel financing (like the Global Fund) changed the narrative. Activists asked what "What will it cost to bring this treatment to all? How do we finance it?"

The third version of the Disease Control Priorities (DCP3) project is being released as a series of nine volumes between 2015 and 2017. As global health has evolved, so too has the notion of priority-setting based on old cost-effectiveness methods. The DCP3 now embraces equity and the progressive financing of health as important factors:

[DCP3] will introduce new extended cost-effectiveness analysis methods for assessing the equity and financial protection considerations of health and macroeconomic policies for extending coverage of proven effective interventions to prevent and treat infectious and chronic diseases, including conditions related to environmental health, trauma and mental disorders.[41]

Conclusion

As discussed in this chapter, measuring the burden of disease is critical to the study and practice of global health delivery. The GDB project, housed at the WHO, quantifies and analyzes the disease burden and investigates trends to support health planning. The concept of the epidemiological transition is useful in anticipating shifts that may occur in the disease burden during economic development. Yet it presents an incomplete picture of the complexity of population health in impoverished countries. To progressively achieve Universal Health Coverage and the right to health, care must be delivered to address the entirety of the disease burden. The DCP project works to support priority-setting to address the burden of disease and now supports equity and more robust financial protection. The global health era has brought a focus on equity and progressive financing to tackle the entirety of the disease burden and achieve the right to health.

References

1. Rosenfield A, Maine D. Maternal mortality—A neglected tragedy: Where is the M in MCH? *Lancet.* 1985;326(8446):83–85.
2. World Health Organization. Everybody's business—strengthening health systems to improve health outcomes: WHO's Framework for Action. 2007. Available from: http://www.who.int/iris/handle/10665/43918.
3. World Health Organization. Global burden of disease. Available from: http://www. who.int/topics/global_burden_of_disease/en/. Accessed Oct 18, 2016.
4. Martinez L. Global infectious disease surveillance. *Intl J Infect Dis.* 2000;4(4):222–228.
5. Thacker SB, Choi K, Brachman PS. The surveillance of infectious diseases. *JAMA.* 1983;249(9):1181–1185.
6. Mathers CD, Ezzati M, Lopez AD. Measuring the burden of neglected tropical diseases: The global burden of disease framework (review). *PLoS Neglected Trop Dis.* 2007;1(2):e114.
7. Lea RA. World development report 1993: "Investing in health." *Forum Dev Studies.* 1993;20(1):114–117.

8. Murray CJ, Lopez AD, Jamison DT. The global burden of disease in 1990: Summary results, sensitivity analysis and future directions. *Bull World Health Org.* 1994;72(3):495–509.

9. Murray CJL, Lopez AD. Global mortality, disability, and the contribution of risk factors: Global burden of disease study. *Lancet.* 1997;349(9063):1436–1442.

10. Murray CJL, Lopez AD. Mortality by cause for eight regions of the world: Global burden of disease study. *Lancet.* 1997;349(9061):1269–1276.

11. Murray CJ. Quantifying the burden of disease: The technical basis for disability-adjusted life years. *Bull World Health Org.* 1994;72(3):429–445. Available from: http://www-ncbi-nlm-nih-gov.ezp-prod1.hul.harvard.edu/pubmed/8062401.

12. Murray CJL, Vos T, Lozano R, et al. Disability-adjusted life years (DALYs) for 291 diseases and injuries in 21 regions, 1990–2010: A systematic analysis for the global burden of disease study 2010. *Lancet.* 2012;380(9859):2197–2223.

13. Ezzati M, Lopez AD, Rodgers A, Vander Hoorn S, Murray CJ. Selected major risk factors and global and regional burden of disease. *Lancet.* 2002;360(9343):1347–1360.

14. Lancet. Global burden of disease. Available from: http://thelancet.com/gbd. Accessed Oct 17, 2016.

15. Omran AR. The epidemiologic transition: A theory of the epidemiology of population change. *Milbank Mem Fund Q.* 2005;49(4):509–538.

16. Lazarus RT. Determinants and consequences of high fertility: A synopsis of the evidence. *World Bank.* 2010:11–19.

17. Amiri A, Gerdtham U. *Impact of maternal and child health on economic growth: New evidence based on granger causality and DEA analysis.* Partnership for Maternal, Newborn & Child Health. Geneva: World Health Organization; 2013.

18. Frenk J, Bobadilla J, Sepúlveda J, Cervantes López M. Health transition in middle- income countries—new challenges for health care. *Health Policy Plan.* 1989;4:29–39.

19. Kessler RC, Aguilar-Gaxiola S, Alonso J, et al. The global burden of mental disorders: An update from the WHO World Mental Health (WMH) surveys. *Epidemiol Psychiatr Soc.* 2009;18(1):23.

20. Dara M, Chorgoliani D, de Colombani P. *TB prevention and control care in prisons.* Geneva: World Health Organization, Regional Office for Europe; 2013. p. 1–17.

21. World Bank. GDP per capita (current US$). Data. Available from: http://data.worldbank.org/indicator/NY.GDP.PCAP.CD. Accessed Oct 17, 2016.

22. Farmer P. Who lives and who dies. *London Rev Books.* 2015;37(3):17–20.

23. Gostin LO. Ebola: Towards an international health systems fund. *Lancet.* 2014;384(9951):e51.

24. Mayer KH, Krakower DS. Antiretrovirals for HIV treatment and prevention: The challenges of success. *JAMA.* 2016;316(2):151–153. Available from: http://dx.doi.org/10.1001/jama.2016.8902. doi:10.1001/jama.2016.8902.

25. Kendall EA, Azman AS, Cobelens FG, Dowdy DW. MDR-TB treatment as prevention: The projected population-level impact of expanded treatment for multidrug-resistant tuberculosis. *PLoS One.* 2017;12(3).

26. Law M, Wald N, Morris J. Lowering blood pressure to prevent myocardial infarction and stroke: A new preventive strategy. *Intl J Tech Assess Health Care.* 2005;21(1):145. Available from: http://journals.cambridge.org/abstract_S0266462305220196. doi:10.1017/S0266462305220196.

27. Weinstein MC, Stason WB. Foundations of cost-effectiveness analysis for health and medical practices. *N Engl J Med.* 1977;296(13):716.

28. Adam T, Lim SS, Mehta S, et al. Cost effectiveness analysis of strategies for maternal and neonatal health in developing countries. *BMJ.* 2005;331(7525):1107.

29. Hogan DR, Baltussen R, Hayashi C, Lauer JA, Salomon JA. Cost effectiveness analysis of strategies to combat HIV/AIDS in developing countries. *BMJ.* 2005;331(7530):1431.

30. Jamison DT, Mosley WH. Disease control priorities in developing countries: Health policy responses to epidemiological change. *Am J Public Health.* 1991;81(1):15–22.

31. Ubel PA, DeKay ML, Baron J, Asch DA. Cost-effectiveness analysis in a setting of budget constraints—is it equitable? *N Engl J Med.* 1996;334(18):1174–1177.

32. Jamison DT, Breman JG, Measham AR, et al. *Disease control in priorities in developing countries.* 2nd ed. New York: Oxford University Press/World Bank; 2006.

33. Drummond M, Sculpher M. Common methodological flaws in economic evaluations. *Med Care.* 2005;43(7):14.

34. Davis JL, Kawamura LM, Chaisson LH, et al. Impact of GeneXpert MTB/ RIF on patients and tuberculosis programs in a low-burden setting. A hypothetical trial. *Am J Respir Crit Care Med.* 2014;189(12):1551.

35. Forman L, Kohler JC, eds. *Access to medicines as a human right: Implications for pharmaceutical industry responsibility.* Toronto: University of Toronto Press; 2012.

36. Strauss J. Health, nutrition, and economic development. *J Econ Lit.* 1998;36(2):766–817.

37. Bloom DE. *The effect of health on economic growth: Theory and evidence.* Cambridge, MA: Harvard University Press; 2001.

38. Bloom DE, Canning D. The health and wealth of nations. *Science.* 2000;287(5456):1207–1209.

39. Jamison DT, Bank W. *Disease control priorities in developing countries.* Published for the World Bank. New York: Oxford University Press; 1993.

40. Laxminarayan R, Mills AJ, Breman JG, et al. Advancement of global health: Key messages from the disease control priorities project. *Lancet.* 2006;367(9517):1193–1208.

41. DCP3. DCP3: Disease control priorities: Economic evaluation for health. www.dcp-3.org. Accessed Nov 1, 2016.

5

Social Forces and Their Impact on Health

Key Points

- The social determinants of health are risk factors for ill health that are rooted in the political, historical, and social context of society. They include things like poverty, income inequality, food insecurity, gender inequality, and racism.
- The term *structural violence* refers to the architecture of society that creates inequality and that arises from factors such as institutionalized racism, discrimination, and neoliberal policies.
- People constrained by structural violence have less ability (also called *agency*) to fulfill their potential.
- To achieve health equity, social determinants must be understood and addressed.
- Proximity to suffering and giving care to individuals is a way to understand the impact of social forces on health.
- Health education campaigns that focus on an individual's behavior often do not recognize the impact of adverse social forces on the ability of a person to adopt healthy behaviors.
- A biosocial analysis moves beyond the biomedical to include the analysis of and attention to social forces that influence health.

Introduction

In medical school, students are taught about the causal link between genetics and diseases such as cystic fibrosis or muscular dystrophy.[1] Medical research proved that the microbe, the human immunodeficiency virus (HIV), causes AIDS.[2]

Epidemiological studies demonstrate a strong linkage between behaviors such as smoking and lung cancer. Yet the social context in which an individual lives is often more critical to one's health than genetics, infections, or behaviors.[3] Around the world, insufficient food, for example, is related to a host of illnesses from tuberculosis (TB) to anemia.[4] Living without access to clean water dooms many to diarrheal disease and death from dehydration.[5] Discrimination based on race, gender, or ethnicity excludes large portions of people from the resources needed to maintain a healthy life, including jobs, housing, and medical care.[6]

In this chapter, the concept of the *social determinants of health* is introduced. The importance of analyzing and addressing the social forces on individuals as well as local, national, and international levels when designing global health delivery systems is emphasized. The association between social forces and health outcomes is reviewed. The concept of a biosocial analysis to advance the practice of social medicine as an important principle in global health and achieving health equity is also outlined.

Social Forces and Health

The social forces that impact health are collectively known as the social determinants of health.[7] The linkage between social forces and health is deeply rooted in the fields of medicine, nursing, and public health.[8,9] In 2008, the World Health Organization (WHO) held a conference that urged the analysis of social forces as they impact health. The WHO defines the social determinants of health as:

> [T]he unequal distribution of power, income, goods, and services, globally and nationally, the consequent unfairness in the immediate, visible circumstances of peoples lives—their access to healthcare, schools, and education, their conditions of work and leisure, their homes, communities, towns, or cities—and their chances of leading a flourishing life.[10]

An impoverished social environment where people lack human rights, particularly social and economic rights, is associated with poor health outcomes (Table 5.1). From the right to food to the right to housing, paying attention to the social determinants of health is a cornerstone of a human rights approach to global health.

The field of *social medicine* is the study of social forces and their impact on health. It is also the practice of addressing social determinants as part of medical care.[11] The father of modern medicine and of social medicine is Rudolf Virchow,[12] a 19th-century physician. His was one of the most prominent early voices linking social forces with health outcomes.[13] In 1848, Virchow

Table 5.1 Examples of the linkage between the social determinants of health, human rights, risks for disease, and disease states.

Social Determinant	Related Human Right	Risk for Disease	Associated Disease or Condition
Poverty	Food Security (ICESCR – Article 11)	Malnutrition Impaired immunity Anemia Lack of brain growth	Variety of infectious diseases
Overcrowding Poor Housing	Shelter (ICESCR – Article 11)	Inadequate ventilation Indoor cooking fires Lack of access to housing, employment, and social services	Tuberculosis Chronic lung disease Exposure to elements Mental health Malnutrition
Racism	IESCR ICCRP	Violence Rape Lack of access of housing, employment, and social services	Depression Disability Death Incarceration Sexually transmitted infections Mental health Exposure to elements Malnutrition
Gender Inequality	Equal Protection (ICESCR – Article 3) (ICCRP – Article 3)	Violence Rape Early pregnancy	Depression Disability Death Sexually transmitted infections Unwanted pregnancies

This table displays the connection between human rights, social determinants of health, and disease or illness. When delivering care, it is important to understand the external political and social forces that influence a person.

ICCRP, International Covenant on Civil and Political Rights; *IESCR*, International Covenant on Economic, Social and Cultural Rights.

investigated a typhus epidemic (a bacterial disease carried by body lice) in Upper Silesia (now northern Germany). In Virchow's famous work, *Report on the Typhus Outbreak of Upper Silesia,* he wrote about the link between social factors such as lack of access to food, education, employment, as well as political isolation with the spread of disease.[14] He called what he saw an "artificial epidemic," one that spread due to social disruption rather than simply due to the microbe itself.[14,15] In his journal documenting his time in Upper Silesia, Virchow wrote, "Medicine is a social science, and politics (is) nothing but medicine on a grand scale."[8] Virchow became an activist for social change. He was involved in progressive politics in favor of the social inclusion of the poor for much of his life. Other health professionals who connected sickness and suffering with the need for social and political change include Steven Biko, Dr. Salvador Allende, and Dr. Ernesto Che Guevara.[16] Many more have linked politics and advocacy with health, such as Dr. Gro Harlem Brundtland, former Prime Minister of Norway and former Director-General of the WHO[17]; Nurse Clara Barton who founded the Red Cross after witnessing the casualties of US Civil war. Dr. Julius Richmond,[18] a pediatrician and former US Surgeon General helped found Head Start and took on the tobacco industry. Dr. Jack Geiger[19] founded the nongovernmental organization (NGO) Physicians for Human Rights. Nurse Lillian Wald campaigned for suffrage, racial integration and helped to found the National Association for the Advancement of Colored People (NAACP). She is considered the founder of community health nursing.[20]

While the term *social determinants of health* is widely used, it is a mistake to think that these issues are determined or fixed. Rather, active social forces, often rooted in history, continue into the modern era through political and social means. The term "structural violence" was first used by Johan Galtung to describe social structures that cause harm to people by decreasing their ability to achieve their rights.[21] While Galtung wrote about conflict, Dr. Paul Farmer used the term "structural violence" to describe the social forces that create and perpetuate ill health, suffering, and premature death.[22] Structural violence includes poverty, racism, and gender inequality. These forces directly impact who lives and who dies. Structural violence is inherently political and is fundamentally about resources and power.[23] For example, apartheid in South Africa denied millions access to housing, jobs, schools, and medical care. It was associated with significantly poorer health outcomes among black Africans.[24] Widespread housing discrimination in the United States[25] resulted in impoverishment of black communities for generations,[26] which has long-term health impacts.

Across the world, disparities within countries result in suffering and death: the Brazilian favela versus the gated community in Rio,[27] the Beacon Hill mansions of Boston versus the housing projects of Roxbury (Figure 5.1A, B),[28] and the suburbs of Mumbai versus its sprawling slums.[29] Such disparities also exist when one compares wealthy countries with impoverished ones: the life expectancy of Sierra Leone is 50 years compared to 82 years in Norway.[30] These disparities demand us to focus beyond the microbe or gene, beyond

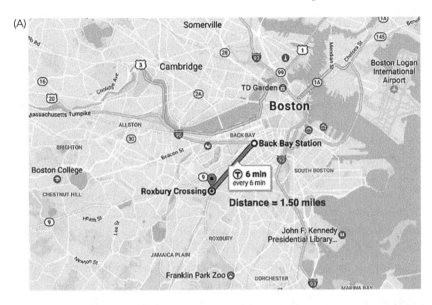

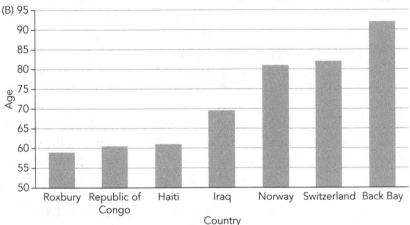

FIGURE 5.1 Comparison of life expectancy between Boston neighborhoods. (A) Distance between Roxbury (low income) and Back Bay (high income), Google maps. (B) Life expectancy in Roxbury, Back Bay, and selected countries.

Compiled with data from: WorldBank Database and http://www.societyhealth.vcu.edu/media/society-health/pdf/PMReport_Boston.pdf.

individual behaviors, and beyond the biomedical model of causation to consider the social forces that impact health. For those on the front lines of care provision, it is impossible to attend to illness without understanding structural violence and the lack of human rights that impact health outcomes and health equity.

The Economic Determinants of Health

The correlation of mortality with social class and income has been documented throughout in the world in a variety of studies.[31,32] Sir Michael Marmot, a British epidemiologist and prominent voice in the study of the social determinants of health, was an investigator in the famous Whitehall study.[33] The study, published in 1984, was carried out in England and followed more than 17,000 civil servants over a period of 10 years. Marmot documented a threefold higher rate of mortality among those in the lowest employment grade of the civil service as compared with those in the highest grade (Figure 5.2).

In a later paper, Marmot provides a useful framing to consider the ways in which income impacts health.[31] First, he reasoned that an individual's income determines his or her capacity to attain the material necessities of life such as food and shelter. The lack of these material necessities results in sickness and death. The clearest example is death due to starvation. On a global scale, acute malnutrition accounts for 10 percent of all child deaths (Figure 5.3).[34] As recently as 2015, nearly half of all deaths in children under five are attributable to malnutrition.[35] In impoverished countries, the most vulnerable lack the material means for survival, spending more than 50 percent of their daily income on food alone (Figure 5.4).[36,37]

The second way that income impacts health, according to Marmot, is at the macroeconomic level—that is, the relationship between health and the gross domestic product (GDP) of a country. Wealthier countries have infrastructure within the public commons that supports the attainment of health. For example, health care is publicly provided in England and Canada through a national network of providers, hospitals, and clinics.[38,39] Wealthier countries also support investments in public goods such as municipal water and sanitation systems, which have direct health benefits. Haiti, for example, has no municipal water supply.[40] Water is largely collected from open and unprotected sources such as rivers and streams. Due to the lack of public infrastructure, when United Nations peacekeeping forces dumped their untreated sewage into the Artibonite River, the source of water for hundreds of thousands of Haitians, a cholera epidemic started.[41] Thousands of people with neither access to treated, municipal water nor the means to purchase water got sick and died of cholera.[42] When cases of cholera reached the neighboring Dominican Republic, a country with municipal water systems and sanitation, the epidemic was rapidly controlled.[43]

The third linkage between economics and health proposed by Marmot is the relationship between income inequality and mortality. Even in wealthy countries, income inequality represents an additional set of concerns. The Whitehall study showed that even with stable employment and relatively homogeneous ethnicity, men had a dramatically different life expectancy based on social class.[44]

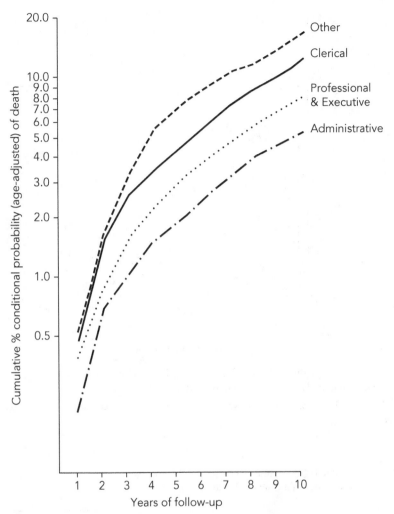

FIGURE 5.2 The Whitehall II study; cumulative conditional probability of death from all causes (age-adjusted) in 10 years, according to civil service grade.

Source: Marmot MG, Stansfeld S, Patel C, et al. Health inequalities among British civil servants: The Whitehall II study. *Lancet*. 1991;337(8754):1387–1393.

Men from the lower social classes suffered premature mortality as compared with those from the highest social class. He found that the clustering of risk within social strata is often more important than an individual's risks or behavior.[45] Communities with lower socioeconomic status have been shown in a variety of studies to have higher rates of accidents, drug use, depression, and anxiety compared to those from higher socioeconomic groups.[46,47] While much of this may seem obvious, understanding and addressing social class and income inequality

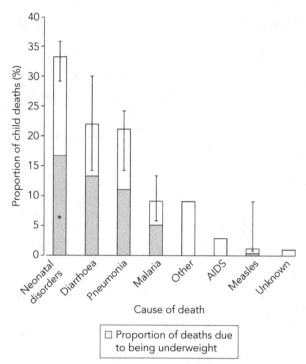

FIGURE 5.3 Graph shows the distribution of child deaths by cause. It also highlights the importance of underlying malnutrition in child mortality.

Source: Black RE, Morris SS, Bryce J. Where and why are 10 million children dying every year? *Lancet*. 2003;361(9376):2226–2234.

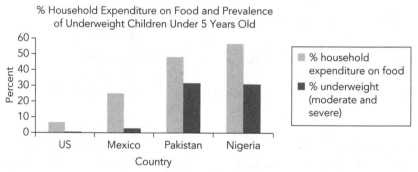

FIGURE 5.4 Percent of household expenditure on food and prevalence of underweight in children under five in selected countries. Percent of household expenditure on food increases with impoverishment. The inability to buy food is an important factor in child health.

Source: https://www.statista.com/statistics/189227/percent-of-disposable-income-spent-on-food-at-home-2009/ and World Bank 2012/2013. Retrieved Feb 27, 2017.

is critical when designing systems of care. It is also important for providers to understand the stresses and prevailing forces against which an individual or community may struggle to achieve health.

Racism, Gender Inequality, and Discrimination

Discrimination based on race, gender, ethnicity, sexual orientation, and other factors has deep historical roots that are perpetuated by active discriminatory policies and unconscious bias. Active discrimination and structural violence compound the stress of income inequality and result in social exclusion from the resources necessary to achieve the right to health. Discrimination impacts health outcomes in a myriad of ways from increasing the risk of ill health to causing poorer health outcomes once a person falls ill.

In the United States, racial discrimination results in poverty and illness. One salient example of increased risk for disease based on racially motivated policies in the United States was the "Planned Shrinkage" policy of Mayor John Lindsay in New York City in the 1970s.[48] Mayor Lindsay removed essential services from poor, mostly African-American communities in an effort to encourage them to move elsewhere. In 1975 and 1976, after "Planned Shrinkage" removed fire brigades, a series of fires in African-American neighborhoods forced many to abandon their homes and move in with family, neighbors, or to become homeless. The overcrowding caused by the policies of Mayor Lindsay correlated with the rise of TB in New York among African-Americans in the 1970s.[49] There are many other case studies of structural violence and health risk. Poverty is often a direct result of discrimination that ranges from unequal access to education to unfair housing policies to wage inequality.[50] In addition, people living in communities that face oppression may have greater exposure to environmental toxins[51] or may be living in overcrowded conditions.[52] Structural violence stems from institutionalized racism and discrimination and is propagated through neoliberal policies.

In the United States, a person's postal Zip Code is a more important correlate of life expectancy than any biologic factors.[53] An example of the impact of social determinants of life and death is the landmark article "Eight Americas: Investigating Mortality Disparities across Races, Counties, and Race-Counties in the United States."[53] In this article, population data from 1997–2001 was analyzed and showed up to a 33-year difference in life expectancy between Americans stratified by county, gender, and race: a subgroup of Asian women from Bergen County, New Jersey (a wealthy area), lived longest, with an average life expectancy of 91 years; a subgroup of Native American men from several very poor counties in South Dakota had an average life expectancy of 58 years. Social, historical, and political factors such as genocide, slavery, Jim Crow laws, mass incarceration, racism, exclusion from health care, and violence track along lines of Zip Codes and result in shorter lifespans.[53]

Discriminatory policies often result in a lack of public health investment in marginalized communities.[54,55] Once a person from a group that is discriminated against falls ill, he or she may face barriers to accessing care, such as a lack of money for transportation to the clinic or a lack of job flexibility for taking time off to seek care.[56,57] Facilities in poorer communities or communities of color may not have adequate equipment or resources to perform diagnostic tests.[58,59] Discrimination also results in poor health outcomes due to bias among health providers. For example, studies have shown racial bias in the treatment of pain among African-Americans.[60] This not only results in increased suffering but is also associated with delays in the diagnosis of serious illness.[61] Similarly, gender bias and sexist views of women's pain has been shown to be associated with delayed treatment and poor outcomes.[62] Language can also be a barrier to accessing care. Studies have shown that non–English-speaking patients have better outcomes if competent interpretation services exist.[63,64]

Choice and Agency

Often, poor outcomes caused by poverty, classism, racism, and sexism are ascribed to bad behavior, cultural differences, or ignorance. Dr. Paul Farmer calls these attributions "immodest claim[s] of causality."[65] To claim that ignorance or an individual's behavior causes an illness is to arrogantly ignore the social factors linked to ill health. Immodest claims of causality are apparent in many health policies that misallocate responsibility for ill health to the person suffering an illness rather than to the systems or structures that oppress people. In disregarding structural violence, many health programs are created to promote behavior change among the poor as a way to improve health. For example, studies have shown that African-American women present with more advanced breast cancer.[66] A behavior change program would ascribe this difference to a lack of knowledge among women of color about the benefits of mammography and would therefore focus on educating these women about the benefits of mammograms and encouraging them to come forward for screening. The immodest claim of causality here is that a lack of knowledge about the benefits of mammography is the main reason for a woman's presentation of advanced breast cancer. Culture and choice are also frequently blamed for the lack of uptake of health services. In truth, many studies have documented that the cause of low mammogram coverage among this population is the lack of access to mammography machines, lack of health insurance coverage for mammography, and the inability of some women to take time off for health care.[67] While individual choice, knowledge, and culture are undoubtedly important elements in the lives of all individuals and communities, it is important to understand how real choice is constrained by social determinants and structural violence.

To understand the limits of ascribing a lack of knowledge, cultural beliefs, or poor choices to the health outcomes of the poor, it is helpful to discuss the concept of agency. *Agency* is a term first described by Jurgen Habermas.[68] Habermas, a German sociologist and philosopher, describes agency as a person's ability to use all of his or her capabilities.[68] That ability, he reasoned, is enabled by adequate resources such as a healthy body, a paying job, or sufficient food. For example, a person may be given the choice of taking a day off without pay if sick. However, if the person depends on a daily wage, he would not have the agency to make this choice. In his famous book *Development as Freedom*,[69] Nobel Prize–winning economist Dr. Amartya Sen addresses the interplay between social and economic freedom and development. Sen acknowledges that agency is central to being truly free but is often severely socially constrained. He writes:

> The freedom of agency that we individually have is inescapably qualified and constrained by the social, political, and economic opportunities that are available to us. There is a deep complementarity between individual agency and social arrangements. It is important to give simultaneous recognition to the centrality of individual freedom and to the force of social influences on the extent and reach of individual freedom.[69]

Exaggeration of an individual's agency is common in development projects that lack an understanding that structural violence constrains the life of the impoverished. For example, many malnutrition programs around the world do not consider the root cause of child malnutrition to be a lack of food.[70] Rather, they claim that the root of child malnutrition is based on the mother's ignorant food choices. Because of this claim of causality, many malnutrition programs involve weighing young children and then educating their mothers about the appropriate food to give.[71,72] Yet if one visits the family's home and talks to the mother, it is generally apparent that the root cause of malnutrition is, tragically and simply, a lack of food and a lack of money to purchase food.[73,74] In wealthy countries, agency is also manipulated by social forces. For example, it is known that habits and behaviors (like smoking and diet) adversely impact health. Yet social forces such as the marketing of cigarettes in African-American neighborhoods[75] or the lack of access to fresh fruits and vegetables in the Navajo Nation[76] result in disproportionate morbidity and mortality related to seemingly modifiable factors.[77] Meanwhile, many public health programs continue to focus significant attention on what are called *information, education, and communication* (IEC) campaigns that seek to modify behavior.[78]

The vignette in Box 5.1 painfully describes the connection between choice and agency. Undoubtedly, access to vital information is important, but poverty constrains choice, often in a brutal fashion. The children in this vignette were forced into accepting money for sex because they did not have true agency to fulfill their potential nor the right to education. When IEC campaigns proceed without understanding the structural violence that traps people in poverty, agency is exaggerated, as is the notion of real choice.

BOX 5.1

Agency and AIDS

HIV prevention provides an ideal example of how choice is constrained by a lack of agency due to poverty. Much of the early HIV epidemic response focused on information, education, and communication (IEC) messages for children to delay the onset of sexual intercourse. In 1994, HIV peaked in Uganda. In the rural Masaka district, the prevalence of HIV among pregnant women was as high as 33 percent.[1] Globally, there was no effective treatment for HIV. The life expectancy for those infected was about 2 years, and many children were orphans.[2] UNICEF called children aged 5–15 were considered the "window of hope"[3] in that IEC campaigns targeting this group before the onset of sexual activity could change the trajectory of the epidemic. Programs used the child-to-child model to train children between the ages of 11 and 14 years to teach their peers about HIV[3]: what the disease was, how it was transmitted, and how it could be prevented.

In one such program, after several days of interactive and lively discussions that included demonstrations of how to put condoms on plantains, many were optimistic about this strategy: what could go wrong? The children were asked to come up with a list of the top five risks factors they had for HIV. They would use the five risk factors to design a curriculum of songs and drama about HIV prevention for their peers. When they listed their top five risk factors, however, all of the children, across many schools, listed the top risk factor as poverty. When they were asked why, they explained, "School is not free, I am already an orphan. If some man will pay my school fees and wants to play sex with me, it is a choice I have to make. If I don't continue school, I will be forced to become a servant, live family to family, I will certainly contract AIDS. If I learn to read, learn my maths, I can sell things in the market, maybe continue school."[4]

A Biosocial Analysis

How do we move from exaggerating agency to understanding and mitigating structural violence?[79] This linkage is a cornerstone of social medicine. A *Biosocial analysis* was documented by Virchow and most recently promoted by Dr. Paul Farmer.[80] There is no clear formula to evaluate or remediate the impact of the social determinants of health. However, the biosocial approach to global health is an approach in which the health provider attempts to understand the patient's experiences, including the social forces present in the life of the person—hunger, violence, and joblessness, as well as the impact of the illness in the context of his or her daily life. A biosocial analysis also necessitates a deep political, social, and historical understanding of the community. This requires reading and understanding the history and politics of a place, listening deeply to the affected, and spending time in the community. Central to the biosocial approach is the notion of *accompaniment*. The idea of accompaniment is described by Father Gustavo Gutierrez, a Peruvian priest and father of liberation theology, as walking with a person on their journey.[81,82] When caregivers accompany a person with an illness, they directly witness the everyday challenges and barriers faced by their patients. By understanding these challenges and barriers, the caregiver can address the forces at work.

The Social History

Clinicians are taught to ask for and record what is called a *social history*.[83] Unfortunately, the social history is commonly focused solely on biomedical risk factors—such as tobacco, drug, and alcohol use. The movement to practice social medicine has highlighted the need to deepen this social history to include the social context of the patient and his or her community. In 2014, Behforouz et al. proposed an expanded social history that promotes a deeper understanding of the structural barriers faced by patients.[83]

More recently, the Social Medicine Consortium, an international collaboration of social medicine practitioners,[84] drafted a statement on the need to bring social medicine into clinical training. The statement reads:

> We have participated in and been complicit with broken health systems whose principles and systems don't lead to healthier communities. We have heard the voices of patients throughout the world whose tragic stories of sickness plead for more just, equitable health systems and care. We have witnessed politics that tolerate xenophobia, racism, sexism, and unregulated capitalism without any accountability.

We have observed economic and social systems that routinely fail to affirm the dignity of all humans and ignore the tremendous assets of all communities. We have trained in educational systems that acknowledge very little or none of this. We refuse to stand by and let this happen. *Social Medicine is our response.*

The Social Medicine Consortium further defines social medicine as an approach that integrates the following principles[84]:

1. Understanding and applying the social determinants of health, social epidemiology, and social sciences approaches to patient care
2. An advocacy and equity agenda that treats health as a human right
3. An approach that is both interdisciplinary and multisectoral across the health system
4. Deep understanding of local and global contexts, ensuring that the local context informs and leads the global movement
5. The voice and vote of patients, families, and communities

A biosocial analysis and the practice of social medicine is needed not only for the appropriate care for the individual patient. It also should inform the design of systems to meet the needs of populations, understand the difficulties faced by patients and providers, and analyze barriers at the political and community levels.[82,85] Social forces are ever-present vectors often pushing—with historical, political, and economic weight—against achieving health equity. However, social forces are remediable through social and political action. Social movements serve to increase the visibility of marginalized groups, fight against the violation of rights, and overturn unjust practices. Movements are critical in the fight for rights and justice.[86]

Mitigating Adverse Social Determinants

In the practice of global health, addressing social determinants can seem like a daunting task. Yet both civil society and government can change the social context. One of the most famous examples of civil society engagement is the struggle for the right to water that took place in Cochabamba, Bolivia, from 1999 to 2002.[87] In the 1980s and 1990s, Bolivia was under extreme budgetary stress due to the terms of the structural adjustment policies (SAPs) imposed by the World Bank and the International Monetary Fund (IMF). In 1999, under pressure from these institutions, the government leased the rights to the public water system to a multinational consortium led by the American corporation Bechtel.[87] Under the guise of increasing access to clean water, the Bechtel-led consortium, called Aguas del Tunari, raised the price of water by more than 40 percent.[88] A civil society group called the Coalition for the Defense of Water and Life led demonstrations against the privatization.[87] The protests lasted many months and were supported by campaigns across the country and through media and letter-writing campaigns around the world. Under pressure from activists, the Bolivian government granted control of Cochabamba's water to the grassroots coalition in 2002.[87]

In the United States, there are also examples of how political action pushed back the social forces of ill health. Recent struggles such as the civil society protests against the Keystone XL and Dakota Access pipelines are examples of the ongoing work needed to assure the right to water and a clean environment.[89] The long and successful Disability Rights movement sought to end discrimination based on physical disability and increase accessibility for all. The work of activists led to the passage of the Americans with Disabilities Act of 1990, which required nondiscriminatory housing, education practices, and accommodations in all facilities for people with disabilities.[90]

Governments have an important role to play in mitigating inequitable social forces and assisting the most vulnerable (Table 5.2). Local, national, and international programs that address social determinants such as food security, housing, and discrimination can have a profound impact on health. Nutritional programs in many settings are an important example of mitigating the impact of the structural violence that produces hunger, malnutrition, and death. In Massachusetts, for example, in 2014 an estimated 363,000 children faced food insecurity.[91] When it was recognized that the lack of school lunches in the summer time led to an increase in theft by adolescents, the NGO Project Bread extended school breakfast and lunch programs into the summer months to protect these children from hunger.[91]

Conclusion

The mandate of global health is the delivery of care to address the burden of disease and achieve equitable outcomes while developing strong, interdisciplinary systems that achieve the right to health for the long term. In order to achieve this, it is critical to understand and address the social determinants of health. This requires a biosocial analysis and concerted action to change some of the fundamental social forces that result in ill health. Throughout this chapter, the importance of considering the social determinants of health for both individuals and populations is discussed. Social determinants are often connected to human rights. The impacts of income, social class, and discrimination on health are

Table 5.2 Examples of three government programs to protect against malnutrition.

Country	Program	Beneficiary	Explicit Relationship with Health
US	Special Supplemental Nutrition Program for Women, Infants and Children (WIC)[1]	Low-income, nutritionally at-risk women, infants, and children	Allocates funds for nutritious foods, nutrition education, and screens and refers for other health services
Mexico	Prospera[2]	Low-income women and children	Conditional cash transfer program encourages mothers to bring children to clinics for routine services and nutrition counselling
Kenya	NMK Njaa Marufuku Kenya[3]	National school feeding program	Provides 1 hot meal of corn and legumes to children in school

[1] USDA Special Supplemental Nutrition Program for Women, Infants and Children https://www.fns.usda.gov/wic/women-infants-and-children-wic

[2] Prospera programa de inclusion social https://www.gob.mx/prospera

[3] NMK school feeding in Kenya http://socialprotection.org/programme/njaa-marufuku-kenya-nmk%E2%80%94 school-feeding-programme

elucidated. The chapter emphasizes that people must have both the choice and the agency to make healthy decisions. The biosocial approach and the practice of social medicine help to analyze and holistically address health. Social movements play an important role in highlighting injustice and changing adverse social factors that impact health.

References

1. Tsui L, Buchwald M, Barker D. Cystic fibrosis locus defined by a genetically linked polymorphic DNA marker. 1985;230(4729):1054–1057.
2. Gallo RC, Montagnier L. The discovery of HIV as the cause of AIDS. *N Engl J Med.* 2003;349(24):2283–2285.

3. Woolf S, Aron L, Dubay L, Simon S, Zimmerman E, Luk K. How are income and wealth linked to health and longevity? 2015. http://www.urban.org/sites/default/files/publication/49116/2000178-How-are-Income-and-Wealth-Linked-to-Health-and-Longevity.pdf

4. Pelletier DL, Frongillo EA, Schroeder DG, Habicht JP. The effects of malnutrition on child mortality in developing countries. *Bull World Health Org.* 1995;73(4):443.

5. Montgomery M, Elimelech M. Water and sanitation in developing countries: Including health in the equation. *Environ Sci Technol.* 2007;41(1):16–24.

6. Williams D. Race, socioeconomic status, and health—the added effects of racism and discrimination. Socioeconomic status and health in industrial nations. *Ann NY Acad Sci.* 1999;896:173–188.

7. World Health Organization. Social determinants of health. Available from: http://www.who.int/social_determinants/en/. Accessed Oct 19, 2016.

8. Krischel M. "Medicine is a social science"—life and work of Rudolf Virchow (1821–1902). *J Urol.* 2014;191(4):E624.

9. Nightingale F. *Florence Nightingale on public health care.* Waterloo, ON: Wilfrid Laurier University Press; 2004.

10. World Health Organization. *Closing the gap in a generation: Health equity through action on the social determinants of health: Commission on Social Determinants of Health final report.* Geneva: World Health Organization, Commission on Social Determinants of Health; 2008.

11. Social medicine. *BMJ.* 1942;2(4255):101.

12. Turk JL. Rudolf Virchow—father of cellular pathology. *J R Soc Med.* 1993;86(12):688.

13. Eisenberg L. Rudolf Virchow: The physician as politician. *Med War.* 1986;2(4):243–250.

14. Virchow R. *Mittheilungen über die in oberschlesien herrschende typhus-epidemic.* 1848. https://archive.org/details/bub_gb_HmEXAQAAMAAJ

15. Taylor R, Rieger A. Rudolf Virchow on the typhus epidemic in Upper Silesia: An introduction and translation. *Sociol Health Illn.* 1984;6(2):201–217.

16. Waitzkin H, Iriart C, Estrada A, Lamadrid S. Social medicine then and now: Lessons from Latin America (brief article). *Am J Public Health.* 2001;91(10):1592.

17. Yamey G. Interview with Gro Brundtland. *BMJ.* 2002;325(7376):1355.

18. United States Office of the Assistant Secretary for Health. *Healthy people: The Surgeon General's report on health promotion and disease prevention.* Washington, DC: US Dept. of Health, Education, and Welfare, Public Health Service, Office of the Assistant Secretary for Health and Surgeon General; 1979.

19. Geiger J. Caring for the poor in the 21st century: Enabling community health centers for a new era. *J Health Care Poor Underserved.* 2014;25(4):2044–2052.

20. Buhlerwilkerson K. Bringing care to the people: Lillian Wald legacy to public-health nursing. *Am J Public Health.* 1993;83(12):1778–1786.

21. Galtung J. Violence, peace, and peace research. *J Peace Res.* 1969;6(3):167–191.

22. Farmer P. An anthropology of structural violence. *Curr Anthropol.* 2004;45(3): 305–325.

23. Farmer P. Who lives and who dies. *London Rev Books.* 2015;37(3):17–20.

24. Coovadia H, Jewkes R, Barron P, Sanders D, Mcintyre D. The health and health system of South Africa: Historical roots of current public health challenges. *Lancet.* 2009;374(9692):817–834.

25. Coates T. The case for reparations. *Atlantic.* 2014;313(5):54.

26. Williams D, Jackson P. Social sources of racial disparities in health—policies in societal domains, far removed from traditional health policy, can have decisive consequences for health. *Health Affairs.* 2005;24(2):325–334.

27. Szwarcwald C, Bastos FI, Barcellos C, Pina MDF, Esteves MAP. Health conditions and residential concentration of poverty: A study in Rio de Janeiro, Brazil. *J Epidemiol Comm Health.* 2000;54(7):530.

28. Chen J, Rehkopf D, Waterman PD, et al. Mapping and measuring social disparities in premature mortality: The impact of census tract poverty within and across Boston neighborhoods, 1999– 2001. *Am J Epidemiol.* 2006;163(11):S139.

29. Unger A, Riley LW. Slum health: From understanding to action (essay). *PLoS Med.* 2007;4(10):e295.

30. World Health Organization. Life expectancy at birth (years) 2000–2015. Available from: http://gamapserver.who.int/gho/interactive_charts/mbd/life_expectancy/atlas.htm.

31. Marmot M. The influence of income on health: Views of an epidemiologist. *Health Affairs.* 2002;21(2):31–46.

32. Galobardes B, Smith GD, Lynch JW. Systematic review of the influence of childhood socioeconomic circumstances on risk for cardiovascular disease in adulthood. *Ann Epidemiol.* 2006;16(2):91–104.

33. Marmot MG, Shipley MJ, Rose G. Inequalities in death—specific explanations of a general pattern? *Lancet.* 1984;1(8384):1003.

34. Trehan I, Manary MJ. Management of severe acute malnutrition in low-income and middle-income countries. *Arch Dis Child.* 2015;100(3):283.

35. World Health Organization. Causes of child mortality. Global Health Observatory (GHO) data Website. Available from: http://www.who.int/gho/child_health/mortality/causes/en/. Updated 2015. Accessed Apr 4, 2017.

36. FAO. The state of food insecurity in the world 2011: How does international price volatility affect domestic economies and food security? Rome: Food and Agriculture Organization of the United Nations; 2011.

37. Statista. Consumer food at home expenditure share in selected countries, 2013 statistic. The Statistics Portal Website. Available from: https://www-statista-com.ezp-prod1.hul.harvard.edu/statistics/189227/percent-of-disposable-income-spent-on-food-at-home-2009/. Accessed Nov 4, 2016.

38. Xu K, Saksena P, Holly A. *The determinants of health expenditure: A country-level panel data analysis*. Results for Development Institute (R4D). 2011. http://www.r4d.org/sites/resultsfordevelopment.org/files/resources/Transitions%2520in%2520Health%2520Financing%2520-%2520The%2520Determinants%2520of%2520Health%2520Expenditure%5B1%5D.pdf

39. Lameire N, Joffe P, Wiedemann M. Healthcare systems—an international review: An overview. *Nephrol Dial Transplant*. 1999;14:3–9.

40. Gelting R, Bliss K, Patrick M, Lockhart G, Handzel T. Water, sanitation and hygiene in Haiti: Past, present, and future. *Am J Trop Med Hyg*. 2013;89(4):665–670.

41. Piarroux R, Barrais R, Faucher B, et al. Understanding the cholera epidemic, Haiti. *Emerg Infect Dis*. 2011;17(7):1161.

42. Barzilay EJ, Schaad N, Magloire R, et al. Cholera surveillance during the Haiti epidemic—the first 2 years. *N Engl J Med*. 2013;368(7):599–609.

43. Tappero JW, Tauxe RV. Lessons learned during public health response to cholera epidemic in Haiti and the Dominican Republic. *Emerging Infect Dis*. 2011;17(11):2087.

44. Marmot M. Epidemiology of socioeconomic status and health: Are determinants within countries the same as between countries? Socioeconomic status and health in industrial nations. *Ann NY Acad Sci*. 1999;896:16–29.

45. Rose G. Sick individuals and sick populations. *Intl J Epidemiol*. 1985;14(1):32–38.

46. Krug EG. *World report on violence and health: Summary*. Geneva: World Health Organization; 2001.

47. Robert S. Community-level socioeconomic status effects on adult health. *J Health Soc Behav*. 1998;39(1):18–37.

48. Wallace R. Urban desertification, public health and public order: 'Planned shrinkage', violent death, substance abuse and AIDS in the Bronx. *Soc Sci Med*. 1990;31(7):801–813.

49. Mukherjee JS, Smith L. Health care gap. In: Moore JH, editor. *Encyclopedia of race and racism* (pp. 801–813). Detroit, MI: Macmillan Reference USA/Thomson Gale; 2008.

50. Galster G. Housing discrimination and urban poverty of African-Americans. *J Housing Res*. 1991;2(2):87.

51. Bullard, RD. *Unequal protection: Environmental justice and communities of color*. San Francisco, CA: Sierra Club Books; 1994.

52. Smedley BD. The lived experience of race and its health consequences. *Am J Public Health*. 2012;102(5):933.

53. Murray CJL, Kulkarni SC, Michaud C, et al. Eight Americas: Investigating mortality disparities across races, counties, and race-counties in the United States (mortality disparities in the US). *PLoS Med*. 2006;3(9):e260.

54. Amowitz L, Iacopino V. Women's health and human rights needs. *Lancet*. 2000;356:S65.

55. Geiger HJ. Race and health care—an American dilemma? *N Engl J Med.* 1996;335(11):815.

56. Kolarcik P, Geckova AM, Orosova O, van Dijk JP, Reijneveld SA. To what extent does socioeconomic status explain differences in health between Roma and non-Roma adolescents in Slovakia? *Soc Sci Med.* 2009;68(7):1279–1284.

57. Byrd WM. *An American health dilemma: The medical history of African Americans and the problem of race.* New York: Routledge; 2000.

58. Calo WA, Vernon SW, Lairson DR, Linder SH. Area-level socioeconomic inequalities in the use of mammography screening: A multilevel analysis of the health of Houston survey. *Womens Health Issues.* 2016;26(2):201–207.

59. Dailey AB, Brumback BA, Livingston MD, Jones BA, Curbow BA, Xu X. Area-level socioeconomic position and repeat mammography screening use: Results from the 2005 national health interview survey. *Cancer Epidemiol Biomarkers Prevent.* 2011;20(11):2331.

60. Chen I, Kurz J, Pasanen M, et al. Racial differences in opioid use for chronic non-malignant pain. *J Gen Intern Med.* 2005;20(7):593–598.

61. Borum M, Lynn J, Zhong Z. The effects of patient race on outcomes in seriously ill patients in Support: An overview of economic impact, medical intervention, and end-of-life decisions. *J Am Geriatr Soc.* 2000;(5):194–198.

62. Fassler J. How doctors take women's pain less seriously. *Atlantic.* 2015. https://www.the-atlantic.com/health/archive/2015/10/emergency-room-wait-times-sexism/410515/

63. Flores G. The impact of medical interpreter services on the quality of health care: A systematic review. *Med Care Res Rev.* 2005;62(3):255.

64. Jacobs EA, Lauderdale DS, Meltzer D, Shorey JM, Levinson W, Thisted RA. Impact of interpreter services on delivery of health care to limited–English proficient patients. *J Gen Intern Med.* 2001;16(7):468–474.

65. Farmer P. *Infections and inequalities: The modern plagues.* Berkeley, CA: University of California Press; 1999.

66. Lannin DR, Mathews HF, Mitchell J, Swanson MS, Swanson FH, Edwards MS. Influence of socioeconomic and cultural factors on racial differences in late-stage presentation of breast cancer. *JAMA.* 1998;279(22):1801–1807.

67. Dai D. Black residential segregation, disparities in spatial access to health care facilities, and late-stage breast cancer diagnosis in metropolitan Detroit. *Health and Place.* 2010;16(5):1038–1052.

68. Habermas J. *Moral consciousness and communicative action.* Cambridge, MA: MIT Press; 1990.

69. Sen A. *Development as freedom.* New York: Anchor; 1999.

70. Drèze J. *Hunger and public action.* Oxford/New York: Clarendon/Oxford University Press; 1989.

71. Dewey KG, Adu Afarwuah S. Systematic review of the efficacy and effectiveness of complementary feeding interventions in developing countries. *Maternal Child Nutr.* 2008;4:24–85.

72. Scaling up international food aid: Food delivery alone cannot solve the malnutrition crisis (editorial). *PLoS Med.* 2008;5(11):e235.

73. Lynch JW, Smith GD, Kaplan GA, House JS. Income inequality and mortality: Importance to health of individual income, psychosocial environment, or material conditions (education and debate). *BMJ.* 2000;320(7243):1200.

74. Tectonidis M. Crisis in Niger—outpatient care for severe acute malnutrition. *N Engl J Med.* 2006;354(3):224.

75. Hackbarth DP, Silvestri B, Cosper W. Tobacco and alcohol billboards in 50 Chicago neighborhoods: Market segmentation to sell dangerous products to the poor. *J Public Health Policy.* 1995;16(2):213.

76. Eldridge D, Jackson R, Rajashekara S, et al. Understanding food insecurity in Navajo Nation through the community lens. In: Ivers L, editor. *Food insecurity and public health.* Boca Raton, FL: CRC Press; 2015.

77. Hutchinson RN, Shin S, Baradaran HR. Systematic review of health disparities for cardiovascular diseases and associated factors among American Indian and Alaska Native populations. *PLoS One.* 2014;9(1).

78. Biehl JG, Petryna A. *When people come first: Critical studies in global health.* Princeton, NJ: Princeton University Press; 2013.

79. Farmer P. Social scientists and the new tuberculosis. *Soc Sci Med.* 1997; 44(3):347–358.

80. Farmer PE, Nizeye B, Stulac S, Keshavjee S. Structural violence and clinical medicine (policy forum). *PLoS Med.* 2006;3(10):e449.

81. Gutiérrez G. *We drink from our own wells: The spiritual journey of a people.* Maryknoll, NY/Melbourne: Orbis Books; 1984.

82. Westerhaus M, Panjabi R, Mukherjee J. Violence and the role of illness narratives. *Lancet.* 2008;372(9640):699–701.

83. Behforouz HL, Drain PK, Rhatigan JJ. Rethinking the social history. *N Engl J Med.* 2014;371(14):1277–1279.

84. Social Medicine Consortium. Achieving health equity this generation: The case for social medicine. A consensus statement by the Social Medicine Consortium. 2015. https://static1.squarespace.com/static/5666e742d82d5ed3d741a0fd/t/58e6a11e-197aea663f22dc7b/1491509534812/Social+Medicine+Consortium+Consensus+St atement+Final-2.pdf

85. Kleinman A. *The illness narratives: Suffering, healing, and the human condition.* New York: Basic Books; 1988.

86. McAdam D, McCarthy JD, Zald MN, eds. *Comparative perspectives on social movements: Political opportunities, mobilizing structures, and cultural framings.* Cambridge/New York: Cambridge University Press; 1996.

87. Olivera O. *Cochabamba!: Water war in Bolivia.* Cambridge, MA: Revista Panamericana de Salud Publica; 2004. http://www.scielosp.org/scielo.php?script= sci_arttext&pid=S1020-49892006000100004

88. Mulreany JP, Calikoglu S, Ruiz S, Sapsin JW. Water privatization and public health in Latin America. [La privatización del abastecimiento de agua y la salud pública en América Latina.] *Revista Panamericana de Salud Pública.* 2006;19(1):23–32.

89. Gambino L. Native Americans take Dakota Access Pipeline protest to Washington; Mar 10, 2017. Available from: https://www.theguardian.com/us-news/2017/mar/10/native-nations-march-washington-dakota-access-pipeline.

90. ADA. ADA: Information and technical assistance on the Americans with Disabilities Act. Available from: www.ada.gov. Accessed Nov 1, 2016.

91. Project Bread. Summer food service programs kick off across Massachusetts. Available from: http://www.projectbread.org/news-and-events/press-releases/summer-food-service-programs.html?referrer=https://www.google.com/. Accessed Oct 31, 2016.

6

Giving Care, Delivering Value

Key Points

- People value their health, and ill health is not a choice.
- Lack of utilization of services is often related to barriers to care or poor quality of services rather than to lack of knowledge.
- Ill health and health seeking is often rooted in a complex web of structural violence and lack of agency.
- Walking the patient's journey or accompaniment educates the provider, program manager, and other decisionmakers about the barriers faced by patients and should support program design.
- An ongoing, durable system of health care that addresses the continuum of prevention, treatment, and care is the foundation of a rights-based approach to health.
- A holistic approach is needed to deliver value to the patient. Patients value care that is accessible, treats the spectrum of their needs, and results in good outcomes.
- The *care delivery value chain* is a framework with which to evaluate the delivery of care across the spectrum of a condition.

Introduction

In its broadest sense, health is holistic. Good health is foundational in helping people to live to their fullest capacity: "not the absence of disease but a state of physical, mental and emotional well-being."[1] The goal of a health system, then, is to provide the foundation for the realization of good health in the broadest sense. People get sick throughout their lifespan, with acute and chronic problems that may be physical, mental, emotional, or a mix of these factors. Building a foundation for holistic health care requires a systems approach that considers the interplay between biomedical and social forces as well as the various phases of health and illness. For such a system to provide patient-centered, equitable access to high-quality care, it must reduce barriers to care,[2,3] support the most vulnerable,[4] and be adequately resourced to bring value to people when they seek care.[5]

When working to deliver health care, this holistic view can feel overwhelming, especially in impoverished communities that are saddled with underfunded systems, are rife with adverse social conditions, and have a high burden of disease. In many cases, it is indeed easier to give vaccinations to all the children in a village than it is to set up a system that ensures that each individual child's health needs are met. In the face of these obstacles, time-limited vertical interventions that can be measured and neatly costed have been prioritized.[6,7] However, the budgetary and administrative ease of such a project vanishes for those who are most proximate to suffering—the sick and the caregiver.[6] For a child sick with pneumonia, getting a vaccination will not alleviate suffering, provide effective therapy, or prevent death from untreated pneumonia. Furthermore, those who are delivering the vaccination but unable to care for the sick child may feel morally uncomfortable working within the narrow scope of an intervention. Moral discomfort, sadness, and feelings of inadequacy are common among providers who lack the medications, diagnostics, and systems to properly care for the sick. It negatively impacts their mental health.[8,9] One important strategy to overcome these challenges is proximity to the patient. To provide patient centered care means that the patient's struggle and experience must be understood and addressed within the system. This chapter highlights the patient centered approach of global health—that is caregiving, following the patient's journey, and the interface of these two—*accompaniment*. The chapter also introduces the *care delivery value chain*, a framework for program design that incorporates the full continuum of care and addresses barriers within each step.

From Counting to Caring

Professor Arthur Kleinman, a psychiatrist and medical anthropologist at Harvard Medical School, describes caregiving as a reflection of our humanity.[10] Many people drawn to global health seek to alleviate human suffering at the individual, human level.[11,12] But what makes an implementer a caregiver? What allows us to move from counting the numbers of those who receive an intervention to caring for an individual and advocating for humanity? While there is no specific answer to these questions, one approach is to wade into the messiness of the broken, inaccessible systems and vertical projects and to walk with and listen deeply to the needs of one individual.[13] Through caregiving, it is possible to reflect the patient's experience in systems design. A biosocial analysis begins with proximity to suffering and an openness to the whole story. From this vantage point—the patient-centered approach—health systems can be built to respond to people's needs to deliver quality, equity, and value.

As alluded to in earlier chapters, despite a high disease burden, many health centers and hospitals in impoverished countries often stand nearly empty.[14] In response to this low utilization of health services, conventional wisdom held that low attendance at clinics is due to people lacking health-seeking behavior, having cultural barriers, or being ignorant about the benefits of modern medicine.[15,16] With these hypotheses, many public health programs focused on *information, education, and communication* (IEC) campaigns or *behavior change communication* (BCC) to increase the number of people seeking health care.[17,18] The goal of IEC and BCC programs is often to promote clinic attendance, sometimes called *demand creation*.[19] Demand creation programs are implemented when uptake of services is low. Such programs encourage the use of a variety of services from antenatal care[20] to antiretroviral therapy [ART] clinic attendance,[21] to family planning,[22] to male circumcision to prevent the transmission of HIV.[23] While knowledge of the availability and potential benefits of care may increase people's utilization of services, demand creation programs often overestimate a person's agency and underestimate the barriers to care. In addition, demand creation programs presuppose that care is of good quality. Many studies have shown that people may avoid clinics because of poor-quality services or lack of drug supply.[24-26] This was very notable early in the Ebola epidemic, where holding centers without testing or treatment were avoided. Once care was available, more people came forward.[27]

In contrast with the underutilization of poor-quality services, when high-quality, accessible services exist there is great demand.[28] When people are sick, they seek care of good quality, often at great expense.[29] The higher the out-of-pocket expense, the more patients will delay seeking care. In a variety of wealthy, middle, and even some impoverished countries from England to Canada, Cuba to Costa Rica, the majority of the cost of health care is borne by the government and funded through taxes and other government revenues (Figure 6.1).[30-33] Adequately funded public systems minimize the patient's out-of-pocket expenditures at the point of service and have more equitable outcomes than systems in which patients pay at the time of service.[34] While the financing of health will be discussed in more detail in Chapter 12, it is important to note here that when people are sick, the looming cost of care is the most important factor in delaying or forgoing care in every country.[35,36]

As discussed in Chapter 1, in most impoverished countries, user fees at the point of care were implemented in the 1980s after the Bamako Initiative.[37]

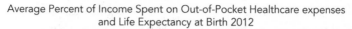

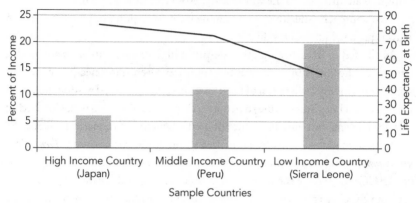

FIGURE 6.1 High (US), middle (Peru), and low (Sierra Leone) income countries. Bar shows percent of income spend on out-of-pocket health expenditures. Line shows life expectancy.

Data compiled from Gallup poll and World Health Organization (WHO)/National Healthcareer Association (NHA) database and WHO life expectancy database. Available from: http://www.gallup.com/poll/166211/worldwide-median-household-income-000.aspx.

Fees were promoted as a way to put money into inadequately funded public systems. There has long been a belief that people value care more if they purchase it.[38] However, there is now overwhelming evidence to show that any fee suppresses utilization and disproportionately affects the poor.[35] The data also shows unequivocally that fee removal increases utilization.[2] Beyond the fees charged, there are also significant financial barriers borne by the patient and family that are unseen by the care provider. Among these hidden, out-of-pocket fees are the cost of transportation to a facility[39] and lost wages or productivity associated with seeking care.[40] Every hour a person waits to be seen, every mile a person walks to gain access, every mode of transport (whether cab, pick-up truck, or donkey) that ferries a person to a facility increases out-of-pocket expenditures.

Understanding and mitigating the catastrophic effects that health expenditures have on patients, families, and communities is central to health equity. Efforts to remove user fees have spread throughout impoverished countries.[2,41] Some programs also provide assistance in the form of transportation vouchers or cash transfers to patients in an effort to curb out-of-pocket expenditure. In every case, removing implicit and explicit fees and barriers increases utilization of services[42,43] and improves patient outcomes and equity.[3,44,45] Addressing barriers has a greater impact on care utilization than education alone.[46]

Reducing the financial burden on patients seeking care is only one piece of the equation to increase the uptake of services. The provision of quality services is also critical.[47] A large program in India that provided cash transfers to women to encourage utilization of maternity services and facility-based delivery demonstrated increased use of services[48] but did not improve maternal health outcomes.[47] The poor maternal outcomes were due to understaffing, lack of supplies, and delays in emergency referral care.[49,50] Therefore, expanding access by reducing barriers must be linked to the provision of quality services (addressed further in Chapter 10). People know which health facilities have the human resources, infrastructure, and medicines to provide quality care. It is not uncommon for people to bypass centers closer to their homes to seek better services, even at higher cost.[24]

The Patient Journey

Tuberculosis (TB) is a severe, airborne infection. Thus, it has a special status in public health. Because TB spreads through the air, diagnosis and treatment are technically offered free in every country, no matter how impoverished.[51,52] Because treatment is free and TB is a disease of impoverished people, the patient journey to seek care and be cured of TB uniquely highlights barriers in access to and quality of care. In the United States, when a person is found to have TB in their sputum (phlegm from a cough), they are put on a cocktail of four drugs that must be taken daily for two months and then multiple times a week for a total of six months. Laboratory tests are done immediately to ensure that the patient's strain is not resistant to any of the drugs prescribed, and, if resistance is detected, the medication is changed. To help patients adhere to this strict regimen, the American public health system employs public health nurses to go into the community and bring the drugs to the patient no matter where they are. Anyone currently living with the patient is also tested and monitored for TB. Given the intense effort that goes into treating TB in a wealthy country, it is easy to imagine how impoverished countries struggle to support TB control. In his paper "Social Scientist and the New Tuberculosis,"[53] Dr. Paul Farmer recounts the story of a patient in Haiti seeking care for TB. He describes, in great detail, the patient journey—both the barriers to accessing care and the under-resourcing of public facilities. The patient's journey continues for many years, eventually finding Farmer's charity clinic (Figure 6.2). These factors underpin tragic outcomes for many around the world.

In the case, the patient is a peasant farmer with no cash income. He first delays seeking therapy because his only option is a distant public clinic, and the

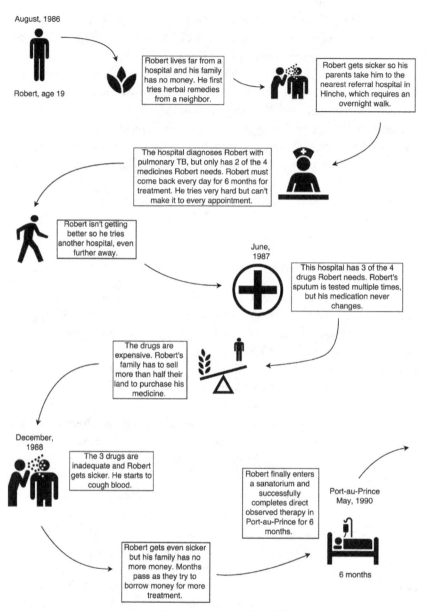

FIGURE 6.2 In his paper, Social Scientists and the New TB, Dr. Paul Farmer describes the journey of one patient to seek care for tuberculosis in Haiti. The patient's journey is a long and arduous path marked by obstacles from out-of-pocket costs, to long geographic distances and health system inadequacies such as medication stock outs and lack of diagnostic capability. Proximity to the patient and accompaniment on his journey can reveal these challenges to the care giver and support systems design that minimizes this barriers.

Source: Data abstracted from Farmer P. Social scientists and the new tuberculosis. *Soc Sci Med.* 1997;44(3):347–358.

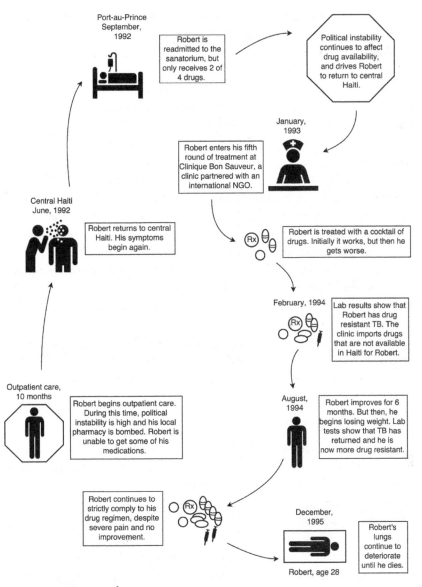

FIGURE 6.2 Continued

transportation is too costly. Instead, he chooses a less costly, local traditional healer. He continues to be ill—coughing and losing weight—until he seeks care in a public facility. However, although the pills and consultation are offered free of charge, the out-of-pocket costs like transportation fees (in this case for a donkey) and so-called opportunity cost (such as lost wages from missing two days of farming per visit) present significant barriers to completing his therapy. He stops taking his medications. He remains ill and continues to seek care, progressively impoverishing himself and his family. After multiple incomplete treatments, he develops a drug-resistant form of TB (resistance to common drugs yet treatable with so-called second-line drugs). The local facilities do not have the laboratory tests necessary to make the appropriate diagnosis nor the drugs to provide the correct treatment. He eventually finds his way to a charity clinic where he is finally diagnosed with and dies of drug-resistant TB.[53]

Often, public health or medical professionals will claim that the cause of a patient's development of drug resistance and eventual death is the patient's lack of understanding about treatment or willful noncompliance to the prescribed medicine.[54,55] Farmer urges against exaggerating the agency of a patient trapped in poverty.[53] Rather it is important to perform a biosocial analysis of the patient's journey—to understand and interrogate the barriers faced by the patient and the poor quality of care available. A social medicine approach would entail lessening the barriers and improving the quality of care. This places the onus of good outcomes on the health system rather than the patient. Patients may refer to their journeys to care as "pilgrimages."[56] The pilgrimage is a painful combination of financial impoverishment and inadequate care that is often fatal. It leaves families and communities with the dual burden of grief and debt. Reducing barriers to care and resourcing systems adequately to deliver quality care are two fundamental aspects of creating a health system that is effective in delivering value to patients.

Health Systems and Value

In 2001, the US-based Institute for Medicine's report on health care quality defined patient-centered care as "providing care that is respectful of and responsive to individual patient preferences, needs, and values and ensuring that patient values guide all clinical decisions."[57] In the medical literature, a formal metric known as the *health-related quality adjusted life year* (QALY) builds on the disability-adjusted life year (DALY) (discussed in Chapter 4) and attempts to capture the patient perspective on quality of life attributed to an illness.[58,59] The patient perspective must also include stress placed on the patient and family.[60,61]

In global health delivery, care should be evaluated based on value, quality, and health outcome. This is different than choosing a single intervention because it is cheap and then analyzing the effectiveness of the discrete intervention. Returning to the example of the child with pneumonia in a vaccination campaign, the goal of global health delivery is a healthy child, not a vaccinated child. For a child to be healthy, vaccinations are important but so is care for illness such as pneumonia. To prevent pneumonia, it is important that the child be breastfed, has adequate nutrition, and is not exposed to indoor cooking smoke [62] Yet the family and child may not have the agency to carry out all these forms of pneumonia prevention. Even if they do, the child may still fall sick. Furthermore, each of the elements needed by the child is often delivered in different and unrelated vertical programs—a group working on child nutrition here, a vaccination program there, a clinic for pneumonia elsewhere. With each fragmented piece, the out-of-pocket and opportunity costs for the child's caregiver increase and the odds of having a healthy child decrease. The fragmentation of the system due to these vertical programs results in discoordination of the human resources, supply chain, and infrastructure needed to achieve the outcome that will have the most value—a healthy child.

In their article "Redefining Global Health-Care Delivery," published in 2013 in *The Lancet*,[5] Partners in Health co-founders Drs. Jim Kim and Paul Farmer, working with the US health care management and strategy expert Professor Michael Porter, proposed that those engaged in global health delivery use of a framework called the *care delivery value chain*. The value chain is a multi-step analysis of the interrelated tasks that are needed to deliver health care and achieve good outcomes. The care delivery value chain is created by elaborating the steps needed throughout the continuum of care, from prevention to diagnosis to follow-up and palliation. The care delivery value chain is developed by gleaning information on the steps of care and patient needs through proximity to the community, accompaniment of the patient, and knowledge of the existing system. To design systems with the value chain, it is necessary to coordinate the various system inputs, including human resources, infrastructure, and supply chain, across the continuum of care.[63] The value chain is different than the cost-effectiveness approach historically favored in public health programs. Cost effectiveness assumes first a fix amount of money is available and within that fixed amount, the least costly intervention is chosen. In contrast, Porter describes value in health care as placing the patient outcome first and then building the system needed to deliver care and cost of achieving the desired outcome:

> Value should always be defined around the [patient] . . . value depends on results, not inputs, value in health care is measured by the outcomes achieved, not the volume of services delivered. . . . Nor is value measured by the process of care used; process measurement and improvement are important tactics but are no substitutes for measuring outcomes and cost.[63]

Delivering value for patients in impoverished settings cannot be done without simultaneously advocating for larger and more effective investments in care delivery. This approach necessarily rejects the extreme cost constraints and fragmentation of funds that are the starting point of many programs.[64]

The concept of the care delivery value chain allows for a systems-based analysis.[65] Developing the value chain requires understanding the continuum of care—from the literature, from providers, and from patients' experience. This concept has been used to analyze a variety of health care systems.[66] One example of the use of the care delivery value chain is to develop and analyze HIV programs (Figure 6.3).[67]

The movement for AIDS treatment access highlighted the linkage of prevention, care and treatment as a continuum of care or value chain.[68–70] Many of the early programs for HIV services focused case finding through isolated testing programs.[71] If patients were found to be positive, they were referred to care in a different place.[72] If a patient also had TB (commonly associated with AIDS), they had to get their TB treatment at yet another location. At each

	Screening/preventing	Diagnosing/Staging	Delaying progression	Initiating antiretroviral therapy	Ongoing disease management	Management of clinical deterioration
Informing and engaging	• Prevention counselling on modes of transmission and condom use	• Explanation of diagnosis and the implications • Explaining the course of HIV and the prognosis	• Explanation of the approach to forestalling progression	• Explanation of medication instructions and side-effects	• Counselling about adherence; understanding factors for non-adherence	• Explanation of the comorbid diagnoses and the implications • End-of-life counselling
Measuring	• HIV testing • Screen for sexually transmitted infections • Collect baseline demographics	• HIV testing for others at risk • Clinical examination CD4+ count and other labs • Testing for common co-morbidities such as tuberculosis and sexually transmitted diseases • Pregnancy testing	• CD4+ count monitoring (continuous staging) • Regular primary care assessment • HIV testing for others at risk • Laboratory evaluation for medication initiation	• HIV staging and medication response • Highly frequent primary care assessments • Assessing/managing complications of therapy • HIV testing for others at risk (bi-annually) • Laboratory evaluation	• HIV staging and medication response • Regular primary care assessment • Laboratory evaluation	• HIV staging and medication response • Regular primary care assessment • Laboratory evaluation
Accessing	• Testing centres • High risk settings • Primary care clinics • Prenatal services	• Primary care clinics • On-site laboratories at primary care clinics • Testing centres • Prenatal clinics	• Primary care clinics • Laboratories (on-site at primary clinic) • Pharmacy • Food centres • Community health workers/home visits • Support groups	• Primary care clinics • Laboratories (on-site at primary clinic) • Pharmacy • Food centres • Community health workers/home visits • Support groups	• Primary care clinics • Laboratories (on-site at primary clinic) • Pharmacy • Food centres • Community health workers/home visits • Support groups	• HIV Staging and medication response • Regular primary care assessment • Laboratory evaluation • Primary care clinics • Pharmacy • Laboratories (on-site at primary clinic) • Community health workers/home visits • Hospitals & hospice facilities • Support groups • Food centres
	Screening/preventing • Connect patients with primary care system • Identify high-risk individuals • Test at-risk individuals • Promote appropriate risk reduction strategies • Modify behavioural risk factors • Create a medical record • Prevent mother-to-child transmission of HIV	**Diagnosing/Staging** • Formal diagnosis and staging • Determine method of transmission and others at potential risk • Identify others at risk • Screen for tuberculosis, syphilis, and other sexually transmitted diseases • Pregnancy testing and contraceptive counselling • Create management plan, including scheduling of follow-up visits • Formulate a treatment plan	**Delaying progression** • Initiate therapies that can delay onset, including vitamins and food • Treat comorbidities that affect progression of disease, especially tuberculosis • Improve patient awareness of disease progression, prognosis, and transmission • Connect patient to care team, including community health work	**Initiating antiretroviral therapy** • Initiate comprehensive anti-retroviral therapy and assess medication readiness • Prepare patient for disease progression and side-effects of associated treatment • Manage secondary infections and associated illnesses	**Ongoing disease management** • Manage effects of associated illnesses • Manage side-effects of treatment • Determine supporting nutritional modifications • Prepare patient for end-of-life management • Provide primary care and health maintenance • Provide psychosocial support	**Management of clinical deterioration** • Identify clinical and laboratory deterioration • Initiate second-line, third-line drug therapies • Manage acute illness and opportunistic infection either through aggressive outpatient management or hospitalisation • Provide additional community/social support if needed • Ensure access to hospice care

FIGURE 6.3 HIV/AIDS care delivery value chain in resource-poor settings. The care delivery value chain elucidates the inputs needed along the continuum of care. This framework decreases system fragmentation and increases value for the patient.

Source: Kim JY, Farmer P, Porter ME. Redefining global health-care delivery. *Lancet*. 2013;382(9897):1060–1069.

step, care was fragmented and patients, facing an additional set of barriers, were lost to follow-up and had poor outcomes. In contrast, to deliver timely and effective care to a person living with HIV throughout the continuum of the disease, the care delivery value chain for HIV begins with the diagnosis of infection and lasts until death. Along this chain, the goal is to logically sequence and integrate needed services, decrease barriers, and facilitate care from the patient's perspective. This logic informs the design of a facility, the leveraging of human resources, and the flow of information. The alignment of services should be straightforward and streamlined to achieve positive health outcomes.

Assumptions within the value chain can be changed with evolving protocols and technologies. For example, when the preceding value chain was created for HIV, there was a long period between the staging of HIV disease and the initiation of ART. Today, as the recommendation is to test and begin ART immediately, this value chain would be modified. The innovation that led to the recommendation of pre-exposure prophylaxis (PrEP) (a once-a-day dose of ART that decreases the risk of contracting HIV through sexual transmission by 90 percent)[73,74] could be added into the value chain after testing if a high-risk person is negative. The care delivery value chain has proved to be a useful tool in program design and evaluation. It has been used in assessing and implementing different kinds of programs in a way that attends to the needs of the individual and maximizes outcomes.

Conclusion

Patient centered care should be delivered based on an understanding of the patient's experience. This experience can be gleaned through caregiving and accompaniment. Barriers to care and poor quality of care are major factors that reduce utilization of services. Barriers faced by patients in accessing and adhering to care should be minimized to assure health equity. Value for the patient and patient centered care should drive health system design and care delivery. Sufficient resources to mitigate barriers and provide high quality of care will result in high utilization of services. In the era of global health, it is important to move beyond narrow interventions to build health systems that effectively deliver care to individuals. The care delivery value chain is a tool that can be used to harmonize the elements of care delivery to minimize barriers, maximize value, and achieve excellent health outcomes. The value chain is informed by best practices and evidence-based medicine as well as by proximity and listening to the challenges faced by an individual in seeking care.

References

1. World Health Organization. *Chronicle of the World Health Organization.* Geneva: World Health Organization, 1947.

2. Yates R. Universal health care and the removal of user fees. *Lancet.* 2009;373(9680):2078–2081.

3. Mukherjee J, Ivers L, Leandre F, Farmer P, Behforouz H. Antiretroviral therapy in resource-poor settings: Decreasing barriers to access and promoting adherence. *JAIDS.* 2006;43:S126.

4. Rich M, Miller A, Niyigena P, et al. Excellent clinical outcomes and high retention in care among adults in a community-based HIV treatment program in rural Rwanda. *JAIDS.* 2012;59(3): E42.

5. Kim JY, Farmer P, Porter ME. Redefining global health-care delivery. *Lancet.* 2013;382(9897):1060–1069.

6. Biehl JG, Petryna A. *When people come first: Critical studies in global health.* Princeton, NJ: Princeton University Press; 2013.

7. Wisner B. GOBI versus PHC? Some dangers of selective primary health care. *Soc Sci Med.* 1988;26(9):963–969.

8. Dieleman M, Biemba G, Mphuka S, et al. We are also dying like any other people, we are also people: Perceptions of the Impact of HIV/AIDS on health workers in two districts in Zambia. *Health Policy Plann.* 2007;22(3):139–148.

9. Raviola G, Machoki M, Mwaikambo E, Good M. HIV, disease plague, demoralization and burnout: Resident experience of the medical profession in Nairobi, Kenya. *Cult Med Psychiatry.* 2002;26(1):55–86.

10. Kleinman A. The art of medicine caregiving as moral experience. *Lancet.* 2012;380(9853):1550–1551.

11. Kerry VB, Ndung'u T, Walensky RP, Lee PT, Kayanja VF, Bangsberg DR. Managing the demand for global health education. *PLoS medicine.* 2011;8(11):e1001118.

12. Merson MH, Page KC. *The dramatic expansion of university engagement in global health: Implications for US policy.* Washington, DC: Center for Strategic and International Studies; 2009.

13. Westerhaus M, Finnegan A, Haidar M, Kleinman A, Mukherjee J, Farmer P. The necessity of social medicine in medical education. *Acad Med.* 2015;90(5):565–568.

14. Kim JY, Porter M, Rhatigan J, et al. Scaling up effective delivery models worldwide. In: Farmer P, Kim JY, Kleinman A, Basilico M, editors. *Reimagining global health.* Berkeley: University of California Press; 2013.

15. Herbert B. In America; refusing to save Africans. *The New York Times.* Jun 11, 2001. Available from: http://www.nytimes.com/2001/06/11/opinion/in-america-refusing-to-save-africans.html. Accessed Nov 4, 2016.

16. Harrison A, Smit J, Myer L. Prevention of HIV/AIDS in South Africa: A review of behaviour change interventions, evidence and options for the future. *S Afr J Sci.* 2000;96(6):285–290.

17. Shaikh B, Hatcher J. Health seeking behaviour and health service utilization in Pakistan: Challenging the policy makers. *J Public Health.* 2005;27(1):49–54.

18. Adane M, Mengistie B, Mulat W, Kloos H, Medhin G. Utilization of health facilities and predictors of health-seeking behavior for under-five children with acute diarrhea in slums of Addis Ababa, Ethiopia: A community-based cross-sectional study. *J Health Pop Nutr.* 2017; 36.

19. World Health Organization. *Generating demand and community support for sexual and reproductive health services for young people.* Geneva: Department of Child and Adolescent Health and Development, World Health Organization; 2009.

20. Darmstadt GL, Bhutta ZA, Cousens S, Adam T, Walker N, de Bernis L. Evidence-based, cost-effective interventions: How many newborn babies can we save? *Lancet.* 2005;365(9463):977–988.

21. Simoni J, Amico K, Pearson C, Malow R. Strategies for promoting adherence to antiretroviral therapy: A review of the literature. *Curr Infect Dis Rep.* 2008;10(6):515–521.

22. Kesterton AJ, Cabral M. Generating demand and community support for sexual and reproductive health services for young people: A review of the literature and programs. Research report. *Reprod Health.* 2010;7:25.

23. Maibvise C, Mavundla TR. Reasons for the low uptake of adult male circumcision for the prevention of HIV transmission in Swaziland. *Afr J AIDS Res.* 2014;13(3):281–289.

24. Leonard KL, Mliga GR, Haile Mariam D. Bypassing health centres in Tanzania: Revealed preferences for quality. *J Afr Econ.* 2002;11(4):441–471.

25. Peters DH, Garg A, Bloom G, Walker DG, Brieger WR, Hafizur Rahman M. Poverty and access to health care in developing countries. *Ann N Y Acad Sci.* 2008;1136(1):161–171.

26. Kruk ME, Hermosilla S, Larson E, Mbaruku GM. Bypassing primary care clinics for childbirth: A cross-sectional study in the Pwani Region, United Republic of Tanzania. [Contournement des cliniques de soins primaires pour l'accouchement: Une Etude Transversale dans la region de Pwani, en Republique-unie de Tanzanie.] *Bull World Health Org.* 2014;92(4):246.

27. Hofman M, Au S. *The politics of fear: Médecins sans Frontières and the West African Ebola epidemic.* New York: Oxford Universtiy Press; 2017.

28. Farmer P, Kim JY, Kleinman A, Basilico M. *Reimagining global health: An introduction.* Berkeley: University of California Press; 2013.

29. Farmer P. Who lives and who dies. *London Rev Books.* 2015;37(3):17–20.

30. Storch JL. Canadian Healthcare System. In: McIntyre M, McDonald C, editors. *Realities of Canadian nursing, professional, practice, and power issues.* 3rd edition. Philadelphia: Wolters Kluwer Health, Lippincott Williams & Wilkins; 2010. p. 34–55.

31. Casas A, Vargas H. The health system in Costa Rica: Toward a national health service. *J Public Health Policy.* 1980;1(3):258.

32. De Vos P. No one left abandoned: Cuba's national health system since the 1959 revolution. *Intl J Health Serv: Plan, Admin, Eval.* 2005;35(1):189.

33. Basu S, Andrews J, Kishore S, Panjabi R, Stuckler D. Comparative performance of private and public healthcare systems in low- and middle- income countries: A systematic review. *PLoS Med.* 2012;9(6):e1001244.

34. Xu K, Evans DB, Kawabata K, Zeramdini R, Klavus J, Murray CJL. Household catastrophic health expenditure: A multicountry analysis. *Lancet.* 2003;362(9378):111–117.

35. Gilson L. The lessons of user fee experience in Africa. *Health Policy Plan.* 1997;12(4):273–285.

36. Creese A, Kuznets J. Lessons from cost recovery in health: Forum on health sector reform. WHO/SHS/NHP/95.5; Geneva: National Health Systems and Policies Unit, Div. of Strengthening Health Services, World Health Organization; 1995. http://apps.who.int/iris/bitstream/10665/58525/1/WHO_SHS_NHP_95.5.pdf

37. Kanji N. Charging for drugs in Africa: UNICEF's "Bamako initiative." *Health Policy Plan.* 1989;4(2):110–120. Available from: http://heapol.oxfordjournals.org. ezp-prod1.hul.harvard.edu/content/4/2/110. Accessed Sep 29, 2016. doi:10.1093/heapol/4.2.110.

38. Minakawa N, Dida GO, Sonye GO, Futami K, Kaneko S. Unforeseen misuses of bed nets in fishing villages along Lake Victoria. *Malaria J.* 2008;7:165.

39. Harris B, Goudge J, John EA, et al. Inequities in access to health care in South Africa. *J Public Health Policy.* 2011;32:S102.

40. Lenore M, Sokrin K. Poverty, user fees and ability to pay for health care for children with suspected dengue in rural Cambodia. *Intl J Equity Health.* 2008;7(1):10.

41. Gilson L, Mcintyre D. Removing user fees for primary care in Africa: The need for careful action. *BMJ.* 2005;331(7519):762.

42. Ridde V, Morestin F. A scoping review of the literature on the abolition of user fees in health care services in Africa. *Health Policy Plan.* 2011;26(1):1–11.

43. Wilkinson D, Gouws E, Sach M, Karim SSA. Effect of removing user fees on attendance for curative and preventive primary health care services in rural South Africa;79(7):665–671.

44. Rawlings LB, Rubio GM. Evaluating the impact of conditional cash transfer programs. *World Bank Res Observ.* 2005;20(1):29–56.

45. Lagarde M, Haines A, Palmer N. The impact of conditional cash transfers on health outcomes and use of health services in low and middle income countries. Cochrane Effective Practice and Organisation of Care Group. *Cochrane DB Syst Rev.* 2009;(4). http://onlinelibrary.wiley.com/doi/10.1002/14651858.CD008137/pdf

46. Gupta I, Joe W, Rudra S. Demand side financing in health: How far can it address the issue of low utilization in developing countries? *World Health Report, Background Paper 27.* 2010. http://www.who.int/healthsystems/topics/financing/healthreport/27DSF.pdf

47. Powell-Jackson T, Mazumdar S, Mills A. Financial incentives in health: New evidence from India's Janani Suraksha Yojana. *J Health Econ.* 2015;43:154–169.

48. Murray S, Hunter BM, Bisht R, Ensor T, Bick D. Effects of demand-side financing on utilisation, experiences and outcomes of maternity care in low-and middle-income countries: A systematic review. *BMC Pregnancy Childbirth.* 2014;14.

49. Chaturvedi S, Randive B, Diwan V, De Costa A. Quality of obstetric referral services in India's JSY cash transfer programme for institutional births: A study from Madhya Pradesh Province. *PLoS One.* 2014; 9(5).

50. Sanjay KR, Dasgupta R, Das MK, Singh S, Devi R, Arora NK. Determinants of utilization of services under MMJSSA scheme in Jharkhand "client perspective": A qualitative study in a low performing state of India. *Indian J Public Health.* 2011;55(4):252–259.

51. International Union Against Tuberculosis and Lung Disease (IUATLD). Available from: http://www.theunion.org/. Updated 2016. Accessed Nov 8, 2016.

52. World Care Council. *The Patients' Charter for Tuberculosis care—Patients' Rights and Responsibilities.* National Tuberculosis Center: University of California; 2006. http://www.who.int/tb/publications/2006/istc_charter.pdf

53. Farmer P. Social scientists and the new tuberculosis. *Soc Sci Med.* 1997;44(3):347–358.

54. Lawn SD, Wilkinson R. Extensively drug resistant tuberculosis. *BMJ.* 2006;333:559–560.

55. Zhao P, Li XJ, Zhang SF, Wang XS, Liu CY. Social behaviour risk factors for drug resistant tuberculosis in mainland China: A meta-analysis. *J Int Med Res.* 2012;40(2):436–445.

56. Belizaire N. A Qualitative study exploring the experience of women seeking care for breast cancer in Haiti. MMSc [thesis]. Boston (MA): Harvard Medical School; 2015.

57. IOM. *Crossing the quality chasm: A new health system for the 21st century.* Washington, DC: National Academy Press; 2001.

58. Zeckhauser R. Where now for saving lives? *Law Contemp Prob.* 1976;40(4):5–45.

59. Murray CJ. Quantifying the burden of disease: The technical basis for disability-adjusted life years. *Bull World Health Org.* 1994;72(3):429–445. Available from: http://www-ncbi-nlm-nih-gov.ezp-prod1.hul.harvard.edu/pubmed/8062401.

60. Gibson T, Ozminkowski R, Goetzel R. The effects of prescription drug cost sharing: A review of the evidence. *Am J Manag Care.* 2005;11(11):730–740.

61. Eaddy MT, Cook CL, O'Day K, Burch SP, Cantrell CR. How patient cost-sharing trends affect adherence and outcomes: A literature review. *PT.* 2012;37(1):45.

62. Ezzati M, Lopez AD, Rodgers A, Murray CJL. *Comparative quantification of health risks: Global and regional burden of disease attributable to selected major risk factors.* Geneva: World Health Organization; 2004.

63. Porter ME. What is value in health care? *N Engl J Med.* 2010;363(26):2477–2481. doi:10.1056/NEJMci1101108.

64. Gostin LO, Mok EA. Grand challenges in global health governance. *Br Med Bull.* 2009;90(1):7–18.

65. Porter ME, Teisberg EO. *Redefining health care: Creating value-based competition on results.* Boston: Harvard Business Review Press; 2006.

66. Gamble J, Icenogle M, Savage G. Value-chain analysis of a rural health program: Toward understanding the cost benefit of telemedicine applications. *Hosp Top.* 2004;82(1):10–17.

67. Rhatigan J, Jain S, Mukherjee JS, Porter ME. *Applying the care delivery value chain: HIV/AIDS care in resource poor settings.* Boston: Harvard Business School; 2009. http://www.hbs.edu/faculty/Publication%20Files/09-093.pdf

68. Hull MW, Wu Z, Montaner JSG. Optimizing the engagement of care cascade: A critical step to maximize the impact of HIV treatment as prevention. *Curr Opin HIV AIDS.* 2012;7(6):579.

69. Deeks SG, Lewin SR, Havlir DV. The end of AIDS: HIV infection as a chronic disease. *Lancet.* 2013;382(9903):1525–1533.

70. Gardner EM, Mclees MP, Steiner JF, Del Rio C, Burman WJ. The spectrum of engagement in HIV care and its relevance to test-and-treat strategies for prevention of HIV infection. *Clin Infect Dis.* 2011;52(6):793.

71. Summers T, Spielberg F, Collins C, Coates T. Voluntary counseling, testing, and referral for HIV: New technologies, research findings create dynamic opportunities. *JAIDS.* 2000;25(Suppl 2):S128.

72. Nsigaye R, Wringe A, Roura M, et al. From HIV diagnosis to treatment: Evaluation of a referral system to promote and monitor access to antiretroviral therapy in rural Tanzania. *JAIDS.* 2009;2(1):6.

73. Grant RM, Lama JR, Anderson PL, et al. Preexposure chemoprophylaxis for HIV prevention in men who have sex with men. *N Engl J Med.* 2010;363(27):2587–2599.

74. Glazek C. Why is no one on the first treatment to prevent HIV? *The New Yorker.* 2013. http://www.newyorker.com/tech/elements/why-is-no-one-on-the-first-treatment-to-prevent-h-i-v

PART THREE

Health Systems Strengthening

Human Resources for Health

Key Points

- A strong and well-trained health workforce is needed to deliver care that addresses the burden of disease and achieves good health outcomes.
- Increasing the number of health workers in areas of highest need is a critical component to effectively deliver health care.
- Decades of underinvestment in health education has resulted in too few health workers. Those present are often inadequately trained.
- Due to the short-term nature of foreign assistance, training programs in impoverished countries are generally centralized, didactic workshops that do not provide the long term clinical mentoring needed to build capacity.
- Public sector workers are severely underpaid due to the impoverishment of governments and the externally imposed restrictions on public sector spending.
- Better compensation, training, and improved working conditions are needed to retain health professionals in countries and regions where the disease burden is highest.

Introduction

Decades of underinvestment in health have resulted in severe shortages in all cadres of health workers in impoverished countries.[1] This difficult state is rightfully called the "human resources for health crisis."[2] To compound this problem, the scant numbers of health workers available are often inadequately trained to address the disease burden. Health workers in impoverished countries are trained without tools for diagnosis, medicines for treatment, or sufficient clinical mentoring.[3] This difficult situation often leaves public workers demoralized or even fearful.[4] The public wage bill, which is the budgetary envelope used to cover the salaries of public-sector workers, remains constrained since the era of structural adjustment.[5] Thus, health workers in public facilities are too few in number, are insufficiently trained, do not have the tools to perform their work, and are woefully underpaid. As a result, many health workers seek additional income within the private sector or leave the country entirely.

A better trained, larger workforce is needed to support internationally agreed upon targets and achieve the United Nations Sustainable Development Goals (SDGs).[6,7] The global health era brought about a renewed focus on developing a long-term professional workforce to address the disease burden, deliver good health outcomes, and achieve health equity (Figure 7.1). There is clear evidence that shows the correlation between available workforce and health outcomes.[1] This chapter reviews the causes of the inadequate workforce, the need to build the capacity of the health workforce, and the attempts in the global health era to remediate these gaps.

The Health System

Within an effective care delivery system, the skill mix of the health workforce should be based on the burden of disease and needs of the patients.[8] Significant research has been done to understand what is needed to develop an adequate workforce to achieve Universal Health Coverage by 2030.[9] When a value chain (Chapter 6) is mapped out for a disease or sets of conditions, care is generally delivered at four levels: in the community, at primary health care clinics, at district hospitals, and at the national or subnational hospitals for specialty care. As compared to wealthy countries, impoverished countries have fewer workers at each institutional level, and the workers have less training.[2] This chapter will focus on formally trained and publicly supported health workers (doctors, nurses, pharmacists, midwives, etc.) who work within the facilities.

In general, health workers and systems are hierarchically interrelated and supervised (Figure 7.2). Community health workers, an important part of the community-based workforce, will be addressed in Chapter 8. In the hierarchy, CHW are usually supervised by a clinic nurse. Community health workers often carry out prevention programs and may find sick or vulnerable people. If they do, the CHW will refer a patient to the health center. The primary health facility, or health center is the first point of contact within the formal health system. The local health center is where sick people come to receive care general care, deliver babies, and receive preventive services such as vaccination or prenatal services. Health centers in impoverished countries are generally staffed by nurses, nursing assistants, medical assistants, or medical officers. The primary care nurse will, if necessary, refer a patient to a hospital with inpatient medical, maternity, pediatric,

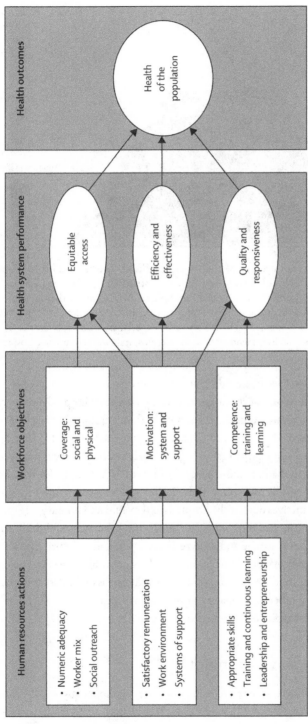

FIGURE 7.1 The global health era brought about renewed focus the human resource crisis. This schematic outlines the actions needed to strengthen human resources so that health workers can meet the objectives of quality care delivery and achieve better health outcomes.

Source: Chen L, Evans T, Anand S, et al. Human resources for health: Overcoming the crisis. *Lancet.* 2004;364(9449):1984–1990.

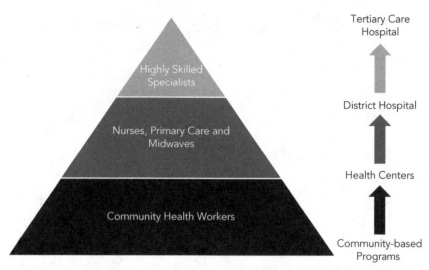

FIGURE 7.2 Pyramid structure shows the typical health system workforce in impoverished countries. The health workforce is generally structured and supervised hierarchically. Community health workers make up the bulk of the workforce. They are supervised by nurses and midwives who work in health centers and district hospitals. Nurses and midwives are in turn supervised by highly skilled specialists who make up the smallest portion of the workforce and who work at district hospitals and tertiary care hospitals.

or surgical services. Even outstanding primary care does not alleviate the need for a capable health workforce at the hospital level. District-level hospitals are generally staffed by more educated cadres of health workers, including physicians, medical officers, and registered or advanced nurses. Hospitals are key points in the health system to ensure quality and access to high-value, life-saving interventions such as basic surgical, orthopedics, and emergency obstetrical services.[10] District hospitals are also strategically important nodes in the health system to advance quality improvement initiatives both at the hospitals and in affiliated primary care centers. District health teams are responsible for supervising the primary health centers in the district. They organize and analyze data on population health that are provided by first-line providers. District-level workers generally supervise the health centers in each district.[11] As the provision of health care is expanded, it important to increase the number and capacity of professional health care workers at each level to ensure equitable access to health care for all.[12]

Challenges and Constraints

The health workforce in impoverished countries is shockingly small given the high burden of disease.[3,13–15] For example, World Bank data from 2010 shows a physician density of 67 per 10,000 people in Cuba and a more than twenty-fold lower physician density, just 3 physicians per 10,000 people, in Botswana even though the countries have relatively similar gross domestic product (GDP) levels per capita (Figure 7.3).[16] Not surprisingly, access to medical care and life expectancy is much higher in Cuba (78.9 years in Cuba vs. 63.4 in Botswana).[16] The World Health Organization (WHO) recommends 22.8 skilled, professional health workers per 10,000 people.[17] A skill professional health worker can be any cadre of worker—nurse, doctor, medical assistant etc., who is formally educated. That standard is quite low as compared with wealthy countries. In 2011, wealthy countries had on average 115 skilled health professionals per 10,000 people, five-fold more than recommended by the WHO.[16]

Health Workforce in Cuba   Health Workforce in Botswana

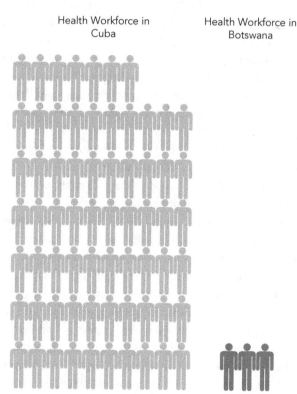

FIGURE 7.3 Physician density in Cuba and Botswana (2010). The World Health Organization (WHO) calls for 22.8 skilled professionals per 10,000 people. Some countries, like Cuba, far exceed this number, whereas other countries, like Botswana, are severely lacking. Cuba has 67 physicians per 10,000 people; Botswana has 3 physicians per 100,000 people.

Source: Data abstracted from World Bank. Health Nutrition and Population Statistics. http://data.worldbank.org/data-catalog/health-nutrition-and-population-statistics. Accessed June, 2017.

As discussed in Chapter 1, the impoverishment of the public sector in post-colonial countries was exacerbated by structural adjustment programs (SAPs) in the 1980s and 1990s.[18] The amount of available resources for public expenditures, set by the World Bank and the International Monetary Fund (IMF), is sometimes referred to as the *public-sector spending cap*.[19] SAPs and neoliberal economic policies imposed severe public spending caps, restricting the amount of money a government could use for the public provision of services. The largest portion of the public sector budget is generally the salary support for teachers, medical personnel and the recurrent operating cost of facilities.[20,21] The public-sector spending caps led to fewer health workers being trained (owing to weak systems of higher education),[22,23] poor pay for public-sectors workers,[20] and under-resourced public facilities.

Higher education for health professionals in impoverished countries is generally provided free of charge and supported by the government. This is provided for free because the need is great. Yet spending caps make it impossible for a government to provide the tools for proper training, pay the faculty, or hire the graduates.[24] When health professionals are hired, the government cannot pay a good salary. Underpaid government health personnel are often considered part-time workers.[20] It is not uncommon for publicly paid health professionals to work until midday and have a private practice to supplement their income.[20,25,26] This part-time commitment to the public sector is often perceived from the outside as corrupt or even a sign of laziness. However, it is often necessary for health workers to have a private practice to support themselves, their families, and their extended family. Low wages create perverse incentives: underfunded public workers may use public resources, such as clinic time and space, to recruit more affluent patients who can pay consultation fees, or they may use private laboratories or pharmacies from which the physician may receive a kickback.[27] Another unintended consequence of low wages is that health workers look for the opportunity to attend training programs for which they will receive payment.[27] The practice of having training programs that give a trainee a per diem, allowance, or sitting fee is very common in impoverished countries. Some donors, particularly the United States, will not support salaries or recurrent costs because of the anti–public sector philosophy of neoliberalism. Instead, nongovernmental organizations (NGOs) supported by such grants will often only offer short-term, centralized training or workshops. In fact, a significant portion of US overseas development assistance is for the per diem fees for lecture-based training.[28] Not only do such training programs pull health workers from their posts in search of more compensation,[29,30] but, without on-site support or mentoring, the training does not improve health care worker performance.[31]

Brain Drain

Inadequate training and compensation result in "brain drain."[32,33] Brain drain describes the movement of trained professionals from impoverished settings to affluent ones.[34] Wealthy countries contribute to the brain drain with the promise of high wages and better working conditions often using incentives to actively recruit professionals away from impoverished countries.[32,35] There is discussion on how to enact international conventions to limit the recruitment of physicians and nurses away from impoverished settings. One example is the WHO Global Code of Practice on the International Recruitment of Health Personnel.[36,37] This policy, introduced in 2010, is a voluntary code to decrease the active recruitment of health professionals from impoverished countries. This voluntary effort was not effective.[36] People continue to search for ways to support their families. Fair compensation and better working conditions in impoverished countries are the most important ways to alleviate the push factor[38] of health workers toward wealthier countries. Brain drain encompasses more than simply the loss of health care workers. Most sub-Saharan African countries heavily subsidize medical and nursing schools. Thus, the emigration of a doctor or nurse who has been trained with government money represents a significant loss of the investment of public funds (Figure 7.4). Internal brain drain is another loss of public-sector investment. Because of better salaries and working conditions, health workers are drawn to NGOs and the private sector rather than remaining in the public sector.[39]

As the global health era brought new focus to the delivery of care, a variety of strategies were used to address the human resource crisis. Strategies to address both the absolute shortage of health professionals and their insufficient training include task shifting, improvements in preclinical training, on-site mentoring, and formal advanced training.

Task Shifting

The practice of delegating tasks from one cadre to another is known as *task shifting*. The need to deliver care in the face of a dearth of health professionals prompted the training of lower cadres of workers to perform tasks that were previously considered the purview of doctors or nurses. Task shifting is not a new phenomenon: it is seen in many settings, in both wealthy and impoverished countries.[40–42] However, the pressure to rapidly scale up HIV services in the setting of profoundly constrained human resources resulted in a new prominence in delegating tasks to less trained workers—from doctors to nurses, nurses to community health workers, and psychologists to lay counselors.[43]

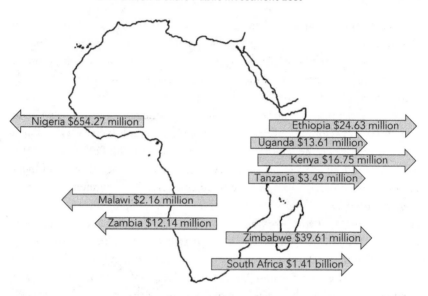

2.17 Billion Dollars Public Investment Lost

Nigeria $654.27 million

Ethiopia $24.63 million

Uganda $13.61 million

Kenya $16.75 million

Tanzania $3.49 million

Malawi $2.16 million

Zambia $12.14 million

Zimbabwe $39.61 million

South Africa $1.41 billion

FIGURE 7.4 Schematic of the public investment lost due to physician brain drain in selected sub-Saharan African countries to Australia, Canada, the United Kingdom, and the United States. Impoverished countries suffer from the loss of skilled health workers to wealthier countries. This brain drain both decreases access to quality health care and represents a loss of monetary investment. In much of sub-Saharan Africa, the government subsidizes clinical education. When physicians trained in country leave, the government loses its investment.

Data adapted from: Mills EJ, Kanters S, Hagopian A, et al. The financial cost of doctors emigrating from sub-Saharan Africa: Human capital analysis. *BMJ.* 2011;343.

There have been many studies looking at the effect of task shifting on the initiation and follow-up of antiretroviral therapy (ART) for people living with HIV. A study by Partners in Health investigators as part of a WHO working group on task shifting quantified the clinical tasks needed to care for HIV patients. It documented the tasks done by different cadres of health workers in the United States. The researchers then studied which health workers carried out each of these tasks in Haiti.[44] Their findings, shown in Figure 7.5, suggest that many tasks could be successfully shifted to lower cadres of workers without harming patient outcomes. A review of the literature, published in 2015,[45] demonstrated that task shifting the care of HIV patients from doctors to nurses or community health workers was safe and did not increase HIV-related mortality. Task shifting has, in some studies, even demonstrated better outcomes because nurses and community health workers are closer to the patients and have a greater knowledge of their journey (Chapter 6), needs, and barriers to care.[46]

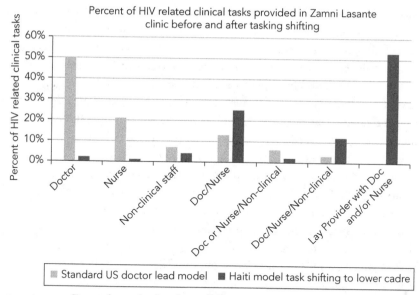

FIGURE 7.5 Figure shows the distribution of responsibilities in HIV care in the United States and Haiti. Haiti has a much smaller professional health workforce and so must shift tasks from highly skilled professionals, such as doctors and nurses, to lay health care providers.

Source: Data abstracted from Ivers LC, Jerome JG, Lambert W, Celletti F, Samb B. Task shifting in HIV care. PEPFAR implementers meeting Kigali, Rwanda, 2007; Ivers L, Jerome JG. Task-shifting in HIV care: A community-based model for scale up of care in rural Haiti and Rwanda. A report to the World Health Organization. Partners in Health/Harvard Medical School, Boston, MA; 2007.

Another review evaluated different models of decentralization and found that task shifting of HIV care from hospitals to primary health care centers also showed better outcomes.[47] Task shifting has been used to compensate for gaps in human resources in other areas as well. Studies have documented the use of task shifting for a variety of health delivery issues, from mental health to antenatal care to non-communicable diseases.[48–50] Despite the persistent limitations in absolute numbers of health workers,[43,45] task shifting can help improve outcomes and optimally use scarce resources. Yet task shifting alone does not obviate the need for a larger number of well-trained, supported, and adequately compensated health workers.

Innovations in Clinical Education

An important factor contributing to the human resource crisis is the lack of funding for health education.[51] There are 2,420 medical schools in the world. The United States has more than 150 medical schools, but 36 impoverished countries do not have any medical schools.[51] A 2010 *Lancet* Commission on

Medical Education for the 21st Century called for major reforms. One major reform identified was the enhancement of global "interdependence in education."[52] Global "interdependence" refers to the shared responsibility of all countries to support medical education in impoverished countries. Modern medical and nursing education in impoverished counties is not possible without such international support. Such collaborations and investment in clinical education have increased in the global health era. A 2011 assessment of health education found that impoverished countries are increasing clinical training: 33 out of 100 medical schools in sub-Saharan Africa had inaugural classes between 2000 and 2009, and 76 percent of medical schools in the region reported greater numbers of first-year students.[22] While ongoing restrictions on public-sector spending often undermine impoverished government's efforts to matriculate more health workers, international coalitions are responding to these limitations. One way that coalitions can respond is to use *twinning* a form of educational collaboration in which an institution from an impoverished country is paired with an institution from a wealthy country.[51] Since the earliest twinning programs in 1948 between Nigeria and the United Kingdom, many schools in impoverished countries have paired with schools in wealthy countries. Moi University School of Medicine in Kenya is paired with the University of Indiana, the Makarere Health Sciences schools in Uganda are paired with Johns Hopkins University in Baltimore, Rwanda's new University of Global Health Equity is paired with Harvard and Tufts Universities, and a new medical school in Botswana is paired with the University of Pennsylvania.[51]

In 2010, the President's Emergency Plan for AIDS Relief (PEPFAR) began formal higher education support through the Medical Education Partnership Initiative (MEPI) and the Nursing Education Partnership Initiative (NEPI) with the aim of training 140,000 health professionals.[53] MEPI granted $130 million over five years to 13 African medical schools, the George Washington University School of Public Health, and Health Services and the African Centre for Global Health and Social Transformation.[54] MEPI programs have three overarching principles: (1) increasing capacity by enhancing the quality and quantity of medical education through visiting professors and up-to-date curriculum; (2) retaining both faculty and graduates in their home country as educators to further build local capacity; and (3) supporting regionally relevant research to both generate new knowledge and incentivize faculty and graduate retention.

MEPI-supported programs include the use of e-learning, curriculum revision, and distance learning to train more students. They also expand training outside the academic center into hospitals, clinics and communities to emphasize proximity to those with poor access to health care. The MEPI consortium has established research support centers to build African research capacity as well.[54] Similarly,

NEPI aims to strengthen the quality and capacity of nursing and midwifery institutions.[53] NEPI partners with Ministries of Health and Education to conduct assessments of national training capacity and to identify schools to receive funding for provide training. Current NEPI programs are in place in Lesotho, Malawi, and Zambia. In 2016, NEPI conducted needs assessments in the Democratic Republic of Congo and Ethiopia as well.[55]

As countries move to address the entirety of the disease burden, medical and nursing specialists are also needed.[1] Rwanda developed a model of long-term workforce training in 2013 with its flagship Human Resources for Health program (HRH Rwanda).[56] The government asked donors (including the Global Fund and PEPFAR) to shift some of their funds from short term didactic training to long-term medical residencies, managerial trainings, and the support of advanced nursing. HRH Rwanda partnered with 26 US medical and nursing schools.[56,57] Over seven years, HRH Rwanda will train 557 physicians, 2,800 nurses and midwives, and 157 health managers. HRH Rwanda will additionally assume responsibility for future training without international staff.[56] Similar human resource programs exist in Liberia,[58] Botswana,[59] Malawi,[60] and other impoverished countries. Importantly, these programs train not only clinicians but also clinical educators who can then support the ongoing expansion of the health workforce.[61] The Clinton Health Access Initiative (CHAI) is one organization that works with governments on HRH programs. CHAI partners with governments to identify the root causes of the health worker shortage and uses these insights to map out a long-term plan to strengthen local capacity to recruit, train, manage, and retain health workers.[62] For example, CHAI and the Malawi Ministry of Health implemented a health worker education program in 2013. This program has enrolled 701 nurse midwife technicians, 30 registered nurse midwives, 26 nursing students, and 435 community midwife assistants.[63]

Mentoring

Mentored supervision is a key element of clinical training. In wealthy countries, nurses and physicians receive years of mentoring before they can see patients on their own (Table 7.1), but there is minimal mentoring in impoverished countries. In the absence of mentoring, training occurs through lectures. Reallocating the money used for centralized, didactic-only training to on-the-job mentoring can have a profound impact on patient outcomes and quality of care. In Rwanda, Partners in Health created a program to mentor primary care nurses on national protocols. This program was especially important when new protocols were introduced with money for AIDS, malaria, and child health. The Mentoring and Enhanced Supervision for Health and Quality Improvement (MESH-QI)

Table 7.1 Typical clinical education.

Preclinical Studies (Undergraduate and Graduate)		Clinical Studies	Specialization	Continuing Education and Professional Development
Classroom learning, Basic Science		Supervised clinical learning	Supervised clinical learning	Responsible for patients
Medicine				
United States	4–6 years	2 years	4–10 years	
Rwanda	2 years	3 years		
Nursing				
United States	2 years	2 years		
Malawi	2 years			

The structure of clinical education differs between wealthy and impoverished countries. In wealthy countries, health professionals undergo years of study and are heavily supervised before they are allowed to practice independently. In impoverished countries, the resources are not available to provide the same level of training.

program supported the Rwandan Ministry of Health's efforts to decentralize care but assured that nurses would stay on the front lines, rather than be pulled to the capital for training.[64] It also gave young, less educated nurses (at that time, just high school graduates) a sense of support in an often overwhelming job. The MESH-QI program provided intensive, on-site supervision and mentorship. Advanced nurses mentored less-experienced nurses. The MESH-QI program used structured checklists to collect data on health facilities and quality of care. MESH mentors helped nurses advance their skills and improved patient flow, charting, and the integration of services. Nurses saw serial improvement with each mentoring visit. They witnessed positive progression in the system and not only in their knowledge base. Empowering health workers strengthens health systems by increasing job satisfaction and therefore worker retention. Based on the successes of the MESH-QI project, Rwanda adopted nurse mentoring as a primary strategy to build a quality health workforce.[65]

The importance of mentoring is noted at all levels, as a student-led lawsuit in Kampala, Uganda illustrates. In September 2016, the Ugandan Minister of Health, Dr. Ruth Aceng, changed the internship policy to include mandatory two-year service at a government health facility. The intention behind this policy was to use new graduates to cover rural and underserved areas as part of their public pay back for the government subsidized medical education. However, it left interns isolated with no mentors, meager stipends, and working in crumbling facilities. The medical students and interns believed that the government should properly support trainees and provide the work environment necessary to deliver care. Consequently, 1,000 medical students, led by Emma Amadriyo, are suing the government on the grounds that they are entitled to postings complete with mentoring, payment, and adequate training facilities.[66]

Conclusion

Long-standing impoverishment of government health budgets has led to critical shortages in human resources for health. Donor-driven training programs historically use didactic programs because they are easier to administer and count. Yet centralized workshops pull health workers away from their posts and do not provide the type of clinical training that is most effective in improving the quality of care. In addition, low pay, poor work environments, and the recruitment of health professionals from impoverished nations to wealthier ones have led to a massive brain drain of physicians, nurses, and other health professionals out of the countries and regions the need them most. Preclinical service is poorly funded and produces insufficient numbers of health workers. Formal training programs lack the faculty and tools needed to provide high-quality training. A critical component of global health delivery is reversing this tide of underinvestment, poor training, and lack of mentorship. New programs that provide long-term, mentored training are replacing sporadic, centralized didactic programs. More resources and innovative programs are needed to train and retain health professionals in their home countries.

References

1. Narasimhan V, Brown H, Pablos-Mendez A, et al. Responding to the global human resources crisis. *Lancet*. 2004;363(9419):1469–1472.
2. WHO. *The world health report 200: Working together for health*. Geneva: World Health Organization; 2006.
3. Mtonga C, Anyangwe SC. Inequities in the global health workforce: The greatest impediment to health in sub-Saharan Africa. *Intl J Environ Res Public Health*. 2007;4(2):93–100.
4. Raviola G, Machoki M, Mwaikambo E, Good M. HIV, disease plague, demoralization and "burnout": Resident experience of the medical profession in Nairobi, Kenya. *Cult Med Psychiatry*. 2002;26(1):55–86.

5. Ooms G, Schrecker T. Expenditure ceilings, multilateral financial institutions, and the health of poor populations. *Lancet.* 2005;365(9473):1821–1823.

6. Anand S, Bärnighausen T. Human resources and health outcomes: Cross-country econometric study. *Lancet.* 2004;364(9445):1603–1609.

7. Kober K, Van Damme W. Scaling up access to antiretroviral treatment in southern Africa: Who will do the job? *Lancet.* 2004;364(9428):103–107.

8. Buchan J, Dal Poz MR. Skill mix in the health care workforce: Reviewing the evidence. *Bull World Health Org.* 2002;80(7):575–580.

9. World Health Organization. *Global strategy on human resources for health: Workforce 2030.* Geneva: World Health Organization 2016.

10. Van Lerberghe W, Lafort Y. *The role of the hospital in the district: Delivering or supporting primary health care?* Antwerp: Public Health Research and Training Unit, Institute for Tropical Medicine; 1990.

11. Nkomazana O, Mash R, Wojczewski S, Kutalek R, Phaladze K. How to create more supportive supervision for primary healthcare: lessons from Ngamiland district of Botswana: co-operative inquiry group. Global Health Action, [S.l.], v. 9, jun. 2016. ISSN 1654-9880. Available at: <http://journals.co-action.net/index.php/gha/article/view/31263>. Date accessed: 04 Aug. 2017.

12. Naicker S, Plange-Rhule J, Tutt RC, Eastwood JB. Shortage of healthcare workers in developing countries: Africa. *Ethn Dis.* 2009;19(1):S1.

13. World Health Organization. Global health workforce shortage to reach 12.9 million in coming decades. 2013. Available from: http://www.who.int/mediacentre/news/releases/2013/health-workforce-shortage/en/. Accessed Nov 30, 2016.

14. Tsolekile L, Abrahams-Gessel S, Puoane T. Healthcare professional shortage and task-shifting to prevent cardiovascular disease: Implications for low- and middle-income countries. *Curr Cardiol Rep.* 2015;17(12):1–6.

15. Kerry VB, Ndung'u T, Walensky RP, Lee PT, Kayanja VF, Bangsberg DR. Managing the demand for global health education. *PLoS Med.* 2011;8(11):e1001118.

16. World Bank. Health nutrition and population statistics. http://data.worldbank.org/data-catalog/health-nutrition-and-population-statistics. Accessed June, 2017.

17. Campbell J, Dussault G, Buchan J, et al. *A universal truth: No health without a workforce.* Geneva: World Health Organization, Global Health Workforce Alliance.;2014.

18. Windisch R, Wyss K, Prytherch H. A cross-country review of strategies of the German development cooperation to strengthen human resources. *Hum Resources Health.* 2009;7.

19. Heller P. Back to basics—fiscal space: What it is and how to get it. *Finance Dev Q.* 2005;42(2). http://www.imf.org/external/pubs/ft/fandd/2005/06/basics.htm. Accessed June, 2017.

20. Mccoy D, Bennett S, Witter S, et al. Salaries and incomes of health workers in sub-Saharan Africa. *Lancet.* 2008;371(9613):675–681.

21. Kim JY, Millen JV, Irwin A, eds. *Dying for growth: Global inequality and the health of the poor.* Monroe, ME: Common Courage Press; 2000.

22. Mullan F, Frehywot S, Omaswa F, et al. Medical schools in sub-Saharan Africa. *Lancet.* 2011;377(9771):1113–1121.

23. Celletti F, Buchse E, Samb B. Medical education in developing countries. In: Kieran Walsh, editor. *Oxford textbook of medical education.* New York: Oxford University Press; 2013:671–695.

24. Cometto G, Tulenko K, Muula AS, Krech R. Health workforce brain drain: From denouncing the challenge to solving the problem. *PloS Med.* 2013;10(9):e1001514.

25. Hagopian A, Ofosu A, Fatusi A, et al. The flight of physicians from West Africa: Views of African physicians and implications for policy. *Soc Sci Med.* 2005;61(8):1750–1760.

26. Hipgrave DB, Hort K. Dual practice by doctors working in South and East Asia: A review of its origins, scope and impact, and the options for regulation. *Health Policy Plan.* 2014;29(6):703–716.

27. Roenen C, Ferrinho P, Van Dormael M, Conceição MC, Van Lerberghe W. How African doctors make ends meet: An exploration. *Trop Med Intl Health.* 1997;2(2):127–135.

28. Grants.gov. Grants: All agency for international development. 2017. Available from: https://www.grants.gov/search-grants.html?agencyCode=USAID. Accessed May 31, 2017.

29. Ridde V. Per diems undermine health interventions, systems and research in Africa: Burying our heads in the sand: Editorial. *Trop Med Intl Health.* 2010. Jul;15(7):E1–E4.

30. Vian T, Miller C, Themba Z, Bukuluki P. Perceptions of per diems in the health sector: Evidence and implications. *Health Policy Plan.* 2013;28(3):237–246.

31. Anatole M, Magge H, Redditt V, et al. Nurse mentorship to improve the quality of health care delivery in rural Rwanda. *Nurs Outlook.* 2013 May-Jun;61(3):137–144.

32. Mullan F. The metrics of the physician brain drain. *N Engl J Med.* 2005;353(17):1810–1818.

33. Dussault G, Franceschini MC. Not enough there, too many here: Understanding geographical imbalances in the distribution of the health workforce. *Hum Resources Health.* 2006;4:12.

34. Dodani S, Laporte RE. Brain drain from developing countries: How can brain drain be converted into wisdom gain? *J R Soc Med.* 2005;98(11):487.

35. Bundred PE, Levitt C. Medical migration: Who are the real losers? *Lancet.* 2000;356(9225):245–246.

36. Edge JS, Hoffman SJ. Empirical impact evaluation of the WHO global code of practice on the international recruitment of health personnel in Australia, Canada, UK and USA. *Globalization Health.* December 2013;9:60.

37. World Health Organization. *WHO Global Code of Practice on the International Recruitment of Health Personnel.* Geneva: World Health Organization; May 21, 2010.

38. Kuehn BM. Global shortage of health workers, brain drain stress developing countries. *JAMA.* 2007;298(16):1853–1855.

39. Larsson EC, Atkins S, Chopra M, Ekstrm AM. What about health system strengthening and the internal brain drain? *Trans R Soc Trop Med Hyg.* 2009;103(5):533–534.

40. Hermann K, Van Damme W, Pariyo G, et al. Community health workers for ART in sub-Saharan Africa: Learning from experience—capitalizing on new opportunities. *Hum Resources Health.* 2009;7:31. https://doi.org/10.1186/1478-4491-7-31

41. Way D, Jones L, Busing N. Implementation strategies: Collaboration in primary care: Family doctors and nurse practitioners delivering shared care. Discussion paper. Ontario College of Family Physicians; 2000.

42. Merkle F, Ritsema TS, Bauer S, Kuilman L. The physician assistant: Shifting the paradigm of European medical practice? *HSR Proc Intensive Care Cardiovasc Anesth.* 2011;3(4):255–262.

43. Lehmann U, Van Damme W, Barten F, Sanders D. Task shifting: The answer to the human resources crisis in Africa? *Hum Resources Health.* 2009;7:49.

44. Ivers LC, Jerome J, Cullen KA, Lambert W, Celletti F, Samb B. Task-shifting in HIV care: A case study of nurse-centered community-based care in rural Haiti (task-shifting in HIV care in rural Haiti). *PLoS One.* 2011;6(5):e19276.

45. Kredo T, Adeniyi F, Bateganya M, Pienaar E. Task shifting from doctors to non-doctors for initiation and maintenance of antiretroviral therapy. *Cochrane Database Syst Rev.* 2014 Jul 1;(7):CD007331. doi: 10.1002/14651858.CD007331.pub3.

46. Zachariah R, Ford N, Philips M, et al. Task shifting in HIV/AIDS: Opportunities, challenges and proposed actions for sub-Saharan Africa. *Trans R Soc Trop Med Hyg.* 2009;103(6):549–558.

47. Lazarus J, Safreed-Harmon K, Nicholson J, Jaffar S. Health service delivery models for the provision of antiretroviral therapy in sub-Saharan Africa: A systematic review. *Trop Med Int Health.* 2013;18:17.

48. Jennings L, Yebadokpo AS, Affo J, Agbogbe M, Tankoano A. Task shifting in maternal and newborn care: A non-inferiority study examining delegation of antenatal counseling to lay nurse aides supported by job aids in Benin. *Implement Sci.* 2011;6:2.

49. Lekoubou A, Awah P, Fezeu L, Sobngwi E, Kengne AP. Hypertension, diabetes mellitus and task shifting in their management in sub-Saharan Africa. *Intl J Environ Res Public Health.* 2010;7(2):353–363.

50. Agyapong VIO, Farren C, McAuliffe E. Improving Ghana's mental healthcare through task-shifting: Psychiatrists and health policy directors perceptions about government's commitment and the role of community mental health workers. *Globalization Health.* 2016;12:57. https://doi.org/10.1186/s12992-016-0199-z

51. Frenk J, Bhutta ZA, Chen LC, et al. Health professionals for a new century: Transforming education to strengthen health systems in an interdependent world. *The Lancet.* 2010;376(9756):1923–1958.

52. The Lancet. Commissions from the Lancet journals: Medical education for the 21st century. 2010. Available from: http://www.thelancet.com/commissions/education-of-health-professionals. Accessed April 20, 2017.

53. PEPFAR. Medical and nursing education partnership initiatives. The United States President's Emergency Plan for AIDS Relief Web site. 2017. Available from: https://www.pepfar.gov/partnerships/initiatives/index.htm. Accessed April 20, 2017.

54. Mullan F, Frehywot S, Omaswa F, et al. The medical education partnership initiative: PEPFAR's effort to boost health worker education to strengthen health systems. *Health Aff (Millwood)*. 2012;31(7):1561.

55. Middleton A, L., Howard M, A., Dohrn M, J., et al. The nursing education partnership initiative (NEPI): Innovations in nursing and midwifery education. *Acad Med*. 2014;89(8):S28.

56. Binagwaho A, Kyamanywa P, Farmer PE, et al. The human resources for health program in Rwanda: A new partnership. *N Engl J Med*. 2013;369(21):2054–2059.

57. Republic of Rwanda. Human resources for health strategic plan 2011–2016. Kigali: Ministry of Health; 2011.

58. Varpilah ST, Safer M, Frenkel E, Baba D, Massaquoi M, Barrow G. Rebuilding human resources for health: A case study from Liberia. *Hum Resources Health*. 2011;9:11.

59. Ministry of Health Government of Botswana. Integrated health service plan: A strategy for changing the health sector for healthy Botswana 2010–2020. 2010. http://www.moh.gov.bw/Publications/policies/Botswana%20IHSP%20Final%20HLSP.pdf. Accessed June, 2017.

60. Palmer D. Tackling Malawi's human resources crisis. *Reprod Health Matters*. 2006;14(27):27–39.

61. Doris Duke Charitable Foundation (DDCF). PHIT partnership implementation research framework. 2017. Available from: http://www.ddcf.org/what-we-fund/african-health-initiative/goals--strategies/phit-partnership-implementation-research-framework/. Accessed May 9, 2017.

62. Clinton Health Access Initiative (CHAI). Human resources for health. 2017. Available from: http://www.clintonhealthaccess.org/program/human-resources-for-health/. Accessed May 9, 2017.

63. Gunda A, Sadri-zadeh R. Human resources for health infrastructure project transition in Malawi. Accessed June, 2017. http://www.clintonhealthaccess.org/blog-hrh-malawi-transition/

64. Magge H, Anatole M, Cyamatare FR, et al. Mentoring and quality improvement strengthen integrated management of childhood illness implementation in rural Rwanda. *Arch Dis Child*. 2015;100(6):565.

65. Binagwaho A, Scott KW. Improving the world's health through the post-2015 development agenda: Perspectives from Rwanda. *Intl J Health Policy Mgmt*. 2015;4(4):203–205. doi:10.15171/ijhpm.2015.46.

66. Anderah R. Medical students take minister to court over internship. *Daily Monitor*. Sept 23, 2016. Available from: http://www.monitor.co.ug/News/National/Medical-Students-minister-court-internship/688334-3392140-f7preoz/index.html. Accessed May 9, 2017.

8

Community Health Workers

Key Points

- Community Health Workers (CHW) are members of the communities they serve.
- CHWs have been involved in health delivery for decades.
- CHWs are most effective when linked to a system of care.
- Historically, CHWs were asked to work as volunteers due to limited health budgets and used to address the shortages of health workers.
- CHWs can deliver preventive and curative services, refer patients to higher levels of care, and accompany patients on their journey to health.
- To maximize the impact of this cadre, CHWs should be compensated, well-trained, and part of an integrated health care system.

Introduction

The term "community health worker" (CHW) generally refers to lay (non-professionally educated) workers who are trained in and have responsibility for health at the community level (i.e., outside the clinic).[1] CHWs are members of the communities they serve. They are proximate to patients, families, and communities. For many decades, CHWs have performed a variety of roles in the health care system, including delivering preventive and curative services, finding the sick and vulnerable, referring patients to health centers, and accompanying patients on their journey to health. Yet this cadre is rarely considered a formal part of the health system. Historically, CHWs were deployed in areas where there was no medical system[2,3] and asked to volunteer to deliver a narrow package of preventive services.[4] The concept of the volunteer CHW was a cornerstone of the elective primary health care in the 1980s and 1990s. Yet, most CHWs are people with little financial means, often peasant farmers or small-scale vendors. It is therefore difficult for them to work without pay and volunteer cadres have high rates of attrition.[5] In addition, it is difficult to hold volunteers accountable within the health system.[6]

The movement for AIDS treatment access and the promise of the United Nations Millennium Development Goals (MDGs) and Sustainable Development Goals (SDGs) renewed calls for CHWs as a necessary component in reaching ambitious health targets.[7] Payment, profession development, and recognition by governments are increasingly discussed. This chapter focuses on the cadre of CHWs. It includes the history, importance, and evolution of CHWs as key players in the workforce needed for global health delivery. The chapter also addresses the training, supervision, and remuneration of CHWs. The importance of advocacy to include this cadre into the formal health workforce in order to achieve Universal Health Coverage is also addressed.

The History of Community Health Workers

Community members who are trained to deliver health education, disease prevention, basic treatment, and long-term support to patients have a long history in health systems around the world. Lay (or nonprofessional) community workers go by a variety of different names from "auxiliaries" to "frontline health workers" to "lay health workers" to "community health workers."[1] For the purpose of this chapter, the cadre that includes all workers who are providing health-related services in the community but who do not have training in a professional school (as a doctor, nurse, nursing assistant, etc.) will be called community health workers (CHWs). Such workers are generally trusted people with some level of literacy who are selected by or with input from the community.[1] Their training varies from a few days to a few months depending on the tasks assigned to them.[8]

Historically, CHWs were trained to provide services in areas where insufficient numbers of doctors, nurses, or other health professionals existed to provide care.[3,9] But CHWs are also critical in extending services closer to patients and providing linkages with facilities.[10] The grandmother of modern CHW programs is China's Barefoot Doctor (BFD) program.[3] This program began with the rural reconstruction of China in the 1920s and 1930s, which preceded the Cultural Revolution of the 1960s. In the 1920s, the population of China was about 80 percent rural. Without modern infrastructure, rural people suffered from many infectious diseases caused by unsanitary conditions.[11] The BFDs trained villagers in the general principles of hygiene and sanitation.[12] In the late 1950s, in addition to educating the population about infectious diseases, BFDs also built latrines and provided some basic medical treatment. The intention of the program was to improve the health of the population so that people could work more productively as farmers.

In 1965, Chairman Mao Zedong officially supported the BFD program saying that in "health and in medical work, put stress on the rural areas."[11–13] Mao expanded the program 1970s not only as a strategy to bring medical care to the rural poor but also to decrease the power of the urban elite medical system.[3] The World Health Organization (WHO) and others credited the BFD program with significantly improving health in China.[14] Massive societal change was also occurring, which undoubtedly had health impacts as well, yet the BFD program's use of lay community workers was promoted by international actors as a means of providing health for all at the Alma Ata conference of 1978.[14]

In the United States, CHWs played an important role in decentralizing health care as well. In the 1960s, many medical programs were launched as part of President Lyndon Johnson's War on Poverty.[15] These programs, such as Medicaid, Medicare, and the Indian Health Service, significantly expanded services to people who had previously been without care.[16–18] With this expansion, a larger workforce was needed. Community workers were trained to follow patients with mental illness, tuberculosis (TB), and high blood pressure. They also supported their patients' continued follow-up with medications and clinic appointments.[19,20] Rural populations—most notably indigenous communities in Alaska—looked to CHWs to alleviate the geographic burden on patients by bringing care to people who lived far from health facilities.[21]

During the same era when the BFD model was accelerating in China and CHWs were active in the United States, African liberation struggles were resetting expectations on that continent.[22] Governments of newly independent countries like Tanzania and Ghana sought to provide modern health care for their citizens as an important part of liberation and self-governance. Emerging from colonialism, however, meant that there were few indigenous professional medical staff.[23] Therefore, in the initial postcolonial period, many CHWs were trained to fill this gap as newly sovereign governments worked to establish new medical and nursing schools to train professional health workers.[24] However, as discussed extensively in previous chapters, with the World Bank and the International Monetary Fund (IMF) promoting neoliberalism, African countries had little money for the expansion of public education. This left the goal of growing an indigenous cadre of professional health workers unrealized. Instead, in the face of constrained public-sector health budgets, the narrowly focused selective primary health care became the norm and a good fit for the CHW cadre. To child-focused growth monitoring, oral rehydration, breastfeeding, and immunization (GOBI) programs,[25] CHWs were asked to volunteer their time and became the key human resource for selective primary health care in many impoverished settings.

CHWs and the Health System

In the global health era, as resources were mobilized and targets were set for health coverage, the importance of CHWs grew.[26–29] CHWs represented a pre-existing cadre and lower cost option for the expansion of essential services.[30] In 2010, it was estimated that 1 billion people would never see a health care professional in their lifetime because of dire poverty and insufficient health system coverage.[31] Given this reality, CHWs are increasingly seen as part of the solution need to deliver care and achieve equity and are engaged in a wide variety of health systems and programs.

The role of CHWs is not monolithic. They perform a variety of functions including health education, prevention, active case finding, referral of patients, and follow-up of chronic conditions (Figure 8.1).[32–34] CHWs are also increasingly relied upon in rural impoverished countries for the diagnosis and treatment of illnesses, particularly of childhood diseases.[33,35] Most importantly, the CHW fosters a meaningful connection between the patient and the health system, delivering messages and relaying information in a way that is understandable and relevant for communities.[36,37] In these ways, CHWs are a unique and critical part of the health workforce needed to achieve Universal Health Coverage.

CHWs are most effective when they are well-trained, linked with a system of care, and supervised regularly.[38,39] Yet, in previous decades, because of the lack of human resources and basic health infrastructure, CHWs often had only basic education and delivered selective primary health care programs without any supervision or connection to a health system.[40,41] Even in the global health era, training programs for CHWs lack standardization and tend to wax and wane with donor funding.[40] Programs are of inconsistent in duration, content, and methodology throughout the world.[42] Moreover, as mentioned in Chapter 7, CHWs often receive didactic teaching, and supported by a per diem. Such financial incentives pull CHWs away from their communities and privilege classroom-based theoretical knowledge over practical in-service and mentored training.[43] Often didactic training sessions are offered to the top CHWs so as to *train-the-trainer* (TOT) or plan for *cascade training* anticipating that the person who received the new information will then train others.[44] This strategy often fails. Particularly when the workforce is not compensated and the cascade of knowledge from one person to the next is inadequately mentored.[45]

While an ideal training package has not been defined for CHWs, their training is generally tied to their scope of work and may be in support of a short term, donor program.[46] In 2013, UNICEF analyzed the CHW training programs and identified 37 cadres of CHWs across 21 East and Southern countries. Most of the CHW programs were externally funded (by USAID, the World Bank, WHO, etc.). Training programs lasted seven days on average.[47] CHWs have been used to perform AIDS education, administration of TB therapy, case finding of children with malnutrition, provision of therapies for childhood illnesses, and even the education and contact tracing related to Ebola.[48-52]

Supervision and ongoing support is an important aspect of CHW programs. Generally, there is stepwise supervision starting with a CHW leader or higher level lay worker.[53,54] Increasingly, supervision of CHWs is done at the health center level, often by a government health worker. This helps to integrate the work of CHWs into the health system.[28] At this level, nurses, often trained in public health, supervise the work of CHWs by monitoring the number of patients they visit, evaluating the CHWs' adherence to established protocols, and confirming their attendance at follow-up meetings.[28] These managerial evaluations may be tied to the CHWs' salary support in what is called *performance-based financing*.[55] Supervision and mentorship have been cited in many studies as a major challenge to CHW performance. In addition, when clinics are understaffed and poorly functioning, the ability of the CHW to provide good care is weakened.[56]

CHW Compensation

Compensation of CHWs also remains an ongoing challenge. If governments are unable to pay the salaries of professionally trained staff, they certainly cannot pay lay workers.[57] As a result, volunteer or part-time CHW programs have proliferated.[58] Nonmonetary incentives for performance including altruism, autonomy, mastery, purpose, and connectedness have been documented to have a positive impact on CHW performance.[59-61] Yet the attrition rate of CHWs in voluntary programs is quite high.[5] The majority of CHWs want to be paid[1] and want a salary as opposed to a stipend.[62] Programs in which CHWs are encouraged to sell products to provide income are often promoted because they can sustain a volunteer health worker. Yet, in such programs, the CHW activities are generally focused more on the income-generating work than on the uncompensated work of health promotion or disease prevention.[63]

Fair compensation for work is a basic human right. Governments, NGOs, and communities around the world are fighting for living-wage compensation for this cadre of workers. Many NGOs, such as PIH, pay CHWs a salary linked to the country's minimum wage.[55] Because this is done by an NGO, the practice is often critiqued as unsustainable, given the restricted ability of governments to assume the cost. However, NGO programs may serve as a pilot for achieving better outcomes that can be adapted by governments.[10] Governments and others are increasingly looking for ways to compensate CHWs. For example, Rwanda developed a system of cooperatives in which each group of CHWs is given start-up

(A)   Prevention and Eduction

A village health worker visits a pregnant women in Neno District, Malawi. She uses counselling cards to explain the warning signs of preeclampsia

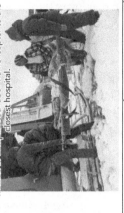

(C)   Treatment

In Rwanda, CHWs carry a box filled with supplies for diagnostics and treatment of childhood illnesses. The box contains: antimalarials, ORS, pneumonia antibiotics, rapid tests for malaria, tools for assessing malnutrition and a stop watch to measure respiratory rate.

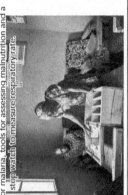

(E)   Referral

Lesotho is a very mountainous country, creating geographical barriers to emergency healthcare services. This community health worker is helping evacuate a woman in complicated labor via helicopter to the closest hospital.

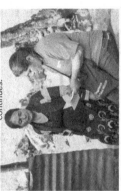

Community Health Workers have the potential to provide support throughout the continuum of care

(B)   Case Finding

Community agents in Carabayllo, Peru, conduct monitoring sessions to identify children with nutritional problems that affect their overall development

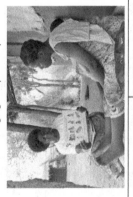

(D)   Support and Follow Up

A community health worker in Chiapas, Mexico, meets with a patient with hypertension. This is one of regular visit the CHW makes to ensure the patient's treatment continues.

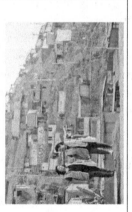

FIGURE 8.1 This schema shows the many areas along the care continuum that are supported by community health workers. Prevention; (A) Partners in Health (2015). Jeanel Drake. Neno District, Malawi: Manyamba (*left*), uses illustrated counseling cards/job aids to explain warning signs. Paulo exhibits swollen ankles, which is a danger sign. Village Health Worker Enelesi Manyamba, 67, visits Violet Paulo, 40, at her home in Felemu, Neno District, Malawi. Paulo is in the third trimester of her pregnancy. Case finding; (B) Partners in Health (2016). William Castro Rodriguez. San Gabriel, Peru: Community agents, who are involved voluntarily in childhood development projects, conduct monitoring sessions in the area around the Lois and Thomas Community Center in San Gabriel, Carabayllo. These activities are meant to identify children with nutritional problems that affect their overall development. On this day, the community health workers (CHWs) just finished an educational session for caretakers/mothers. Dina Gomez, community agent/health worker; Inela Espinoza, community agent/health worker. Provision of community based care: (C) Partners in Health (2015). Cecille Joan Avila. Twibanire, Rwinkwavu, Rwanda: Mukamana gives a walkthrough of the contents of her CHW box. Athanasie Mukamana has been a CHW with PIH/IMB since 2005. She has been a CHW for the MOH since 1995. Accompaniment of patients with chronic conditions: (D) Partners in Health (2016). Aaron Levenson. Chiapas, Mexico: CHW Magdalena Gutierrez chats with Nicomedes Lopez, a patient with hypertension, as part of her regular visits to ensure that her treatment continues. Referral to higher levels of care (E) Partners in Health (2011). Mojela Masupha. Nohana, Lesotho: A helicopter evacuation of a woman in labor.

money to form a cooperative business to fund their work.[64] Some cooperatives have been successful in generating revenue; other have not. Among the groups without an income, the turnover is high. In 2005, the WHO task force for the achievement of the MDGs also focused on the important role of CHWs and the need for compensation.[65] Recently, the United Nations' MDG task force created the Financing Alliance for Health,[66] which is charged with investigating and piloting novel financing mechanisms such as social impact bonds and cooperatives to pay for CHWs at the national level.[67,68]

Scope of Work

Despite the ongoing challenge of compensation, CHWs are effective in a variety of roles. Task-shifting work to CHWs has successfully improved the reach of a wide variety of global health interventions.[31,33,69] CHWs are still central in performing selective primary health activities known as GOBI[33,36] and other preventive services such as the distribution of vitamin A (to prevent blindness), deworming tablets (to prevent anemia), prenatal vitamins, and family planning.[33]

CHWs also help patients adhere to long-term therapies. Their roles in TB programs to ensure patients' completion of six-month regimens of therapy have long been appreciated.[76] This work of *accompaniment* or walking with a patient throughout the duration of their illness to provide emotional support (Figure 8.2) produces high rates of retention in care for both TB and HIV treatment.[77,78] CHWs have been critical in the global scale-up of AIDS treatment[79] and also support diabetes care and mental health services.[80,81]

Other CHWs support pregnant women to assure antenatal care, facility-based delivery, and postpartum care.[82] The CHW in the case of pregnancy support also plays an important role in referral to care. Maternal health workers are trained to recognize danger signs and facilitate transport to a health center or even hospital if a woman has an obstetrical emergency.[83]

In the global health era, CHWs are increasingly relied upon to perform more complex tasks such as the *integrated community case management of childhood illness* (iCCM).[51] In iCCM programs, CHWs provide diagnostic and curative services to children.[52,84] For iCCM, CHW use simple algorithms to detect and treat diarrhea, pneumonia, and malaria as well as novel tools such as rapid malaria diagnostic tests. Putting these tools in the hands of trained and supervised CHWs has been shown to impact the timely diagnosis, treatment, and referral of sick children. It also decreases child mortality.[33,54] Finally, the role of CHWs as cultural agents and ambassadors in contact tracing and case finding has been

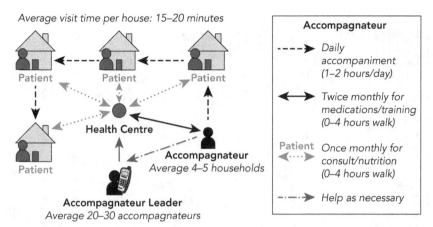

FIGURE 8.2 Schematic of the Partners in Health (PIH) model of accompaniment of patients with HIV, tuberculosis, or chronic illness. PIH employs community health workers (CHWs) that are supervised in the community but report to the public facility. One of the main responsibilities of CHWs is accompaniment. The CHW walks with and listens to the patient on his or her journey, thereby gaining perspective of the patient's life and decreasing barriers to accessing care.

Source: Mukherjee JS, Barry D, Weatherford RD, Desai IK, Farmer PE. Community-based ART programs: Sustaining adherence and follow- up. *Curr HIV/AIDS Rep.* 2016;13(6):359.

documented in sensitive situations from HIV to mental health to the Ebola crisis of 2014.[85] A trusted local person is critical in combatting stigma and maintaining confidentiality. In an evaluating the work of CHWs in the national health reform Lesotho in 2016, CHWs had a documented impact at every stage of the value chain and for a variety of conditions (Figure 8.3).[36,70,71] CHWs significantly expand the coverage of these important interventions.[72–75]

National-Scale Programs

Some governments, such as Rwanda, Ethiopia, and Pakistan, are making progress in incorporating CHWs into the care delivery value chain.[31,33,86] In Rwanda, the Ministry of Health endorsed a volunteer-based system of community health workers in 1995. Once the government succeeded in securing money from the Global Fund and other sources, the cadre grew to over 45,000 by 2005. After 2005, compensation schemes were launched and capacity building programs targeted toward the major diseases were codified. In 2009, each village elected a man and a woman to be CHW binomes. The CHW binomes deliver health promotion, disease prevention, and curative services throughout the country. Each village has two types of CHWs. One type specializes in iCCM. In iCCM programs

| CHW overall role | Serve as an extension of the health center into the community | | | | | |
| CHW competency-based activities | Prevention | Diagnosis/assessment | | Treatment | Management | |
Care Delivery Value Chain	Community-based demand creation and health facility support	Patient identification and community-based diagnosis	Patient accompaniment	Patient accompaniment	Patient accompaniment and tracking	Community-based care support
HIV/AIDS	• Educate community on HIV prevention and treatment; promote "Test & Treat" campaign	• Track which patients have been diagnosed as HIV-positive	• Accompany patients to facility for HIV testing	• After patient receives diagnosis from nurses, link with patient for ongoing care	• Track and record patients, including defaulters; • Accompany (defaulted) ART and pre-ART patients to health center for refills, appointments • Report community deaths	• Provide DOT for ART and ensure that the patient has sufficient food to take medication. • Answer basic treatment-related questions (e.g. drug side effects) and provide psychosocial support • Promote adherence for people in denial of status
Tuberculosis	• Educate community about TB prevention and treatment	• Identify suspected TB patients (i.e. cough, night sweats, weight loss, chest pains, bloody sputum) by going door-to-door • Conduct contact tracing (i.e. check whether other household members have cough)	• Accompany patients to facility for testing (i.e. sputum collection)	• Stay with patient during treatment initiation • Answer basic treatment-related questions (e.g. drug side effects)	• Track and record patients, including defaulters; • Accompany patients to health center for refills, appointments, and sputum collection after 2 months of treatment • Report community deaths	• Provide DOT for TB medications, record DOT, and ensure that the patient has sufficient food to take medication • Answer basic treatment-related questions (e.g. drug side effects) and provide psychosocial support
Maternal/Newborn Health	• Educate patients about common problems during pregnancy; benefits of HIV-testing and PMTCT, and family planning	• Identify suspected pregnancies (i.e. women with a missed menstrual cycle) by going door-to-door • Screen pregnant women in community for symptoms of high-risk pregnancy (i.e. bleeding, regular vomiting, decreased fetal movement)	• Accompany women for pregnancy test and four ANC visits	• Accompany women and ensure they enter maternal waiting home as directed by nurse-midwife (typically at 38th week of pregnancy)	• Accompany HIV-exposed infants to facility for DNA-PCR; • Accompany mothers for PNC at one, six, and 14 weeks; • Record patient accompaniments • Report community deaths	• Conduct follow-up visits at home to mother/neonate during first seven days after delivery • Check to see if mothers are properly breastfeeding and burping • Check for danger signs for maternal and infant health
Child Health	• Educate communities about child health and importance of nutrition • Mobilize the community for National Immunization Days	• Identify under-5 children that should attend Under-5 Clinics (i.e. for immunization) • Monitor growth of children in the community using salter scale every month • Identify malnourished children in the community using growth tread graphs		• Accompany children for vaccines and growth monitoring during scheduled appointments • Accompany malnourished children for treatment	• Track patients and number of accompaniments • Report community deaths	
Other activities	• Convene community meetings for health facilities ("pitsos") • Participate in health outreach campaigns by health facilities • Report health hazards in the community	• Participate in investigations of communicable disease outbreaks				• Provide counseling/ bereavement support as needed

FIGURE 8.3 Figure shows the mapping of the different functions of community health workers along the value chain of health care delivery based on work in Lesotho.

Community health workers function along the continuum of care. They are a key member of the delivery strategy for a number of diseases and conditions, including: newborn, child, and maternal health; HIV, and tuberculosis.

Source: Seidman et al. Village health worker activities along the care delivery value chain: The case of Lesotho. 2017. Paper forthcoming.

in Rwanda, community members with a sick child seek care at the binome's home. iCCM binomes are also taught to recognize when a sick child must be sent to a clinic. They also lead educational campaigns to promote health. The second type of CHW is an *agente santé maternelle* (ASM). ASMs are responsible for maternal and neonatal health. They encourage clinic-based antenatal and postnatal care.[53] Ethiopia employs a similar model. The country has 38,000 CHWs called *health extension workers* (HEWs).[87] Each village selects two HEWs. They focus on health promotion, disease prevention, and iCCM and are based at fixed health posts in every village.[88]

Despite the successful scale-up of CHW programs in Rwanda and Ethiopia, challenges in these systems remain. Some programs struggle with low utilization of CHW services. Studies have shown that low utilization of CHWs performing iCCM is due to lack of drug availability, user fees for CHWs services, and long geographic distance to CHW homes or fixed health posts.[43,89] In Burkina Faso, people bypassed CHWs to seek consultations at facilities they deemed superior and that offered professional health services.[90] These impediments to the success of CHW programs mirror the structural challenges and social determinants that undermine the utilization of health care in general. Such studies are a potent reminder that CHW programs alone cannot leapfrog over broken systems. Adequate support for supply chains, mentoring, and the minimization of out-of-pocket costs is sorely needed to improve health care utilization.

Conclusion

CHWs are an important part of the health workforce. Their proximity to and knowledge of communities is critical to achieving health equity. The work of CHWs has been associated with positive health outcomes, particularly for vulnerable populations. CHWs perform a variety of functions across the value chain. They deliver health promotion, disease prevention, and education. Additionally, they can provide treatment, care, and follow-up. CHWs fill essential gaps in the professional health workforce and play an essential role in the successful scale-up of HIV treatment and child health services in impoverished settings. Yet much work remains. CHWs are not adequately compensated in most health systems. Moreover, the inadequate supply of drugs, economic barriers to care, and lack of mentorship inhibit the work of CHWs. Investments are needed to support this cadre through mentoring and compensation. If they receive adequate support, CHWs will be critical to the achievement of Universal Health Coverage.

References

1. Glenton C, Colvin CJ, Carlsen B, et al. Barriers and facilitators to the implementation of lay health worker programmes to improve access to maternal and child health: Qualitative evidence synthesis (review). *Cochrane Database Syst Rev.* 2013;(10):CD010414.
2. Koplan JP, Himna AR, Parker RL, You-Long G, Ming-Ding Yang. The barefoot doctor: Shanghai County revisited. *Am J Public Health.* 1985;75(7):768–770.
3. Rosenthal MM, Greiner JR. The barefoot doctors of China: From political creation to professionalization. *Hum Org.* 1982;41(4):330–341.
4. Zhang D, Unschuld PU. China's barefoot doctor: Past, present, and future. *Lancet.* 2008;372(9653):1865–1867.
5. Nkonki L, Cliff J, Sanders D. Lay health worker attrition: Important but often ignored. *Bull World Health Org* 2011;89(12):919.
6. Olang'o CO, Nyamongo IK, Aagaard-Hansen J. Staff attrition among community health workers in home-based care programmes for people living with HIV and AIDS in Western Kenya. *Health Policy.* 2010;97(2):232–237.
7. Tulenko K, Mogedal S, Afzal MM, et al. Community health workers for universal health-care coverage: From fragmentation to synergy. *Bull World Health Org.* 2013;91(11):847.
8. Viswanathan M, Kraschnewski J, Nishikawa B, et al. *Outcomes of community health worker interventions.* Rockville, MD: Agency for Healthcare Research and Quality, US Department of Health and Human Services; 2009.
9. Werner D, Thuman C, Maxwell J. *Where there is no doctor: A village health care handbook.* Berkeley, CA: Hesperian Foundation; 1992.
10. Mukherjee JS, Barry D, Weatherford RD, Desai IK, Farmer PE. Community-based ART programs: Sustaining adherence and follow-up. *Curr HIV/AIDS Rep.* 2016; 13(6):359.
11. Wen C. Barefoot doctors in China. *Lancet.* 1974; 303(7864):976–978.
12. Yip K. Health and nationalist reconstruction: Rural health in nationalist China, 1928– 1937. *Mod Asian Stud.* 1992;26:395–415.
13. Valentine V. Health for the masses: China's "Barefoot Doctors." NPR Global Health. 2005. Available from: http://www.npr.org/templates/story/story.php?storyId=4990242. Accessed Dec 7, 2016.
14. Weiyuan C. China's village doctors take great strides. *Bull World Health Org.* 2008;86(12):914.
15. Matthews D. Everything you need to know about the War on Poverty. *The Washington Post.* Jan 8, 2014. Available from: https://www.washingtonpost.com/news/wonk/wp/2014/01/08/everything-you-need-to-know-about-the-war-on-poverty/?utm_term=.b6761353071c. Accessed Apr 9, 2017.
16. Witmer A, Seifer SD, Finocchio L, Leslie J, O'Neil EH. Community health workers: Integral members of the health care work force. *Am J Public Health.* 1995;85(8):1055.

17. Kunitz SJ. The history and politics of US health care policy for American Indians and Alaskan Natives. *Am J Public Health*. 1996;86(10):1464–1473.

18. Moore JD, Smith DG. Legislating Medicaid: Considering Medicaid and its origins. *Health Care Financ Rev*. 2005;27(2):45–52.

19. Richter R, Bengen B, Alsup P, Bruun B, Kilcoyne M, Challenor B. The community health worker: A resource for improved health care delivery. *Am J Public Health*. 1974;64(11):1056.

20. Moodie AS, Rogers G. Baltimore uses inner city aides in a tuberculosis control program. *Public Health Rep (1896–1970)*. 1970;85(11):955–963.

21. Morgan MT. Alaskan community health aides. *Am J Public Health*. 1975;65(4):411–411.

22. Gibson R. *African liberation movements: Contemporary struggles against white minority rule*. Published for the Institute of Race Relations. New York: Oxford University Press; 1972.

23. Coovadia H, Jewkes R, Barron P, Sanders D, Mcintyre D. The health and health system of South Africa: Historical roots of current public health challenges. *Lancet*. 2009;374(9692):817–834.

24. Norman-Taylor W. Some principles in the training of auxiliary health personnel for work in tropical rural areas. *Public Health*. 1960;74(11):413–418.

25. UNICEF. *The state of the world's child*. New York: UNICEF; 1983.

26. Zachariah R, Ford N, Philips M, et al. Task shifting in HIV/AIDS: Opportunities, challenges and proposed actions for sub-Saharan Africa. *Trans R Soc Trop Med Hyg*. 2009;103(6):549–558.

27. Schneider H, McIntyre D, Birch S, Eyles J. Access challenges in TB, ART and maternal health services. Phase 1 results, REACH. 2009. Available from: http:// uct-heu.s3.amazonaws.com/wp-content/uploads/2010/02/USER-REPORT.pdf.

28. Hermann K, Van Damme W, Pariyo G, et al. Community health workers for ART in sub-Saharan Africa: Learning from experience—capitalizing on new opportunities. *Hum Resources Health*. 2009;7:31. https://doi.org/10.1186/1478-4491-7-31.

29. Lehmann U, Van Damme W, Barten F, Sanders D. Task shifting: The answer to the human resources crisis in Africa? *Hum Resources Health*. 2009;7:49. https://doi. org/10.1186/1478-4491-7-49.

30. Berman PA, Gwatkin DR, Burger SE. Community-based health workers: Head start or false start towards health for all? *Soc Sci Med*. 1987;25(5):443–459.

31. Bhutta Z, Lassi Z, Pariyo G, Huicho L. *Global experience of community health workers for delivery of health related millennium development goals: A systematic review, country case studies, and recommendations for integration into national health systems*. Geneva: World Health Organization; 2010.

32. Witmer A, Seifer SD, Finocchio L, Leslie J, O'Neil EH. Community health workers: Integral members of the health care work force. *Am J Public Health*. 1995;85(8):1055.

33. Haines A, Sanders D, Lehmann U, et al. Achieving child survival goals: Potential contribution of community health workers. *Lancet*. 2007;369(9579):2121–2131.

34. Mukherjee JS, Eustache FE. Community health workers as a cornerstone for integrating HIV and primary healthcare. *AIDS Care.* 2007;19:73–82.

35. UNICEF. *Caring for the sick child in the community.* Geneva: World Health Organization;2011.

36. Lewin S, Munabi-Babigumira S, Glenton C, et al. Lay health workers in primary and community health care for maternal and child health and the management of infectious diseases. *The Cochrane Library*; 2010. Available from: http://www.chw-central.org/sites/default/files/Lewin-Effectiveness%20of%20lay%20health%20workers.pdf.

37. Rosenthal EL, Brownstein JN, Rush CH, et al. Community health workers: Part of the solution. *Health Aff (Millwood).* 2010;29(7):1338

38. Gilson L, Walt G, Heggenhougen K, et al. National community health worker programs: How can they be strengthened? *J Public Health Policy.* 1989;10(4):518.

39. Palazuelos D, Ellis K, DaEun Im D, et al. 5-SPICE: The application of an original framework for community health worker program design, quality improvement and research agenda setting. *Glob Health Action.* 2013 Apr 3;6:19658. doi:10.3402/gha.v6i0.19658.

40. Walt G, Gilson L, editors. *Community health workers in national programmes: Just another pair of hands?* Milton Keynes, UK; Philadelphia: Open University Press; 1990.

41. Perry H, Zulliger R. *How effective are community health workers? An overview of current evidence with recommendations for strengthening community health worker programs to accelerate progress in achieving the health-related Millennium Development Goals.* Baltimore, MD: Johns Hopkins Bloomberg School of Public Health; 2012.

42. O'Brien MJ, Squires AP, Bixby RA, Larson SC. Role development of community health workers: An examination of selection and training processes in the intervention literature. *Am J Prev Med.* 2009;37(6): S269.

43. Lehmann U, Sanders D. *Community health workers: What do we know about them?* Geneva: World Health Organization; 2007.

44. Aitken I. Training community health workers for large-scale community-based health care programs. Maternal and Child Health Integrated Program (MCHIP). Washington, DC: USAID; 2013. Available from: http://www.mchip.net/sites/default/files/mchipfiles/CHW_ReferenceGuide_sm.pdf.

45. Pallas SW, Minhas D, Perez-Escamilla R, Taylor L, Curry L, Bradley EH. Community health workers in low- and middle-income countries: What do we know about scaling up and sustainability? *Am J Public Health.* 2013;103(7):e74.

46. ACF International. *Community management of acute malnutrition in Nigeria: Training manual on data management and reporting.* Yobe State: European Commission Humanitarian Aid;2011.

47. Kumar M, Nefdt R, Ribaira E, Diallo K. *Access to healthcare through community health workers in east and southern Africa.* Maternal, newborn and child health working paper. New York: UNICEF; 2014.

48. Adams J, Lloyd A, Miller C. *The Oxfam Ebola response in Liberia and Sierra Leone.* Oxford: Oxfam; 2015.

49. UNFPA. Community health workers respond to Ebola outbreak in Sierra Leone. UNFPA West and Central Africa Web site. 2014. Available from: http://wcaro.unfpa.org/news/community-health-workers-respond-ebola-outbreak-sierra-leone?page=2%2C4.

50. Partners in Health (PIH). How contact tracing can stop Ebola. 2014. Available from: http://www.pih.org/media/need-to-know-contact-tracing.

51. World Health Organization/UNICEF. *Caring for the sick child in the community: A training course for community health workers.* Geneva: World Health Organization; 2011.

52. Friedman L, Wolfheim C. *Review of integrated community case management training and supervision materials in ten African countries.* Maternal and Child Health Integrated Program (MCHIP). Washington, DC: USAID; 2013.

53. Olaniran A, Smith H, Unkels R, Bar-Zeev S, van den Broek N. Who is a community health worker? A systematic review of definitions. *Glob Health Action.* 2017;10(1):1272223.

54. Johnson AD, Thomson DR, Atwood S, et al. Assessing early access to care and child survival during a health system strengthening intervention in Mali: A repeated cross sectional survey. *PLoS One.* 2013;8(12):e81304.

55. Ayeh GA. The role of village health workers (VHW) in the prevention of mother to child transmission (PMTCT) care in Lesotho – a mixed methods study. MMSc [thesis]. Boston (MA): Harvard Medical School; 2017.

56. Rowe AK, de Savigny D, Lanata CF, Victora CG. How can we achieve and maintain high-quality performance of health workers in low-resource settings? *Lancet.* 2005;366(9490):1026–1035.

57. Perry H, Sierra-Esteban F, Berman P. Financing large-scale community health worker programs. Maternal and Child Health Integrated Program (MCHIP). Washington, DC: USAID; 2013.

58. Perry HB, Zulliger R, Rogers MM. Community health workers in low-, middle-, and high-income countries: An overview of their history, recent evolution, and current effectiveness. *Ann Rev Public Health.* 2014;35:399–421.

59. Pink DH. *Drive: The surprising truth about what motivates us.* New York: Penguin; 2011.

60. Dawnay E, Shah H. *Behavioural economics: Seven principles for policy makers.* London: New Economics Foundation; 2005.

61. Kasteng F, Settumba S, Kllander K, Vassall A, and SCALE Study Group. Valuing the work of unpaid community health workers and exploring the incentives to volunteering in rural Africa. *Health Policy Plan.* 2015:42.

62. B-Lajoie M, Hulme J, Johnson K. Payday, ponchos, and promotions: A qualitative analysis of perspectives from non-governmental organization programme managers on community health worker motivation and incentives. *Hum Resources Health.* 2014;12:66.

63. Perry H, Zulliger R, Scott K, Javadi D, Gergen J, Shelley K. Case studies of large-scale community health worker programs: Examples from Afghanistan,

Bangladesh, Brazil, Ethiopia, India, Indonesia, Iran, Nepal, Pakistan, Rwanda, Zambia and Zimbabwe. In: *Developing and strengthening community health worker programs at scale: A reference guide and case studies for program managers and policy-makers.* Maternal and Child Health Integrated Program (MCHIP). Washington, DC: USAID; 2014.

64. Condo J, Mugeni C, Naughton B, et al. Rwanda's evolving community health worker system: A qualitative assessment of client and provider perspectives. *Hum Resources Health.* 2014;12(1):1.

65. Task Force on Health Systems Research. *The Millennium Development Goals will not be attained without new research addressing health system constraints to delivering effective interventions: Report of the Task Force on Health Systems Research.* Geneva: World Health Organization; 2005.

66. Finance Alliance for Health. Finance Alliance for Health. 2017. Available from: http://www.financingalliance.org/. Accessed Apr 19, 2017.

67. Dahn B, Woldemariam AT, Perry H, et al. *Strengthening primary health care through community health workers: Investment case and financing recommendations.* Geneva: World Health Organization; 2015.

68. Jackson ET. Evaluating social impact bonds: Questions, challenges, innovations, and possibilities in measuring outcomes in impact investing. *Comm Dev.* 2013;44(5):608–616.

69. Lewin S, Munabibabigumira S, Glenton C, et al. Lay health workers in primary and community health care for maternal and child health and the management of infectious diseases. *Cochrane Library.* 2010.

70. Mannan I, Rahman SM, Sania A, et al. Can early postpartum home visits by trained community health workers improve breastfeeding of newborns? *J Perinatol.* 2008;28(9):632–640.

71. Rahman A, Malik A, Sikander S, Roberts C, Creed F. Cognitive behaviour therapy-based intervention by community health workers for mothers with depression and their infants in rural Pakistan: A cluster-randomised controlled trial. *Lancet.* 2008;372(9642):902–909.

72. Berman PA. Village health workers in Java, Indonesia: Coverage and equity. *Soc Sci Med.* 1984;19(4):411–422.

73. Viswanathan K, Hansen PM, Rahman MH, et al. Can community health workers increase coverage of reproductive health services? *J Epidemiol Comm Health.* 2012;66(10):894–900.

74. Mullany LC, Lee TJ, Yone L, et al. Impact of community-based maternal health workers on coverage of essential maternal health interventions among internally displaced communities in Eastern Burma: The MOM project. *PLoS Med.* 2010;7(8):e1000317.

75. Patel AR, Nowalk MP. Expanding immunization coverage in rural India: A review of evidence for the role of community health workers. *Vaccine.* 2010;28(3):604–613.

76. Chowdhury AMR. Community health workers role in DOTS. *Health Action.* 1999;24:13.

77. Thomson D, Rich M, Kaigamba F, et al. Community-based accompaniment and psychosocial health outcomes in HIV-infected adults in Rwanda: A prospective study. *AIDS Behav.* 2014;18(2):368–380.

78. Farmer P, Léandre F, Mukherjee JS, et al. Community-based approaches to HIV treatment in resource-poor settings. *Lancet.* 2001;358(9279):404–409.

79. Kredo T, Adeniyi F, Bateganya M, Pienaar E. Task shifting from doctors to non-doctors for initiation and maintenance of antiretroviral therapy. *Cochrane Library.* 2014. doi: 10.1002/14651858.CD007331.pub3

80. Eustache E, Oswald C, Belkin GS, Raviola GJ. Mental health response in Haiti in the aftermath of the 2010 earthquake: A case study for building long-term solutions. *Harv Rev Psychiatry.* 2012;20(1):68–77.

81. Fedder DO, Chang RJ, Curry S, Nichols G. The effectiveness of a community health worker outreach program on healthcare utilization of West Baltimore City Medicaid patients with diabetes, with or without hypertension. *Ethn Dis.* 2003;13(1):22.

82. Satti H, Motsamai S, Chetane P, et al. Comprehensive approach to improving maternal health and achieving MDG 5: Report from the mountains of Lesotho (Comprehensive Maternal Health Program in Lesotho). *PLoS One.* 2012;7(8): e42700.

83. Kerber KJ, de Graft-Johnson JE. Bhutta ZA, Okong P, Starrs A, Lawn JE. Continuum of care for maternal, newborn, and child health: From slogan to service delivery. *Lancet.* 2007;370(9595):1358–1369.

84. Kalyango JN, Rutebemberwa E, Alfven T, Ssali S, Peterson S, Karamagi C. Performance of community health workers under integrated community case management of childhood illnesses in Eastern Uganda. *Malaria J.* 2012;11(1):282.

85. Dhillon RS, Kelly JD. Community trust and the Ebola endgame. *N Engl J Med.* 2015;373(9):787–789.

86. Liu A, Sullivan S, Khan M, Sachs S, Singh P. Community health workers in global health: Scale and scalability. *Mt Sinai J Med.* 2011;78(3):419–435.

87. Kok MC, Kea AZ, Datiko DG, et al. A qualitative assessment of health extension workers' relationships with the community and health sector in Ethiopia: Opportunities for enhancing maternal health performance. *Hum Resource Health.* 2015;13(1):80.

88. Admassie A, Abebaw D, Woldemichael AD. Impact evaluation of the Ethiopian Health Services Extension Programme. *J Dev Effect.* 2009;1(4):430–449.

89. Stekelenburg J, Kyanamina SS, Wolffers I. Poor performance of community health workers in Kalabo District, Zambia. *Health Policy.* 2003;65(2):109–118.

90. Sauerborn R, Nougtara A, Diesfeld H. Low utilization of community health workers: Results from a household interview survey in Burkina Faso. *Soc Sci Med.* 1989;29(10):1163.

Evolution in Drug Access

Key Points

- Both availability and accessibility of pharmaceutical products are critical to the delivery of health care.
- Due to high prices and market failures, access to essential drugs remains a critical challenge for individuals and governments around the world.
- The World Health Organization (WHO) Essential Medicines List serves as a guide to drug procurement for impoverished countries and as signal to generic drug manufacturers that there will be a market.
- Quality generic drugs are important components of delivering medical care.
- Novel systems for drug development and distribution are needed to assure the equitable availability of drugs.
- There is a growing movement to decrease costs, increase supply, and advance development of drugs for diseases affecting impoverished people.

Introduction

The global health era has brought about a renewed commitment to the treatment of disease. Thus, the focus on what drugs are needed and how to assure a reliable supply chain of medications is an important area of global health work. The discovery of penicillin by Alexander Fleming in 1928 turned diseases like pneumonia from often fatal conditions to curable ones.[1] The 1940s development of the first drug for tuberculosis (TB), streptomycin, gave hope to patients with the stigmatized and chronic disease.[2] Despite the remarkable discoveries of these and other life-saving medicines in the 20th and 21st centuries, unequal access to drugs is a persistent cause of health disparities between rich and poor, both within and between countries.

Both access to medical treatment and to the fruits of scientific advancement are part of the Universal Declaration of Human Rights[3] and the charter of the World Health Organization (WHO).[4] Yet people in impoverished countries have always suffered from a lack of access to even basic antibiotics. Drugs needed for chronic conditions like diabetes or schizophrenia are in even scarcer supply. This chapter focuses on the concept of the Essential Medicines List, the challenges faced in accessing drugs, and some methods of expanding drug availability. The chapter also focuses on the role of social movements in expanding access to drugs.

What Is an Essential Drug?

At the World Health Assembly in 1975, the WHO and its member states first addressed the challenge of access to drugs for people living in impoverished countries.[5] Dr. Halfdan Mahler, then Director-General of the WHO, called for the creation of drug policies that would meet global health needs. In the proceedings of that meeting, the concept of essential drugs was introduced described as "those [drugs and vaccines] considered to be of the utmost importance and hence basic, indispensable, and necessary for the health needs of the population."[6] Essential drugs were, WHO argued, "those most needed for the health care of the majority of the population and, therefore, should be available at all times in adequate amounts and in the proper dosage [and] forms."[6] By 1977, the WHO defined a Model List of Essential Drugs (now the Essential Medicines List or EML),[7] which included 200 drugs and vaccines. Sadly, the aspiration of the EML—that the set of 200 drugs and vaccines be made universally available was not followed by the financing to do so. Still, the creation of the EML was an important step to developing a framework for access to drugs in impoverished countries. It set a standard for what ought to be available to all, even if the reality was remote.

The EML does serve many functions for impoverished countries. First, impoverished countries benefit from the fact that many countries will procure the drugs on list. This creates a reliable, global demand for the specific drugs and encourages large-scale generic production. Large-scale generic production in turn enables countries to procure drugs in bulk at lower prices. Second, the EML enables governments to regulate the import and use of a common set of drugs. The WHO's Essential Drug and Medicines Policy program also supports governments through the procurement process and in setting regulatory policy.[8] Third, the EML specifies a group of drugs around which training can be provided. The EML is updated every two years. The most recent EML was released in 2015 and included new hepatitis C drugs and pediatric formulations of TB drugs.[9]

Access to Essential Drugs

Despite the creation of the EML, unequal access to essential drugs remains a central problem in global health. Procurement of an adequate yearly or quarterly supply of drugs is an important recurring cost of the health care system. Governments of impoverished countries lack the financing to procure and distribute even the most inexpensive drugs.[10] Lack of money for procurement and distribution results in a multitude of problems from chronic stock-outs of some drugs to expiration of others.[11] At the patient level, high out-of-pocket expenditures on drugs (whether at public or private facilities) are a major barrier to care.[12] In the postcolonial period and the Alma Ata era, local production of essential drugs was discussed as a development priority for impoverished country governments. Publically financed factories to produce essential medications would provide jobs, introduce technology, increase drug availability, and decrease cost. However, the for-profit pharmaceutical industry was against this type of expansion of access.[13] Moreover, under the structural adjustment programs of the 1980s, private solutions were favored over government investments and donors were unwilling to invest in government-run manufacturing.[14]

The 1987 UNICEF conference held in Bamako, Mali (discussed in Chapter 1) was in part driven by the need to support the provision of essential drugs. The Bamako Initiative sought to replicate and scale the success of revolving drug fund pilot programs.[15] UNICEF provided an initial injection of capital to supply rural health posts with essential drugs. But the recurring costs needed to maintain the supply of drugs would be funded thereafter by patient user fees.[16] From Bamako forward, encouraging people to pay for drugs became a cornerstone of public health. The theory held that if people were educated about the health benefits of drugs, they would buy them. This work, also called *social marketing*, sought promote the purchase of health-related products through education campaigns.[17] The Bamako Initiative posited that if social marketing was effective, people's health-seeking behaviors would change. They would learn through education to value their health and understand the benefits of medicines and therefore pay for drugs. Public health personnel reasoned that social marketing would increase utilization of services and thus increase payment to facilities. This would assure that there would be sufficient cash to support the recurring costs of drugs. Unfortunately, many social marketing programs did not increase the purchase of drugs. People already understood quite well that medicines were necessary. They simply could not afford them. Social marketing remains a cornerstone of health programs and many millions of dollars are spent on this approach. It has been studied extensively by many groups. One important study by the Poverty Action Lab at the Massachusetts Institute of Technology showed that social marketing to promote the purchase of mosquito nets increased the use of nets by the middle class but not by the poor. The same education was provided for both groups, but the agency of the poor to use the information was constrained by poverty. Since governments had no other options to procure drugs, the Bamako Initiative's user fees became the main avenue for the poor to access essential treatments, and an emphasis on changing behavior through social marketing remained.

Patents, Profits, and Patient Access

AIDS activists again led the way in the evolution of the essential drug list and the fight for equal access to medications. As discussed in Chapter 2, antiretroviral therapy (ART) was life-saving but inaccessible to the majority of patients in impoverished countries.[18] All ARTs were patented by the companies that developed them. The patents were protected by the World Trade Organization's (WTO) international trade agreements. These treaties are governed by a subsidiary body called the Council for Trade-Related Aspects of Intellectual Property Rights (TRIPs). African countries claimed a national emergency and invoked flexibilities in TRIPs to either import the generic version of a patented product (usually from India) or demand a compulsory license to manufacture the drug locally.[19] In addition to supporting governments to use TRIPs flexibilities to obtain or manufacture generic ART, activists pushed for the WHO to include ART on the EML.[20,21] They reasoned that if antiretroviral drugs were included on the EML it would send a signal to generic companies to increase the manufacture of these drugs. Higher volumes would drop prices further. The pressure from activists sparked the release of a discussion paper from the WHO in 2001 entitled "Updating and Disseminating the WHO's List of Essential Drugs: The Way Forward."[22] The paper encouraged the inclusion of newly developed drugs, even those under patent, on the EML when there were no generic options. But powerful pharmaceutical companies lobbied the US government against the inclusion of newer drugs on the EML. The WHO's discussion paper was met by a strongly worded rebuttal from the US government.[23] The companies feared that countries would use the EML as a justification to invoke TRIPs flexibilities and demand access to generic drugs, thus cutting into their profits. But the momentum toward the generic production of ARTs was powerful. At the 2001 meeting of the WTO, activists succeeded in pushing the WTO and influential members, particularly the United States, to allow for TRIPs flexibilities to be used to gain access to generic AIDS drugs. The Doha Declaration of the WTO, penned as a result of the 2001 meeting, stated that the interpretation of TRIPs should allow member states to protect the public health including the purchase or manufacture generic drugs still under patent.[24] In 2002, antiretrovirals were added to the EML. Generic production was massively increased owing to the regulatory change and the new Global Fund to Fight AIDS, TB and Malaria which guaranteed the impoverished countries would have resources to purchase ART. AIDS was the catalyst for this movement to expand the EML. Including ART on the EML encouraged generic companies to increase production and lower price. This was powerful example and a step toward the equitable sharing of scientific advancements with all of humanity as a matter of human rights rather than market forces.

It is important to understand the impact that the profit motive and market forces have on drug access. Pharmaceutical companies often cite the need to be profitable for shareholders[25] and to recuperate the costs of research and development. These are the two stated reasons behind the price of drugs set by companies.[25] However, both profits for shareholders and costs for drug development are debated arguments.[25] Many see drugs as a public good that should be regulated by the needs of society rather than by the market. The fight for broader access to expensive treatments is not limited to impoverished countries. Due to the influence of the pharmaceutical industry in the American political process, US legislators regularly vote against the government's ability to negotiate prices, even for drugs that were developed using public funds.[26-28] The US legislators' arguments against regulating drug prices are rooted in neoliberal economic theory: they argue that market forces spur innovation, whereas price controls slow the pace of drug development.[29] As a result of the prohibition on negotiation, the cost of drugs is significantly higher in the United States than in neighboring Canada.[30] Civil society and some in the US government advocate for negotiating power to lower drug prices (Figure 9.1).

The cost of drugs remains an important impediment to treatment for many. The treatment of hepatitis C is an instructive case. The virus hepatitis C results in severe liver disease in 15–30 percent of those infected[31] and liver cancer in a subset of those with the viral infection. For many years, there was no oral treatment. Intravenous interferon that was used had many side effects and was not always effective. In 2013, new oral drugs were approved that replaced a long and difficult regimen based on injections with a single pill taken daily for 12 weeks. The first drug (sofosbuvir) had few side effects and a much higher cure rate than the previous complicated regimens.[32] The price of sofosbuvir, however, was set by Gilead pharmaceuticals at $1,000 per pill, or $84,000 for a 12-week curative course.[33] In setting the drug's price, Gilead estimated what the paying market would bear. They cited responsibility to shareholders and the need to recuperate the cost of research and development.[29] Given the price tag of sofosbuvir, Medicaid, the US publically supported, state-run medical insurance scheme for the poor, was unable to cover the cost in most states. Sofosbuvir was not put

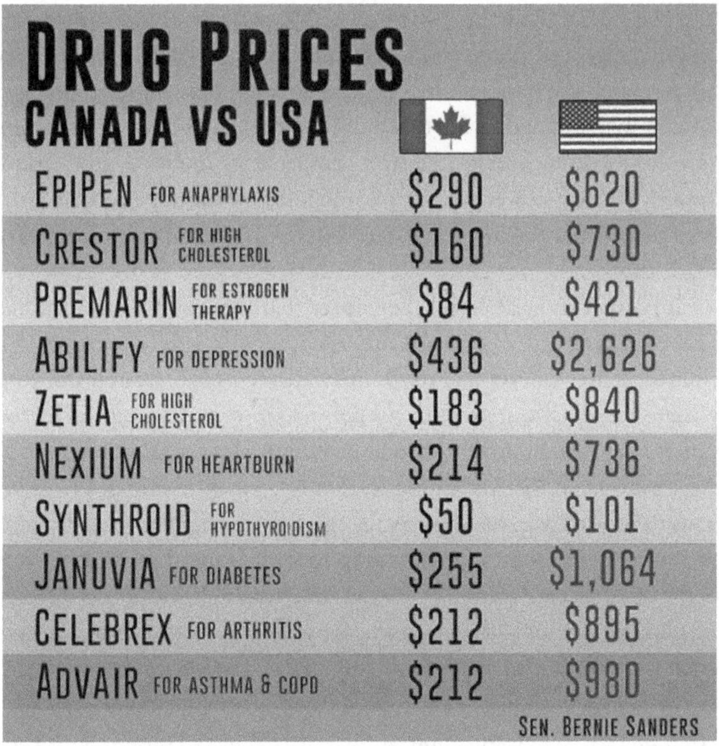

FIGURE 9.1 A campaign advertisement from US Senator Bernie Sanders' presidential campaign in 2016 highlights the difference between drugs prices in the US as compared with Canada. The Senator, advocates for lower prescription drug prices proposing a strategy the includes restoring Medicare's negotiating power, allowing the importation of prescription drugs from Canada, restoring discounts for low-income seniors, prohibiting deals that keep generics off the market, increasing penalties for fraud, and increasing cost and pricing transparency.

Source: Sanders B. Drug prices Canada vs USA. 2016. Available from: https://www.facebook.com/senatorsanders/photos/a.91485152907.84764.9124187907/10155278149797908/?type=3&theater. Accessed May 31, 2017.

on the formulary (the Essential Medicines List for Medicaid).[34] The medicine is therefore rationed based on the resources of each state and made available only to the sickest patients.[35] This rationing causes two problems. First, many patients with a curable disease are becoming sicker and even dying while waiting for treatment. Second, without treatment, there is ongoing transmission of the virus.[36] A 2016 study showed that governments would have to spend from 10.5 percent of total pharmaceutical expenditure (Netherlands) to 190.5 percent (Poland)[37] to treat the entire hepatitis C–infected population. Meanwhile, access to this and other new drugs for hepatitis C remains even further out of reach in impoverished countries. In some cases, pharmaceutical companies implement tiered pricing, which means selling drugs at lower costs in countries with lower gross domestic products (GDPs).[38] While tiered-pricing can expand access, this system results in inequities between and within countries.[39]

In an attempt to address the various issues surrounding access to medicines, UN Secretary-General Ban Ki-moon launched a High-Level Panel in November 2015. The purpose of the panel was to "solicit and assess proposals and recommend solutions to address the policy incoherence between the justifiable rights of inventors, international human rights law, trade rules, and public health in the context of health technologies."[40] On September 14, 2016, the High-Level Panel released its report on promoting innovation and access to health technologies.[41] This report emphasized the need to balance human rights, intellectual property (IP) rights, and public health. The authors provided five key recommendations[41,42]:

1. *Respect and strengthen the legal landscape*: In the words of the authors, "International agreements should be used to improve innovation and access, not hinder it."[42]
2. *Implement additional models for R&D funding*: The authors stress that research and development must be delinked from consumer prices so that both investment and discovery innovations can be rewarded and people can access medicines at a fair price.
3. *Initiate a transparency paradigm shift*: The authors emphasize that marketing, distribution, and pricing of health technologies should be clear to the public.
4. *Increase investment*: The authors call for increased investment from private sources and governments in diseases that affect the poor.
5. *Create a framework for accountability*: The authors call for all stakeholders and shareholders to be accountable for ethical access to health technologies.

The recommendations of the report supported countries that needed medicines to invoke TRIPs flexibilities without retribution from wealthy countries whose interested reflected the private pharmaceutical industry and patent holders. The report urged that the public health impact be taken into account as new drugs were brought to market and that the need to recuperate research and development costs be delinked from the analysis of impact of a drug. Lastly, it urged more public investment in drugs needed for public good rather than profit. Advocates called for the rapid implementation of these plans.

New Avenues to Address Market Failures

Most preclinical drug discovery is done at the academic level and funded by public money (Figure 9.2). This is typically considered the most economically risky stage of drug discovery because there are no assurances that the synthesis of a new compound will be successful.[43] However, once a compound shows promise, it is picked up by the pharmaceutical industry to complete the scientific research and clinical trials and bring the drug to market. Due to the influence of the pharmaceutical industry, drug development is typically not driven by the burden of disease itself but by the potential for profits that company will make from a drug.[44] Are those suffering from a condition those who can pay? What price will the market bear? What profit can be made? What return on investment in research and development can be expected? The market-driven model for drug development stifles innovation for diseases that have a small market share. This includes rare diseases that affect few people and diseases that predominantly affect the poor.[44,45] However, as global health has advanced in the past two decades, so too has the movement to overcome market failures and improve access to drugs for diseases of the poor.

Prior to the development of strategies to address market failures for diseases of the poor, the US addressed market failures in drug discovery for the treatment of rare diseases (defined as diseases that affect fewer than 200,000 Americans). For this purpose, the US Congress authored the Orphan Drug Act (ODA) in 1983. The ODA created incentives for companies to develop treatments for rare diseases. First, grants were awarded for research on rare diseases. Second, market exclusivity was extended for the company once a new product was developed. The ODA's incentives were successful in spurring innovation. For example, Gaucher's disease is a rare genetic condition that is covered under the ODA. In 1994, the US biotechnology company Genzyme developed a treatment called Cerezyme. Preclinical research, clinical trials, and the development of Cerezyme were supported by public, National Institute of Health (NIH) funding under the ODA and a $3 million donation from the US-based charity, the National Gaucher Foundation.[46] Once Genzyme developed and patented Cerezyme, the company set the price at $300,000 per patient per year. As a justification for the high price, the company cited the cost of development and the small market.[47] By 2009, Genzyme was the world's third largest biotechnology company with revenues of about $4.5 billion.[46] In 2014, Genzyme released a new drug to treat Gaucher's disease—Cerdelga—priced at just over $310,000 per patient per year.[47]

The ODA did spur innovation, but did not address market failures with regard to making drugs available for the poor. Even with grants for drug development, companies would never be able to make the kind of profits that drug sales in

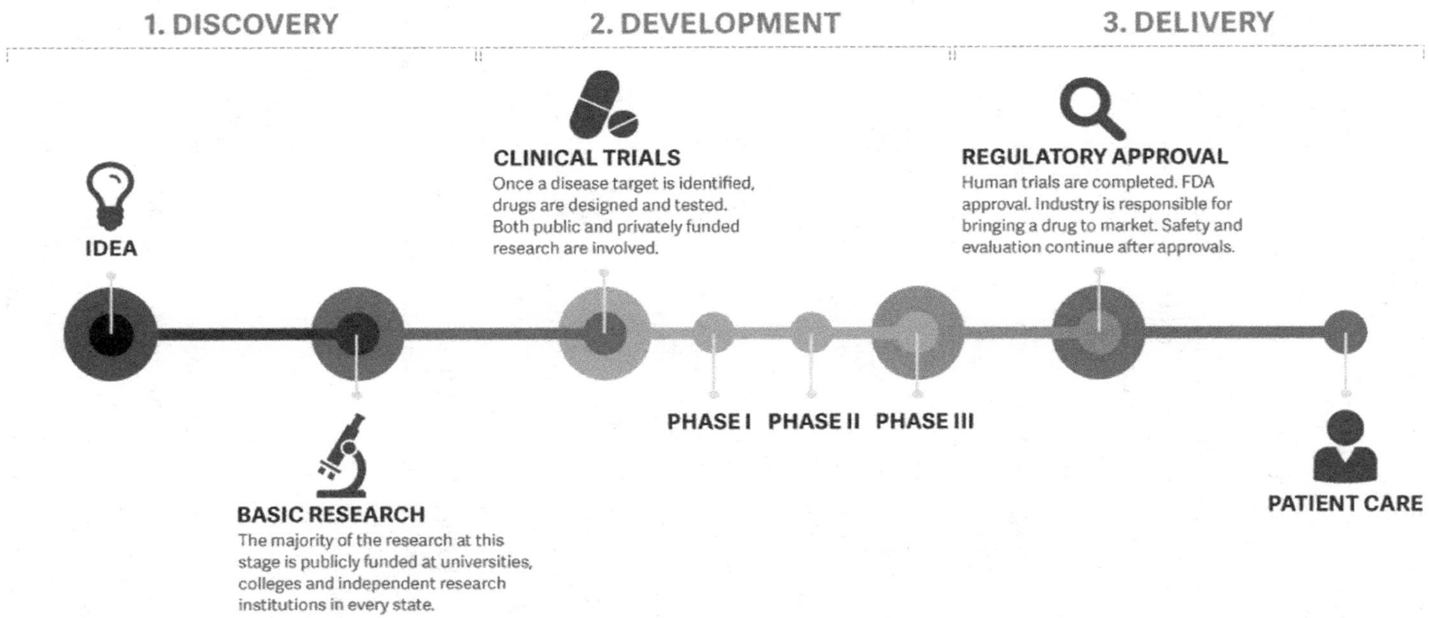

1. DISCOVERY   **2. DEVELOPMENT**   **3. DELIVERY**

IDEA

BASIC RESEARCH
The majority of the research at this stage is publicly funded at universities, colleges and independent research institutions in every state.

CLINICAL TRIALS
Once a disease target is identified, drugs are designed and tested. Both public and privately funded research are involved.

PHASE I   PHASE II   PHASE III

REGULATORY APPROVAL
Human trials are completed. FDA approval. Industry is responsible for bringing a drug to market. Safety and evaluation continue after approvals.

PATIENT CARE

FIGURE 9.2 Example of a drug discovery, development, and delivery timeline.

Source: Research America. Bench to bedside: Drug development pipeline. Research America: An Alliance for Discoveries in Health Web site. 2017. Available from: http://www.researchamerica.org/advocacy-action/issues-researchamerica-advocates/bench-bedside-drug-development-pipeline. Accessed Feb 27, 2017.

wealthy countries garnered. New drug development for TB is a prime example of this type of market failure. TB affects more than 1 billion people on the planet, but most cannot pay for drugs.[48,49] Due to the lack of a paying market, until recently, there were no new TB drugs developed since 1972.[50] In an attempt to correct the lack of profit associated with drug discovery for diseases affecting the poor, the US Food and Drug Administration (FDA) passed the FDA Amendments Act of 2007,[51] which created an incentive system for companies to develop new drugs for one of 16 neglected tropical diseases (NTD) (see Table 9.1). The incentive given by the FDA to the pharmaceutical companies was a voucher that could be redeemed in exchange for the expedited review of other drugs developed for more profitable conditions.[52,53] The voucher's expedited timeline offered a four-month window of earlier access to the market. Four months of market access for a profitable drugs could translate into hundreds of millions of dollars.[54] The FDA Amendments Act was used by Novartis, a Swiss multinational pharmaceutical company. It developed of the antimalarial drug Coartem in 2009.[51] Coartem—a combination of two potent antimalarials—has rapidly become the standard of care in impoverished countries of sub-Saharan Africa and Asia, but, because of the low cost, Novartis does not make a significant profit.[55] In exchange for the development of Coartem, Novartis received a voucher from the FDA that could be used to extend market exclusivity for a more profitable drug.

Philanthropic money and overseas development assistance from wealthy countries have also played a role in the development of new drugs for the poor. For example, the not-for-profit organization the TB Drug Alliance was founded with the goal of developing better TB drugs and making them rapidly available to impoverished countries.[56] Funded by philanthropy and governments, the equity proposition of the Alliance (as opposed to a profit motive) was central to their research and development efforts. In the past five years, the Alliance has developed several new TB drugs, including fixed-dose combination drugs and pediatric TB drugs. Once new formulations were developed, they were rapidly turned over to generic manufacturers to scale-up production.

The international community has also pooled resources to improve access to drugs and vaccines. The Global Drug Facility (GDF), founded in 2001 as part of the Stop TB Partnership,[57] is one example of a nontraditional procurement mechanism with the intention of improving access to TB drugs. The GDF supports national governments in forecasting for TB drug procurement. The GDF acquires drugs through bulk purchases from generic manufacturers, thus assuring the lowest price possible. This helps countries buy at low price, assure quality, and avoid delays during the procurement process. The GDF has also simplified packaging to facilitate drug management. Similarly, the Global Alliance for Vaccines and Immunizations (Gavi) was created in 2000 with a $750 million five-year

Table 9.1 Neglected tropical diseases.

Neglected Tropical Diseases	Description	Burden of Disease
Malaria	• Life-threatening disease transmitted by mosquitos	• Estimated 214 million cases and 438,000 deaths in 2015, >90 percent burden in sub-Saharan Africa
Buruli ulcer	• Chronic necrotizing skin disease	• About 2,600 cases reported in 2013; prevalence decreased after active case finding efforts in 2010
Dengue/Dengue hemorrhagic fever	• Virus transmitted by mosquito • Characterized by high fever, hemorrhage, pneumonia, and circulatory failure	• 390 million infections annually • Majority of deaths in South-East Asia and Western Pacific
Fascioliasis	• Parasite that mainly affects the liver	• Highest burden in Asia and Latin America • In 2005, 7.9 million cases with severe outcomes and 7,000 deaths
Lymphatic filariasis	• Transmitted by mosquitos • Damages the lymphatic system, kidneys; sores on arms, legs, or genitals	• 120 million infected in 2015 • 65 percent of cases found in South-East Asia and 30 percent in Africa
Schistosomiasis	• Transmitted by contact with larvae in contaminated water • Can lead to chronic ill health, including cancer and kidney failure	• 90 percent of cases occur in sub-Saharan Africa • Estimated 207 million cases worldwide in 2010
Yaws	• Poverty-related skin diseases; mainly affects children under 15 • Causes chronic disfigurement and disability	• Gross disfigurement and disability in 10 percent of cases

(*continued*)

Table 9.1 Continued

Neglected Tropical Diseases	Description	Burden of Disease
Blinding trachoma	• Infection causes scarring of eyelids that results in blindness	• More than 21 million active cases worldwide • 85 percent of cases found in 29 African countries
Dracunculiasis (guinea-worm disease)	• Parasitic worm transmitted by drinking contaminated water	• In 2009, 187 countries were declared disease free, but Ethiopia, Ghana, Mali, and Sudan reported cases
Human Africa trypanosomiasis (sleeping sickness)	• Parasite that infects central nervous system and causes neurological and psychiatric disorders leading to death	• Mainly found in impoverished rural Africa
Leprosy	• Left untreated, causes permanent damage to skin, nerves, limbs, and eyes	• 72 percent of cases in 2013 found in South-East Asia
Onchocerciasis (river blindness)	• Transmitted by blackflies • Can lead to permanent blindness	• More than 99 percent of 37 million global infections in sub-Saharan Africa
Soil transmitted helminthiasis (STH)	• Infection amplify malnutrition • Impedes child physical growth and cognitive development	• More than 1 billion people infected • 41 percent of cases found in South-East Asia • 24% of cases found in Africa
Tuberculosis	• Caused by airborne bacteria	• 10.4 million new cases and 1.8 million deaths in 2015 • One of top 10 causes of death worldwide
Leishmaniasis	• Transmitted by sandflies • Causes vital organ failure; ulcers on face, arms, and legs.	• Predominantly rural disease • Estimated 1.3 million new cases annually

Source: Data abstracted from WHO Neglected Diseases and WHO diseases specific epidemiology. Retrieved online Feb 27, 2017.

pledge from the Bill and Melinda Gates Foundation. Gavi is designed to leverage financial resources and expertise to make vaccines more affordable and accessible. The organization tackles a different type market failure. In the past, countries that were unsure about their yearly budgets would order vaccines late, which delayed the manufacturing of the vaccines. The delay also hampered vaccine delivery programs. Gavi was founded to ensure vaccine supply for these countries: by purchasing a buffer stock of vaccines, Gavi enables manufacturers to produce at a steady pace, regardless of country budgetary timelines. This assures that vaccines are immediately available as soon as a country's health budget is approved.

Generic Drugs

India is the most important source of generic drugs.[58] When the country joined the WTO in 1995, it agreed to a 10-year window after which the country would recognize patents for drugs. During this 10-year period, India continued to produce generic options.[58,59] Notably, India is the single largest producer of generic ARTs, accounting for 76 percent of generic ARTs used in impoverished countries.[60] In 2005, India ratified the Patent (Amendment) Act, after which the country recognized patents for the first time. This diminished the ability of the Indian pharmaceutical industry to manufacture drugs that are still on patent.[61]

In countries that are compliant with the WTO, when a drug is off patent or is developed without a patent it can be manufactured generically. If a WTO signatory country uses TRIPs flexibilities it may purchase a generic drug or obtain the patent through a compulsory license and manufacture a drug locally. Generic drug companies are for-profit companies but operate with a smaller profit margin for shareholders and do not carry the cost of research and development. In countries like India, they also have lower operating costs. Due to these lower costs, much of the movement for expanding drug access relies heavily on the use of generic drugs.

One important aspect of generic pharmaceuticals is quality control. India, where most generic pharmaceuticals are produced, is a country with less regulation than wealthier countries, and quality control is not assured.[62] There are several international mechanisms in place to correct for this and ensure the quality of generic drugs. In the United States, the FDA certifies the quality standards for factories and production processes with a standard called Good Manufacturing Process (GMP).[63] This standard is used to evaluate factories around the world. However, some factories that produce drugs may not be GMP-certified because they do not meet the standard, do not have the money to go through the process, or are located in a country that uses a different standard. Internationally, there is work under way to harmonize quality standards.[64] The WHO is currently responsible for assessing the quality of generic manufacturers that are producing drugs for impoverished countries. The WHO's process is called *prequalification*.[65] The prequalification process includes an assessment of the manufacturing facility, a review of the drug dossier, evaluations of drug consistency and performance, and site visits to manufacturers. The WHO's prequalification standard is used by procurement agencies to make purchasing decisions for drugs, vaccines, and other pharmaceutical products. It is therefore a critical step for introducing generic drugs into national formularies. Despite the prequalification process, as drugs are produced, there is no standard mechanism for continuous testing.[66] Some companies, such as the International Dispensary Association (IDA), specialize in the procurement and distribution of generic drugs to impoverished countries. The IDA performs batch testing on generic pharmaceuticals prior to distribution to countries or programs.[67] This extra layer of quality control is done at a small markup in price, and many governments and projects around the world rely on this additional standard of quality.

Country-Level Procurement and Distribution

Most impoverished and middle-income countries have a fairly similar system for procurement and distribution of drugs following a hub-and-spoke model.[68] Generally, the national drug program is in charge of forecasting need, assessing budgetary availability, and putting out a tender (or bid) for the annual drug order. This is often done separately for programs with donor funding (like those for AIDS or malaria) and for programs that have a separate procurement stream (vaccines are supported by UNICEF and TB drugs are supported by the GDF). The government procures drugs for the public system. Upon arrival, drugs are stored in a national drug store. District-level pharmacies and hospitals request the medicines from the national drug store based on utilization over the prior month or quarter. The drugs are then distributed from district depots to health centers, also based on consumption over the prior month or quarter.[69] At each level of procurement and distribution, many problems arise (Figure 9.3) resulting in an inadequate amount of needed medications. First, the impoverished country's available budget may be insufficient to purchase needed drugs to meet the disease burden. Second, a lack of management systems may result in leakage via theft or mismanagement of drugs. Third, it is not uncommon for poorly and erratically paid staff to sell drugs and supplies, even those that are supposed to be free of charge to patients, to supplement their salaries.[70] Fourth, the systems and inputs needed for distribution are inadequate. Vehicles needed to deliver drugs

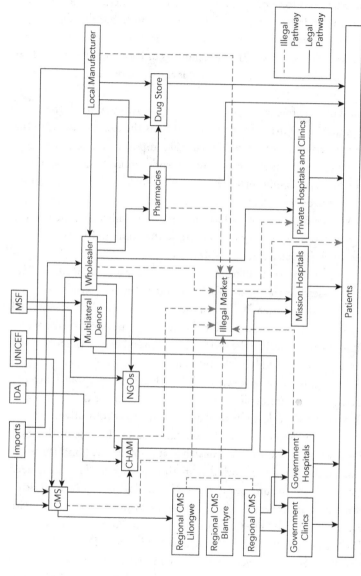

FIGURE 9.3 This figure illustrates the flow of pharmaceutical products in Malawi. The complicated system involves many actors from donors to manufacturers to nongovernmental organizations to health centers. At every level, there is opportunity for mismanagement and loss.

Source: McCabe, Ariane; Seiter, Andreas; Diack, Aissatou; Herbst, Christopher H.; Dutta, Sheila; Saleh, Karima. 2011. Private Sector Pharmaceutical Supply and Distribution Channels in Africa: A Focus on Ghana, Malawi and Mali. Health, Nutrition and Population (HNP) discussion paper; World Bank, Washington, DC. © World Bank. https://openknowledge.worldbank.org/handle/10986/13590 License: CC BY 3.0 IGO

from the national store to districts may be out of fuel or in disrepair, and paper records of utilization may be poorly kept or incomplete.[71] Finally, at each level— national, district and health center, forecasting is done based on the previous years consumption. Since the system is underutilized and experiences frequent stockouts, the true need for a drug is not registered and therefore not ordered. For example, if 10 children need amoxicillin in one month, but the pharmacy is stocked out after just two children receive the drug, the consumption of the drug for the month is registered as two. The next month's order would therefore be for just two courses of amoxicillin. This perpetuates the stock-out and the underuti- lization of services.

This method of drug forecasting is called the *consumption method*. The quan- tity or prior utilization of drugs may be referred to as the *demand signal*.[72] The consumption method of drug forecasting is used in impoverished countries. But, it has major flaws. When clinics are chronically underutilized—because of lack of staff and medicines—significantly lower levels of drugs are dispensed than are actually needed. The demand signal, in this case, is much lower than the disease burden. This vicious cycle of low utilization triggers insufficient procurement in the next cycle. Constant stock-outs also erode the community's trust in the health system which further depresses utilization.

The *morbidity method* is an alternative way to forecast drug needs. It does not depend on assessing the prior year's consumption but rather relies on the anticipated disease burden.[73] This method uses the number of expected cases and the standard regimen used to treat each case. Impoverished govern- ments are often unable to utilize the morbidity method because the forecasted amount of drugs needed to address the burden of disease would greatly exceed the national drug budget.[74] Moreover, weak health systems without Universal Health Coverage often cannot determine the full burden of disease because many people who are ill seek traditional alternatives to chronically underper- forming public health systems. Some experts also worry that use of the mor- bidity method will result in excess drugs that are not utilized and therefore wasted. However, the use of the morbidity method to forecast HIV drug need has proved successful.[75] In June 2006, the UN General Assembly committed to striving for universal coverage of HIV patients with ART by 2010,[76] with funding largely provided by the Global Fund and the President's Emergency Plan for AIDS Relief (PEPFAR).[77] The disease burden of HIV is well-known through ongoing, iterative surveillance. The confluence of money, political will, surveillance, and robust national plans has allowed countries like Rwanda to achieve near-universal coverage of HIV treatment (Figure 9.4). Stock outs of HIV drugs, even in impoverished countries, are rare.

While the global health era has seen improvement in drug access for some drugs,[78] a 2011 review showed that availability of essential drugs varied from as

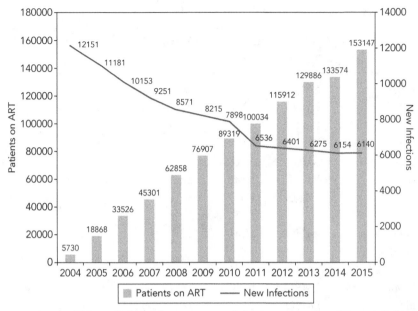

FIGURE 9.4 This graph shows the successes made by the government of Rwanda linking the disease burden of HIV to the supply chain needed to approach full-coverage ART. As coverage of ART has increased, the prevalence of HIV has decreased.

Source: Nsanzimana S, Prabhu K, McDermott H, Karita E, Forrest JI, Drobac P, Farmer P, Mills EJ, Binagwaho A. Improving health outcomes through concurrent HIV program scale-up and health system development in Rwanda: 20 years of experience. *BMC Med.* 2015 Sep 9;13:216. https://doi.org/10.1186/s12916-015-0443-z

low as 29 percent in the WHO African region to 54 percent in the Americas. The availability of drugs needed for chronic diseases was significantly lower.[79] As always, aggregate data hide varying degrees of inequality. Even as impoverished countries have received more external aid for health, committed more of their GDPs to health, and leveraged vertical money to strengthen health systems, there has been insufficient funding to markedly improve access to essential drugs.[79] A variety of approaches for expanding access to essential drugs are used, including fully privatized systems, user fees, revolving drug funds, and disease-specific drug funds.[80] In the resulting struggle, access remains limited and fragmented.

Drugs and Rights

Despite the financial barriers to access, more impoverished countries are guaranteeing the right to essential medicines in their constitutions,[81,82] as seen in Table 9.2. Countries are committing a larger share of their national budgets to the provision of health, and an adequate drug supply is essential for health care delivery. Legal cases in low- and middle-income countries have won verdicts that forced

Table 9.2 Global view of medicines-related rights in national constitutions.

Country	WHO Region	Income Level	Year of Adoption	Respect	Protect	Fulfill
Angola	AFRO	UMI	2010		✓	
Bolivia	PAHO	LMI	2009		✓	✓
Brazil	PAHO	UMI	2014		✓	
Bulgaria	EURO	LMI	2007		✓	
Cape Verde	AFRO	LMI	2010		✓	
Cuba	PAHO	UMI	2002			✓
Czech Republic	EURO	HI	2013			✓
Dominican Republic	PAHO	UMI	2010			✓
Ecuador	PAHO	UMI	2011	✓		✓
Egypt	EMRO	LMI	2014			✓
El Salvador	PAHO	LMI	2009		✓	
Guatemala	PAHO	LMI	1993		✓	
Honduras	PAHO	LMI	2013		✓	
Mexico	PAHO	UMI	2014			✓
Mozambique	AFRO	LI	2007		✓	
Niger	AFRO	LI	2010			✓
Panama	PAHO	UMI	2004			✓
Paraguay	PAHO	LMI	2011	✓		✓
Philippines	WPRO	LMI	1987	✓		✓
Portugal	EURO	HI	2005	✓		✓
Suriname	PAHO	UMI	1992	✓		
Syrian Arabic Republic	EMRO	LMI	2012			✓

Abbreviation used in this table: AFRO: WHO Africa Region: WHO Eastern Mediterranean Region; EURO: WHO European Region; PAHO: WHO Pan American Region; SEARO: WHO South East Asia Region; WPRO: WHO Western Pacific Region; LI: Low income economy; LMI: Lower middle income economy; UMI: Upper middle income economy; HI: High income economy

Source: Perehudoff SK, Toebes B, Hogerzeil H. Essential medicines in national constitutions: Progress since 2008. *Health Hum Rights*. 2016;18(1):141–156.

governments to procure needed drugs. Many such lawsuits about essential drugs were related to ART, as highlighted in Chapter 2, but lawsuits for access to other drugs have also been brought against the governments of Brazil, Thailand, and Ghana by civil society.[83]

Beginning in 2014, a *Lancet* international commission examined access to essential medicines and potential solutions to expand access in order to fulfill the commitment to the Sustainable Development Goals' (SDG) call for Universal Health Coverage.[84] The commission highlighted five areas of international collaboration needed to achieve the SDGs by 2030[85]: (1) paying for a basket of essential medicines, (2) making essential medicines affordable, (3) assuring the quality and safety of medicines, (4) promoting the correct use of medicines, and (5) developing missing essential medicines.

In November 2016, the Lancet Commission on Essential Medicines presented its report entitled "Essential Medicines for Universal Health Coverage." The report calculated that about $13–25 per capita per year was needed for countries to procure and distribute "a basket of essential medicines."[80] To provide a frame of reference, it is generally accepted that about $86 per capita in public financing is needed to achieve Universal Health Coverage.[86,87] This means that, at a rate of $13–25 per capita, governments would need to allot 15–27 percent of their health budget to purchasing medications. This is not that different from Organization for Economic Cooperation and Development (OECD) countries which spent between 6.7 percent (Denmark) to 30.2 percent (Hungary) of their health budgets on pharmaceuticals based on a 2014 study.[88] Proper financing is the critical challenge to assuring drug access for the achievement of Universal Health Coverage.

Conclusion

The access to drugs is a central feature of assuring the right to health. In the global health era, under pressure from activists, the WHO's EML is now continually being expanded to include new drugs. Yet development of new drugs is significantly shaped by market forces and the profit motive. Therefore, new drugs are rarely developed for the poor. The FDA Amendments Act of 2007 attempted to address these issues by incentivizing the development of drugs for neglected tropical diseases. New organizations such as the TB Drug Alliance are attempting to address market failures by philanthropically driven drug development. Other groups, like the GDF and Gavi, support countries through large-scale purchasing and assistance in forecasting. The cost of drugs, however, remains the major barrier to access. At the national level, impoverished countries cannot procure enough drugs to address the burden of disease. At the health center level, low utilization of services results in a woeful underestimate of true need. Some impoverished countries have included access to medicines in their national constitutions, but the international community must commit long term financing to increase drug access as central to the achievement of Universal Health Coverage.

References

1. Fleming A. On the antibacterial action of cultures of a penicillium, with special reference to their use in the isolation of B. influenzae. *Br J Exp Pathol.* 1929;10:226–236.

2. Hinshaw HC, Pyle MM, Feldman WH. Streptomycin in tuberculosis. *Am J Med.* 1947;2(5):429–435.

3. United Nations GA. *Universal declaration of human rights.* New York: United Nations Dept. of Public Information; 1952.

4. World Health Organization. *Chronicle of the World Health Organization.* Geneva: World Health Organization; 1947.

5. World Health Organization. Twenty-eighth World Health Assembly. Geneva: World Health Organization; 1975.

6. World Health Organization Expert Committee. The selection of essential drugs: World Health Organization technical report series 615. Geneva: World Health Organization; 1977.

7. World Health Organization. WHO Model Lists of Essential Medicines. 2015. Available from: http://www.who.int/medicines/publications/essentialmedicines/en/. Accessed Jan 18, 2017.

8. World Health Organization. Essential drugs and medicines policy. WHO African Region Web site. 2017. Available from: http://www.who.int/countries/eth/areas/medicines/en/. Accessed May 10, 2017.

9. World Health Organization. WHO Model List of Essential Medicines, 19th edition. Geneva: World Health Organization; 2015.

10. Reich MR. The global drug gap: drug market in rich and poor countries. *Science.* 2000;287(5460):1979.

11. McCabe A. Private sector pharmaceutical supply and distribution chains: Ghana, Mali and Malawi. *Health Systems for Outcomes: Pharmaceuticals.* 2009. http://documents.worldbank.org/curated/en/745621468270302773/Private-sector-pharmaceutical-supply-and-distribution-chains-Ghana-Mali-and-Malawi

12. Wagner AK, Graves AJ, Reiss SK, Lecates R, Zhang F, Ross-Degnan D. Access to care and medicines, burden of health care expenditures, and risk protection: Results from the world health survey. *Health Policy.* 2011;100(2):151–158.

13. Maciocco G, Stefanini A. From Alma Ata to the Global Fund: The history of international health policy. *Soc Med.* 2008;3(1):36–48.

14. Thomas C, Weber M. The politics of global health governance: Whatever happened to "health for all by the year 2000"? *Glob Govern.* 2004;10(2):187–205.

15. Kanji N. Charging for drugs in Africa: UNICEF's "Bamako Initiative." *Health Policy Plan.* 1989;4:110–120.

16. Chabot J. The Bamako Initiative. *Lancet.* 1988;332(8621):1177–1178. Available from: http://www.sciencedirect.com.ezp-prod1.hul.harvard.edu/science/article/pii/S0140673688902413.

17. Cheng H, Kotler P, Lee N. *Social marketing for public health: Global trends and success stories*. Sudbury, MA: Jones and Bartlett Publishers LLC; 2011.

18. Sawyer E. Remarks at the opening ceremony. ACT UP Web site. 1996. Available from: www.actupny.org/Vancouver/sawyerspeech.html. Accessed Nov 17, 2016.

19. Thoen E. TRIPS, pharmaceutical patents, and access to essential medicines: A long way from Seattle to Doha. *Chicago J Intl L*. 2002;3(1):27–68.

20. Berwick D. "We all have AIDS": Case for reducing the cost of HIV drugs to zero. *BMJ*. 2002;324(7331):214–216.

21. World Health Organization. WHO takes major steps to make HIV treatment accessible. Geneva, Switzerland; 2002. http://www.who.int/mediacentre/news/releases/release28/en/

22. Laing R, Waning B, Gray A, et al. 25 years of the WHO essential medicines lists: Progress and challenges. *Lancet*. 2003;361(9370):1723–1729.

23. Rosenberg T. Look at Brazil. *The New York Times Magazine*. January, 28, 2001.

24. World Trade Organization. *The DOHA declaration explained*. Geneva: World Trade Organization; 2001. Geneva, Switzerland.

25. Forman L, Kohler JC, eds. *Access to medicines as a human right: Implications for pharmaceutical industry responsibility*. Toronto: University of Toronto Press; 2012.

26. Gerth J, Stolberg SG. Medicine Merchants: Birth of a blockbuster. Drug makers reap profits on tax-backed research. *The New York Times*. April 23, 2000. Available from: http://www.nytimes.com/2000/04/23/us/medicine-merchants-birth-blockbuster-drug-makers-reap-profits-tax-backed.html.

27. Lee TT, Gluck AR, Curfman G. The politics of Medicare and drug-price negotiation. Bethesda, MD: Health Affairs Blog; September 19, 2016. http://healthaffairs.org/blog/2016/09/19/the-politics-of-medicare-and-drug-price-negotiation/

28. Hastert DJ. Medicare prescription drug, improvement, and modernization act of 2003. 2003. https://www.congress.gov/bill/108th-congress/house-bill/1

29. Kesselheim AS, Avorn J, Sarpatwari A. The high cost of prescription drugs in the United States: Origins and prospects for reform. *JAMA*. 2016;316(8):858–871.

30. Kounang N. Why pharmaceuticals are cheaper abroad. CNN. Sep 28, 2015. Available from: http://www.cnn.com/2015/09/28/health/us-pays-more-for-drugs/ Accessed Apr 21, 2017.

31. World Health Organization. Hepatitis C. Media Centre Web site. 2016. Available from: http://www.who.int/mediacentre/factsheets/fs164/en/. Accessed Jan 19, 2017.

32. Lawitz E, Mangia A, Wyles D, et al. Sofosbuvir for previously untreated chronic hepatitis C infection. *N Engl J Med*. 2013;369(7):678–679.

33. Smith M. Treating HCV—is the price right? *Medpage Today*. Feb 18, 2014. Available from: http://www.medpagetoday.com/gastroenterology/hepatitis/44357. Accessed Jan 19, 2017.

34. Canary LA, Klevens RM, Holmberg SD. Limited access to new hepatitis C virus treatment under state Medicaid programs. *Ann Intern Med*. 2015;163(3):226.

35. Roubein R. Senators hammer pharma over $84,000 hep. C drug. *The Atlantic.* December 1, 2015. https://www.theatlantic.com/politics/archive/2015/12/senators-hammer-pharma-firm-over-84000-hep-c-drug/456366/

36. Freyer FJ. Hepatitis C costs leave many without care. *Boston Globe.* April 9, 2016. Available from: https://www.bostonglobe.com/metro/2016/04/09/for-hepatitis-patients-cure-for-high-drug-prices/j2X4aVi7BEpU5BSL0YVovN/story.html. Accessed Apr 21, 2017.

37. Marseille E, Kahn JG. A revolution in treatment for hepatitis C infection: Mitigating the budgetary impact. *PLoS Medicine.* 2016;13(5):e1002031.

38. Moon S, Jambert E, Childs M, von Schoen-Angerer T. A win-win solution? A critical analysis of tiered pricing to improve access to medicines in developing countries. *Glob Health.* 2011;7(39). Available from: https://globalizationandhealth.biomedcentral.com/articles/10.1186/1744-8603-7-39.

39. MSF. Access campaign. Medecins Sans Frontieres Web site. 2017. https://www.msfaccess.org/. Accessed May 4, 2017.

40. Dreifuss R, Mogae FG. United Nations Secretary-General's high-level panel on access to medicines. 2017. Available from: http://www.unsgaccessmeds.org/new-page/. Accessed May 10, 2017.

41. Dreifuss R, Mogae F, Al-Khasawneh A, et al. *Report of the United Nations Secretary-General's high-level panel on access to medicines: Promoting innovation and access to health technologies.* United Nations Secretary-General's High-Level Panel on Access to Medicines. Geneva, Switzerland: United Nations Secretary-General's High-Level Panel on Access to Medicines (United Nations); 2016.

42. High-Level Panel on Access to Medicines. *United Nations Secretary-General's high-level panel on access to medicines: Promoting innovation and access factsheet.* Geneva, Switzerland: United Nations Secretary-General's High-Level Panel on Access to Medicines (United Nations); 2016.

43. Dickson M, Jean PG. Key factors in the rising cost of new drug discovery and development. *Nat Rev Drug Discovery.* 2004;3(5):417.

44. Trouiller P, Olliaro P, Torreele E, Orbinski J, Laing R, Ford N. Drug development for neglected diseases: A deficient market and a public-health policy failure. *Lancet.* 2002;359(9324):2188–2194.

45. Mccabe C, Edlin R, Round J. Economic considerations in the provision of treatments for rare diseases. *Adv Exp Med Biol.* 2010;686:211–222.

46. Deegan PB, Cox TM. Imiglucerase in the treatment of Gaucher disease: A history and perspective. *Drug Design Dev Ther.* 2012;6:81–106.

47. Weisman R. New Genzyme pill will cost patients $320,250 a year. *The Boston Globe.* Sep 2, 2014. Available from: https://www.bostonglobe.com/business/2014/09/02/new-genzyme-pill-treat-rare-gaucher-disease-will-cost-patients-year/5thkIb587nKi7zRAb9GgxM/story.html. Accessed May 10, 2017.

48. Gupta R, Kim J, Espinal M, Caudron J. Responding to market failures to tuberculosis control. *Science.* 2001;293(5532):1049–1051.

49. Archibugi D, Bizzarri K. The global governance of communicable diseases: The case for vaccine R& D. *Law Policy*. 2005;27(1):33–51.

50. Zumla A, Nahid P, Cole ST. Advances in the development of new tuberculosis drugs and treatment regimens. *Nat Rev Drug Discovery*. 2013;12(5):388.

51. Robertson AS. Preserving an incentive for global health R& D. *Am J Law Med*. 2016;42(2-3):524–542.

52. Silverstein K. Millions for Viagra, pennies for diseases of the poor. *The Nation*. July 19, 1999. https://www.thenation.com/article/millions-viagra-pennies-diseases-poor/

53. Chu B. Bill gates: Why do we care more about baldness than malaria? *Independent*. Mar 16, 2013. Available from: http://www.independent.co.uk/news/world/americas/bill-gates-why-do-we-care-more-about-baldness-than-malaria-8536988.html. Accessed Apr 21, 2017.

54. Waltz E. FDA launches priority vouchers for neglected-disease drugs. *Nat Biotechnol*. 2008;26(12):1315.

55. Ridley RG. Medical need, scientific opportunity and the drive for antimalarial drugs. *Nature*. 2002;415(6872):686.

56. TB Alliance. Donors. 2017. Available from: https://www.tballiance.org/about/donors. Accessed Jan 23, 2017.

57. UNOPS. Stop TB partnership. 2017. Available from: http://www.stoptb.org/. Accessed Apr 21, 2017.

58. Brenda W, Ellen D, Suerie M. A lifeline to treatment: The role of Indian generic manufacturers in supplying antiretroviral medicines to developing countries. *JAIDS*. 2010;13(1):35.

59. Chaudhuri S. *The WTO and India's pharmaceuticals industry: Patent protection, TRIPS, and developing countries*. New Delhi/New York: Oxford University Press; 2005.

60. Medecins Sans Frontieres. Untangling the web of antiretroviral price reductions. Geneva, Switzerland: Medecins Sans Frontieres Access Campaign, 18th Edition; 2016. https://www.msfaccess.org/sites/default/files/HIV_report_Untangling-the-web-18thed_ENG_2016.pdf

61. Basheer S. India's tryst with TRIPS: The patents (amendment) act, 2005. *Ind J L Tech*. 2005;1.

62. Bate R, Tren R, Mooney L, et al. Pilot study of essential drug quality in two major cities in India. *PLoS One*. 2009;4(6):e6003.

63. US Food & Drug Administration. Facts about the current good manufacturing practices (CGMPs). 2016. Available from: http://www.fda.gov/Drugs/DevelopmentApprovalProcess/Manufacturing/ucm169105.htm. Accessed Jan 23, 2017.

64. World Health Organization. Essential medicines and health products: Production. 2014. Available from: http://www.who.int/medicines/areas/quality_safety/quality_assurance/production/en/. Accessed Jan 24, 2017.

65. World Health Organization. Prequalification. 2017. Available from: http://www.who.int/topics/prequalification/en/. Accessed Apr 21, 2017.

66. Nayyar GM, Breman JG, Newton PN, Herrington J. Poor-quality antimalarial drugs in Southeast Asia and sub-Saharan Africa. *Lancet Infect Dis.* 2012;12(6):488–496.

67. IDA Foundation. Quality assurance of supplies. Available from: http://www.ida-foundation.org/quality/quality-assurance-of-supplies.html. Accessed Jan 23, 2017.

68. Klose A, Drexl A. Facility location models for distribution system design. *Eur J Oper Res.* 2005;162(1):4–29.

69. Ripin D, Jamieson D, Meyers A, Warty U, Dain M, Khamsi C. Antiretroviral procurement and supply chain management. *Antivir Ther (Lond).* 2014;19:79–89.

70. Ferrinho P, Omar MC, Fernandes MDJ, Blaise P, Bugalho AM, Lerberghe WV. Pilfering for survival: How health workers use access to drugs as a coping strategy. *Hum Resources Health.* 2004;2:4.

71. USAID Deliver Project. Using last mile distribution to increase access to health commodities. 2011.

72. Hook J. 6 trends shaking the pharmaceutical market. Arlington, VA: USAID; 2017. http://www.villagereach.org/wp-content/uploads/2011/12/UsinLastMileDist.pdf

73. Griffiths A. *Estimating drug requirements: A practical manual.* Geneva: World Health Organization; 1991.

74. Redditt V, ole-MoiYoi K, Rodriguez J, Weintraub R. Malaria control in Zambia. *Cases in Global Health Delivery.* Harvard Business Publishing; 2012. http://www.globalhealthdelivery.org/files/ghd/files/ghd-024_malaria_control_in_zambia.pdf

75. World Bank NO. *Managing procurement and logistics of HIV/AIDS drugs and related supplies: Report of a regional training workshop.* Washington, DC: World Bank, World Health Organization, Global Fund, MSH, JSI/DELIVER and ESTHER, with support from the National Action Committee on AIDS (NACA); 2005.

76. World Health Organization. *Toward universal access scaling up priority HIV/AIDS interventions in the health sector. Progress report, April 2007.* Geneva: World Health Organization, UNAIDS, UNICEF; 2007.

77. Ravishankar N, Gubbins P, Cooley RJ, et al. Financing of global health: Tracking development assistance for health from 1990 to 2007. *Lancet.* 2009;373(9681):2113–2124.

78. Hogerzeil HV. The concept of essential medicines: Lessons for rich countries. *BMJ.* 2004;329(7475):1169.

79. Nunan M, Duke T. Effectiveness of pharmacy interventions in improving availability of essential medicines at the primary healthcare level. *Trop Med Intl Health.* 2011;16(5):647–658.

80. Wirtz VJ, Hogerzeil HV, Gray AL, et al. Essential medicines for universal health coverage. *Lancet.* 2017;389(10067):403–476.

81. Perehudoff SK, Toebes B, Hogerzeil H. Essential medicines in national constitutions: Progress since 2008. *Health Hum Rights.* 2016;18(1):141–156.

82. Perehudoff SK, Laing RO, Hogerzeil HV. Access to essential medicines in national constitutions. *Bull World Health Org.* 2010;88(11):800.

83. Beall R, Kuhn R. Trends in compulsory licensing of pharmaceuticals since the Doha Declaration: A database analysis (compulsory licensing of pharmaceuticals). *PLoS Med.* 2012;9(1):e1001154.

84. Commissions from the Lancet Journals. Essential medicines. 2016. Available from: http://www.thelancet.com/commissions/essential-medicines. Accessed Jan 17, 2017.

85. Wirtz VJ, Hogerzeil HV, Gray AL, et al. Essential medicines for universal health coverage. *Lancet.* 2016;389(10082):1881–1882.

86. Yates R. Estimate for UHC costs. 2017.

87. Rottingen John-Arne, Ottersen T, Ablo A, et al. *Shared responsibilities for health: A coherent global framework for health financing.* London: Chatham House, The Royal Institute of International Affairs; 2014.

88. OECD Data. Pharmaceutical spending. OECD.org Web site. 2014. Available from: https://data.oecd.org/healthres/pharmaceutical-spending.htm. Accessed May 10, 2017.

Monitoring, Evaluation, Disease Surveillance, and Quality Improvement

Key Points

- Good clinical data is critical to optimizing the care of the individual patient. Data also supports planning and evaluating programs and health systems.
- Paper records are still the main source of health data in impoverished countries. This makes evaluation and quality improvement difficult.
- Health information systems are among the basic building blocks of health systems. They increasingly have an electronic component.
- Investments in electronic medical records are increasingly important as complex care is delivered.
- Standard data sets, such as tuberculosis cohort data and demographic health surveys (DHS), are ways that national programs can be evaluated and compared with one another.
- Quality improvement in health care delivery relies on the collection of high quality data and on monitoring and evaluation frameworks.

Introduction

The first Global Burden of Disease Project in 1990 as well as the Disease Control Priorities report and the World Development Report in 1993,[1-3] highlighted the need for health information. At that time, it was clear that a lack of quality data hampered the understanding of the burden of disease. Furthermore, as disease outbreaks such as AIDS, severe acute respiratory syndrome (SARS), cholera, and Ebola[4-6] moved to the forefront of international attention, robust systems for surveillance, monitoring, and evaluation were needed not only to protect public health but also to deliver quality care to the sick.

In order to meet the targets set by the UN's Millennium Development Goals (MDGs) and benchmark progress, countries required the development of data systems to follow individual patients, evaluate population-level data, and assure that care reached the most vulnerable. To facilitate standardized data collection, a globally agreed-upon set of international metrics was developed to reflect community-, country-, and international-level health information.[7] This chapter addresses the evolution of health data in the global health era. The chapter also outlines the use of monitoring and evaluation for programmatic quality improvement.

Registers, Records, and Health Information Systems

Medical record rooms in impoverished countries are often home to stacks of weather-worn paper categorized by patient name, number, or location. It can be impossible to wade through the morass of papers to find out when a patient's last clinic visit was or what drugs were prescribed. While wealthy countries have electronic systems, in impoverished settings, medical records are generally paper-based, and the systems and personnel needed to adequately maintain them are lacking. The chaotic paper-based systems for medical records limits both the ability to provide high-quality care to the individual patient and to assess the health outcomes of the population.

Prior to the global health era, health systems were not designed to offer continuous, longitudinal care.[8] Thus, patients with chronic diseases were intermittently treated and would eventually return with severe complications of their diseases. High blood pressure is an interesting example of a chronic condition that requires longitudinal management and is often neglected due to a lack of data systems. Most people with high blood pressure do not have symptoms. However, to avoid the long-term consequences of untreated hypertension, such as heart disease, patients need a consistent supply of antihypertensive medication and regular monitoring. They also need education and reminders to refill prescriptions and continue their therapy. Because patients with hypertension are asymptomatic, they generally present at clinics for other complaints (like a cough or a cold), and their high blood pressure is detected incidentally (Figure 10.1). In impoverished settings, it is not uncommon to see a person who has been evaluated many times by different providers for different presenting symptoms but is also found to have high blood pressure at each visit. Such patients are often treated or their acute illness and may or may not be treated for their high blood pressure (depending on what is available). Patients with this chronic condition may experience gaps of months or even years between prescriptions.

		AMBULATORY CARE CARD **Name** *Lovely Smith* **Address**		MINISTRY OF HEALTH **Date of Birth** *64 y.o.* **Village** *Freeland 6*	
Date	**Vital Signs**	**Symptoms**	**Diagnosis**	**Treatment**	**Provider**
9/24/2000	200/100 60kg 37 C	*Cough, SOB, pain* *Chest crackles*	*pneumonia*	*Penicillin po x 10d.* *paracetamol, Vit B12*	*Dr. Patrick*
08/08/2001	190/90	*1 Very itchy rash on hands,* *pustules between fingers*	*Scabies, hypertension*	*Benzoate benzyl apply to whole body* *3 nights, wash clothes in hot water, Miss Carmen* *HCTZ 25 mg po qd*	
4/12/2004	187/85 61kg	Diarrhea x 3 weeks. No vomiting or fever, headache and dizziness	Gastroenteritis	ORS sachets x10	*Dr. Paul*
6/12/2010	200/120	Cannot speak or walk, listless	*Stroke*	*Supportive care*	*Dr. Mary*

FIGURE 10.1 An illustration of a standard outpatient medical record. In this fictional example, the patient, Lovely Smith, who was 64 years old was seen three times in 10 years without a clear follow up plan. While she presented with acute illnesses she also had underlying high blood pressure. She is seen by different providers, whose handwriting is not very legible. There is no space on the medical card to properly follow-up a chronic condition. She returns with symptoms of a stroke from untreated or sporadically treated high blood pressure.

The issue of poor medical records has plagued health delivery in impoverished countries for decades.[9] There have been efforts made to streamline and simplify data collection since the era of selective primary health care. One example of a simplified record for a vertical program is UNICEF's Road to Health card (Figure 10.2).[10] The card is provided to the parents of children under the age of five. It provides space to chart serial weights along a preprinted growth chart so that the child's growth may be followed over time. The card also has space to record the date and type of vaccinations administered. The Road to Health card also has instructional pictures for parents on the use of oral rehydration salts to prevent severe dehydration, on the importance of breastfeeding, and on the milestones of child development. Some countries have more extensive Road to Health cards with information for maternal health records. Generally the mother keeps the card and presents it at vaccination visits which avoids the need for medical record storage at the facility.

In other countries, patient-held booklets are used by adults and children; these booklets feature formatted pages for pregnancy follow-up or HIV treatment and blank pages for general care.[11] These booklets (Figure 10.3) are helpful if the previous care given to the patient has been documented. The limitations of patient-held booklets are that they are easily lost or damaged. Patient booklets

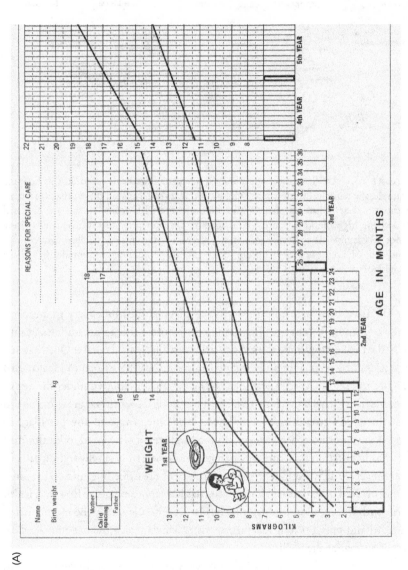

(A)

(B)

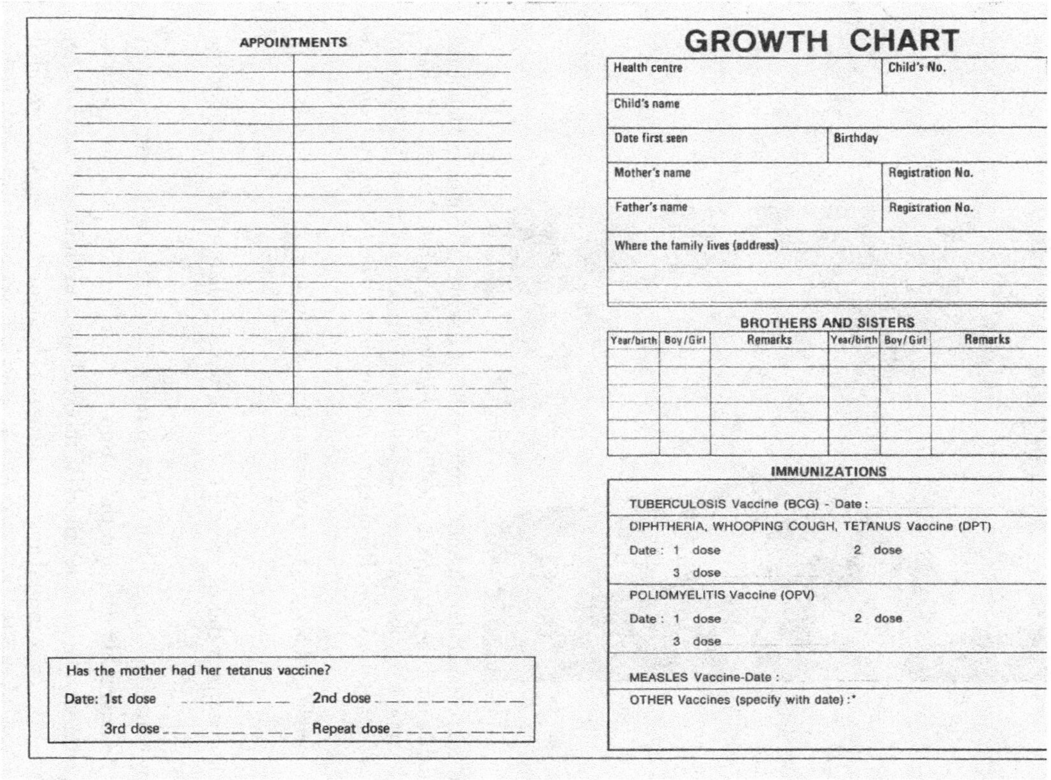

APPOINTMENTS

GROWTH CHART

Health centre	Child's No.

Child's name

Date first seen	Birthday

Mother's name	Registration No.

Father's name	Registration No.

Where the family lives (address)

BROTHERS AND SISTERS

Year/birth	Boy/Girl	Remarks	Year/birth	Boy/Girl	Remarks

IMMUNIZATIONS

TUBERCULOSIS Vaccine (BCG) - Date :

DIPHTHERIA, WHOOPING COUGH, TETANUS Vaccine (DPT)

Date : 1 dose   2 dose

3 dose

POLIOMYELITIS Vaccine (OPV)

Date : 1 dose   2 dose

3 dose

MEASLES Vaccine-Date :

OTHER Vaccines (specify with date) :*

Has the mother had her tetanus vaccine?

Date: 1st dose   2nd dose

3rd dose   Repeat dose

FIGURE 10.2 Photograph of the standard Road to Health Growth Card used throughout the world in child survival programs.

Source: World Health Organization (WHO); received courtesy of UNICEF.

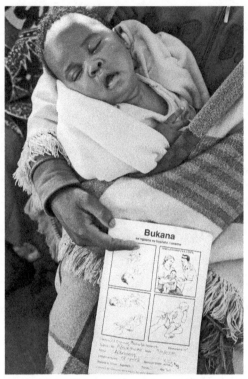

FIGURE 10.3 Malethoko Mohohala waits with her daughter, Sebonoang Mohohala, for postnatal care at the Partners in Health-funded clinic in Bobete, Lesotho. The baby girl was born on December 12, 2012 at 2.25 kilograms. The father of the child is Majoma Mohohala (listed on *bukana*). The mother and baby walked to Bobete from the village of Likomeng.

Source: Partners in Health, 2013; photo courtesy of Rebecca E. Rollins.

also do not support the aggregation of data for surveillance and analysis at the health center level.

Many countries collect health data in registers at each clinic. Basic registers include demographic data and the reason for visit. Vertical programs, such as family planning, maternal health, HIV, tuberculosis, and childhood vaccination, often have separate records demanded by donors.[12] All of these registers are filled in and aggregated by hand. Aggregated data are sent to the Ministry of Health on a regular basis. Given the woeful understaffing of the clinics (as discussed in Chapter 7), it is not uncommon for health center staff to complain about the amount of paperwork and number of registers to be filled out for a single visit. More recently, as donor demand for data has grown, so too has the paperwork and even the sheer size of the registers.[12]

To respond to these demands, better health information systems (HIS) to support data collection and aggregation for health system evaluation and planning are being developed. Large international collaborations are developing and implementing electronic medical records (EMR).[13] Personal devices, such as smartphones and tablets, are also increasingly being used by clinic-based staff and community health workers to record a variety of inputs, including data from community surveillance and medication adherence.[14,15] These new technologies increase the quality and accessibility of patient data and thereby improve patient care. However, they are costly and can disrupt workflow.[16,17] Additional staffing is often required for data entry and maintenance of the system. Regardless of the technology used, strong HIS improve health outcomes (see Figure 3.5)[18] but require more resources.

Data common to most HIS include[19]:

- descriptive statistics of the population (age, gender, address, etc.)
- economic data (household assets, income, etc.)
- the prevalence of various health determinants (access to water, smoking, etc.)
- the health status of the population (frequency of different conditions and associated morbidity and mortality)
- metrics about the health system's performance (the number of health workers, access to drugs, electricity, etc.)

HIS are very costly. For example, in May 2015, the Partners HealthCare, a large medical network in Boston, Massachusetts (comprising 10 hospitals and more than 6,000 doctors) launched a new EMR system in 2014 that cost $1.2 billion.[20] Most hospitals in wealthy countries use private, copyrighted systems that are bought or leased. EMRs are a significant recurrent cost for these health systems. Because of the dire need for electronic systems in the global health era and the exorbitant cost of private systems, a movement arose to significantly decrease the cost of EMRs. An international group of programmers and designers created Open Medical Records System (OpenMRS).[21] OpenMRS began in 2004 as a nonprofit organization led by the Regenstrief Institute in South Africa and Partners in Health, with the mission of creating an open source medical records system for developing countries. The software platform is designed to provide countries the ability to customize their EMRs system with minimal programming knowledge. The use of OpenMRS is free of charge. It is now being used in Kenya, Rwanda, South Africa, Mozambique, Haiti, India, China, Pakistan, the United States, the Philippines, and many other countries around the world.[21] There are other efforts from impoverished countries to implement low-cost HIS. One example is Baobab Health Trust (BHT), a Malawi-based nongovernmental organization (NGO) founded in 2001.[22] BHT designs and develops point-of-care EMRs, with an emphasis on employing and empowering local people. Another example of open-source EMR is Ubuntu, a South African programming enterprise founded in 2004.[23]

Demographic Health Surveys

Countries track health data at the population level on a regular basis to evaluate their progress and to compare progress between countries. Since the mid-1980s, the growing importance of data has led to the development of country-level surveys called Demographic Health Surveys (DHS).[24] These surveys are coordinated with the country and supported by the US Agency for International Development (USAID) with input from UNICEF, the World Health Organization (WHO), and UNAIDS. DHS are now performed in more than 90 countries in Africa, Asia, Latin America, and the Caribbean and generally performed every five years.[25] The information collected includes total fertility (number of children born to a woman), access to family planning and other reproductive health services, maternal health, child health (including immunizations and child survival), HIV/AIDS, malaria, and the nutritional status of pregnant women and children under the age of five.[25] A sample DHS table of contents can be found in Box 10.1. The purpose of the DHS program is to support the collection and use of data at the country level to help with program monitoring and evaluation. DHS data also support the development of evidence-based health policies.[24] When implementing global health programs and analyzing impact, the DHS data are often used as the baseline.

The Development of Common Indicators: Example from Tuberculosis Control

One factor that all the efforts to improve data collection and utilization have in common is the need for standardized health indicators and outcome definitions. Common indicator and outcome definitions are important to evaluate the impact of programs so that strengths and weaknesses can be identified and shared. An *indicator* is defined as a specific, observable, and measurable factor that can be used to track the progress of patients, health systems, and populations.[26] Indicators may measure inputs, processes, outputs, or outcomes. A *health outcome* is the impact that a disease or intervention has on the population.[27]

The treatment and control of tuberculosis (TB) is a useful example to discuss indicators and outcomes. (For historical reasons, TB data are not part of the

---

BOX 10.1

Example DHS Table of Contents (Tanzania)

Demographic and Health Survey—Tanzania 2010

- Chapter 1—Introduction
- Chapter 2—Household Population and Housing Characteristics
- Chapter 3—Characteristics of Respondents
- Chapter 4—Fertility Levels, Trends, and Differentials
- Chapter 5—Fertility Regulation
- Chapter 6—Other proximate Determinants of Fertility
- Chapter 7—Fertility Preferences
- Chapter 8—Infant and Child Mortality
- Chapter 9—Maternal Health
- Chapter 10—Child Health
- Chapter 11—Children's and Women's Nutrition
- Chapter 12—Malaria
- Chapter 13—HIV and AIDS-Related Knowledge, Attitudes and Behaviour
- Chapter 14—Women's Empowerment and Demographic and Health Outcomes
- Chapter 15—Adult and Maternal Mortality
- Chapter 16—Gender-Based Violence
- Chapter 17—Female Genital Cutting

DHS.) Because TB is an airborne disease and treatment prevents transmission, it was among the first conditions to be treated even when public health programs in impoverished countries were focused on prevention only. Treatment of TB, however, is long. It requires multiple drugs given over six to eight months. Patients with TB must adhere to daily treatment to be cured and so as not to develop resistant strains of the bacteria. To manage the long-term, multidrug treatment at national scale, a standardized monitoring and evaluation process was developed.

In 1993, a plan was launched to scale-up TB case finding and treatment.[28] Longitudinal treatment was new in impoverished settings, and the fear of patients developing resistance to the new drugs being introduced in Africa and elsewhere was great. Therefore, the new global TB program called for observation of each dose of medicine for the duration of treatment. This plan was called the directly observed therapy short-course (DOTS).[29] Through this program, TB diagnosis and treatment, previously only done in specialized TB centers, was decentralized to health centers.[30] Laboratories were given microscopes, and personnel were trained to look for the bacteria that causes TB (a test called *sputum microscopy*). Personnel at health centers were trained to initiate and follow-up a multidrug regimen for TB. The staff was instructed to observe each daily treatment for six to eight months. Countries were expected to adhere to five key principles[31] of the DOTS strategy:

1. Sustained political commitment
2. Access to quality-assured TB sputum microscopy
3. Standardized short-course (six-month) chemotherapy (drugs) administered to all patients with TB under proper case management conditions, including direct observation of treatment (DOT)
4. Uninterrupted national supply of quality-assured drugs
5. A recording and reporting system that enables outcome assessment

The fifth principle—that of having a recording and reporting system that enables outcome assessment—was critical to achieving the other strategic components of DOTS. Tracking the number of treatments allowed for accurate drug forecasting to prevent stock-outs. Forecasting based on data was also needed to assure the adequate stock of laboratory supplies to detect people who need treatment. Finally, the data—including the number of people cured and those lost to follow-up—allowed for the analysis of the program.

National TB programs are evaluated by three main indicators: case detection rate, coverage rate, and treatment success rate (Table 10.1).[32] Each of these indicators has a standardized definition. First, a case must be defined. A new case of smear positive TB is defined as a person who has given a sputum sample (usually because they are coughing) in which the TB bacteria is seen under a microscope. The indicator *case detection rate* gauges the strength of case finding in a country. It is reported as the percentage of new cases of smear positive TB divided by the number of cases of smear positive TB expected in a community (based on internationally supported surveillance estimates).[32] *DOTS coverage* refers to a facility with personnel who are trained to perform case detection by smear microscopy, administer treatment, and keep a register of those tested and on treatment. The *DOTS coverage rate* is the number of public facilities that can detect and treat TB under the DOTS strategy as a percentage of the total number of public facilities. Treatment success refers to a patient who has completed TB treatment and no longer has TB bacteria in his or her sputum. The *treatment success rate* number of the patients who achieve treatment success as a percentage of all patients diagnosed with TB and started on treatment within a specific period.[32] Using

Table 10.1 Summary of common indicators for tuberculosis (TB) programs.

Indicator	Definition
Case	A person with TB bacteria in their sputum (smear)
Case Detection Rate	New cases of smear positive TB cases as a percentage of those anticipated in the community
DOTS Coverage Rate	Public facilities that have received the training and tools to provide DOTS as a percentage of the total number of facilities.
Treatment Success Rate	Number of patients who achieved treatment success as a percentage of all patients who were diagnosed with TB and started on treatment

DOTS, Directly observed therapy short-course.

common indicators, it is possible to evaluate the strengths and weaknesses of a national TB program. Common indicators allow for comparison between programs as well (Table 10.2).

At the health center level, personnel in the TB program are trained to use these common indicators. Standardized paper treatment records are used to track the direct observation of each dose of treatment (Figure 10.4). Health centers

Table 10.2 Tuberculosis (TB) case detection rate, DOTS coverage, and treatment success rate Peru and Nigeria 1999.

	Peru		Nigeria	
	GDP per Capita	Life Expectancy	GDP per Capita	Life Expectancy
	1,963	74	299	46
Indicator				
TB case detection rate	80%		7%	
DOTS coverage	100%		45%	
Treatment success rate	90%		79%	

DOTS, directly observed therapy short-course; GDP, gross domestic product.

Source: Data abstracted from Encyclopedia of the Nations. DOTS population coverage, tuberculosis, communicable diseases, World Health Organization. 1999. Available from: http://www.nationsencyclopedia.com/WorldStats/WHO-tb-dots-population-coverage.html. Accessed May 31, 2017.

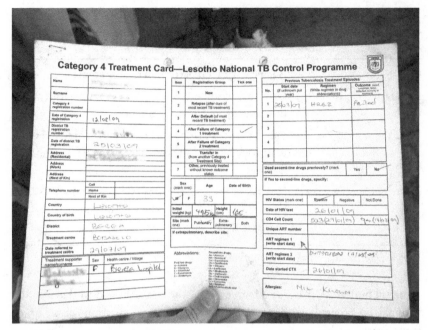

FIGURE 10.4   An example of a Category 4 treatment card for the Lesotho National TB Programme, with patient information blurred out.

Source: Partners in Health; photo courtesy of Jennie Riley.

report on the patients screened and treated on a regular basis.[33] Clinics record standard outcomes for a group of patients (known as a cohort) who received treatment during the previous six months. The outcomes for each cohort analyzed are segregated into five mutually exclusive categories: treatment success (smear negative at the end of treatment), death (of any cause during treatment), default (failure to take drugs for at least two consecutive months), failure (smear positive at the end of treatment or within five months of treatment completion), transferred out (to another location in the TB program), and completed treatment (completed course of medication but does not meet criteria for success or failure).[32] The cohort is analyzed with these five outcomes, and the results are reported to the national TB program twice yearly.[32] While there are many global challenges in TB control and the DOTS strategy is imperfect,[34,35] the use of standardized indicators and outcomes is important.

TB is just one example of the use of standardized indicators and outcomes. Vaccination programs, among the oldest programs in public health, also have a standardized set of indicators and outcomes. Indicators used for vaccination programs included programmatic indictors such as the number of children fully immunized by age one as a percentage of all children who were born in a given year (birth cohort). Indicators can also measure political commitment or government capabilities such as the percentage of routine vaccines financed by the.[36] A more recent example of work to standardize indicators and outcomes is the Primary Health Care Performance Initiative (PHCPI), launched in September 2015 by the Bill and Melinda Gates Foundation, the World Bank, the WHO, and the UN General Assembly. The initiative is led by Ariadne Labs[37] and seeks to facilitate and promote better data measurement and data sharing to evaluate the delivery of primary health care.[38] PHCPI has defined 25 indicators that they call "vital signs" to evaluate a health system. The PHCPI indictors include inputs (such as staffing and supply chain), service delivery (such as number or patients seen), and outputs (such as facility based deliveries performed). The goal of the initiative is to link these indicators with the outcomes of primary health care systems to support planning and quality improvement.

Data for Health as a Human Right

Data used for monitoring, evaluation, disease surveillance, and quality improvement are often aggregated across districts, countries, and even regions. Aggregated data hide inequalities. When equity and the right to health care is the goal, the disaggregation of data is critical to understand who receives an intervention, who has a positive outcome, and why. For example, the aggregated life expectancy of Boston is high (about 80 years), but the disaggregated data shows a 33-year difference in life expectancy between the rich and poor within Boston.[39] Disaggregating the data would reveal discrepancies relating to neighborhood differences in social determinants of health such as a lack of health insurance, poor access to grocery stores, substandard housing, racism, and violence.[39] A rights-based approach demands disaggregating data to assure the needs of the most vulnerable are considered to make progress toward equitable outcomes.

Choosing indicators and outcomes that reflect equity is also important. In the previous example of TB, each target, indicator, and outcome measured tracked the achievement of a program. Yet the WHO set the target of case detection at 70 percent of total cases. In choosing an indicator, it is important to understand what it does and does not represent. When examining that target through a human rights lens, one should question why 70 percent was set as the global target for case detection (rather than 100 percent case detection being the goal). Who was more likely to be reached with these programs? The 70 percent target was chosen because it represented the percent of adult TB patients expected to have a positive smear test (in the era before HIV). A positive smear occurs when the sputum sample from a cough contains enough bacteria to see under a microscope.[40,41] The indicator was chosen because smear-positive TB is considered more infectious from a public health perspective and, therefore, more important for disease control. However, more than 30 percent of people who have TB do not have a positive smear. They, too, have a right to treatment. Children, adults with HIV, and those with malnutrition commonly have TB outside the lungs or insufficiently concentrated to show up in a sputum sample.[41] These people may have forms called *extrapulmonary and smear-negative TB*. People with smear-negative TB are often vulnerable and poor. If smear-positive TB is the only form recognized by the TB program, patients with other forms of TB will get sick and die without a diagnosis or treatment.

One approach to analyze equity is to evaluate subsets of indicators in the most vulnerable population. For example, improvements in the health indicators in the lowest economic quintile would be considered a measure of programmatic success.[42] Another approach is to choose indicators that reflect the severity of disease because the most vulnerable suffer from delayed care. A choice of indicators that captures inequities from the outset is best.

Core Health Indicators

Indicators and outcomes are increasingly important to benchmark the progress of a country toward the Millennium and Sustainable Development Goals. Reports on many different indicators are demanded by a variety of donor-funded and vertical programs. In 2014, the WHO led an effort to harmonize indicators to reduce the burden of reporting on country programs. In 2015, the WHO, along with other major health agencies, published the Global Reference List of 100 Core Health Indicators[7] to help countries select indicators, align with reporting requirements, harmonize global databases, facilitate analytical capacity, and reflect evolving public health priorities. The 100 indicators are grouped into four main areas: health status, risk factors, service coverage, and health systems (Table 10.3).

As health is delivered, it is important for countries and programs to decide where the indicator will be captured (at registration, in the laboratory, in the clinic) and by whom it will be recorded (data clerk, provider). It is also important to know how data will be recorded, aggregated, and archived (by paper system, electronic record, cell phone, or tablet). Training, ongoing mentoring, and supervision regarding the collection, aggregation, analysis, and evaluation of indicators is needed to assure that the data collected are of high enough quality to support patient care and planning efforts.

Table 10.3 Core health indicators by group.

Health Status	Risk Factors	Service Coverage	Health Systems
Mortality by age and sex	Nutrition	Reproductive, maternal, newborn, child and adolescent	Quality and safety of care
Mortality by cause	Infections		Access
	Environmental risk factors	Immunization	Health workforce
Fertility	Noncommunicable diseases	HIV	Health information
Morbidity		HIV/TB	
	Injuries	Tuberculosis	Health financing
		Malaria	Health security
		Neglected tropical diseases	
		Screening and preventative care	
		Mental health	

Source: World Health Organization. *Global reference list of 100 core health indicators*. Geneva: World Health Organization; 2015.

Monitoring and Evaluation Frameworks

While some vertical programs (such as TB control or childhood vaccination initiatives) have standard monitoring and evaluation frameworks, not all global health initiatives have standard frameworks. In the global health era, it is common practice to develop a framework for monitoring and evaluation at the onset of a program. Indicators are selected that can measure input, processes, outputs, and outcomes. They are tracked in a way that reflects the programmatic flow over time. Each indicator should have a clear definition that is easily understandable and, when possible, based on available data. When evaluating the processes and outcomes of a program, it is important to know the baseline value of the indicator prior to the intervention period. It is also helpful to have a target or desired value that will be achieved if the program has its desired effect. As monitoring plans are elaborated, it is important to define the source of the data, frequency of its collection, and the staff person responsible for collecting the data. Monitoring and evaluation frameworks can be developed for a specific intervention (training a community to wash their hands), for a program (national TB program), or for an entire health system.

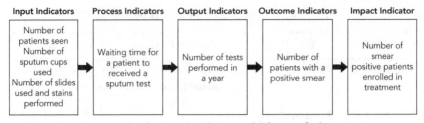

Input Indicators	Process Indicators	Output Indicators	Outcome Indicators	Impact Indicator
Number of patients seen Number of sputum cups used Number of slides used and stains performed	Waiting time for a patient to received a sputum test	Number of tests performed in a year	Number of patients with a positive smear	Number of smear positive patients enrolled in treatment

FIGURE 10.5 An example of tuberculosis logic model for case finding.

One common way for programs to organize a monitoring framework is by using a *logic model* (Figure 10.5). The logic model is a way to describe a system in a stepwise fashion that illustrates the interrelatedness of the elements of the program.[43] The purpose of creating a logic model is to depict the steps of an intervention and to analyze each step. Because problems in global health delivery are increasingly complex, the logic model can be a helpful way to map out a theory of change and analyze the impacts of each component.[44]

Once a logic model or other monitoring framework has been developed, the data recorded for each step may be compared to an expected value. Process improvement depends on this type of analysis. Using TB case detection as an example, if only 10 percent of the expected cases were diagnosed in a year, looking at each step in the logic model for case detection would help define areas of weakness. For example, if the country is stocked-out of sputum cups, fewer tests would be performed nationwide; whereas, if the stain used to prepare the sputum was contaminated, a sufficient number of test would have been done, but the number that were positive would be lower than expected. Another tool which is used to elucidate the details of a program and define monitoring processes is called a *log frame* (Figure 10.6). Log frames describe the system and highlight the linkages between each step in a more thorough manner than a logic model.

Quality Improvement

Monitoring and evaluation frameworks allow for an analysis of quality. When a logic model is outlined with indicators and expected targets, each step presents an opportunity for quality improvement. The focus on quality improvement in health care grew out of industrial practices.[45] These practices examined processes and systems to improve outcomes instead of the actions of an individual. The focus on systems rather than individuals helps to create what improvement specialists call a *blame-free environment.*[46] Multiple studies have shown that a team-based, blame-free environment is critical to improving quality and decreasing medical errors.[47,48] By the 1990s, quality improvement became a standard area of work in health care in the United States and Europe.[49]

	Major Outcomes & Outputs Leading to Ultimate Goal				Activities	Inputs: Staff, Stuff, Space
Ultimate Program Goal	Strategic Objective (Long-term Outcome)	Intermediate Result (Intermediate Outcome)	Sub-Intermediate Result (Outputs)		(What you DO)	(e.g., equipment, medications, staff FTE, etc.)
Reduced morbidity and mortality from TB	At least 70% of expected cases of TB are diagnosed within a year	Increase number of people with TB symptoms are brought to clinic and given smear test	Number of CHWs trained to screen for TB		Hire and train CHWs in TB case finding	20 CHW, 4 CHW supervisors
					Assign CHWs to managable regions and populations	50% FTE Program Manager
					Create M&E tools for CHWs to track their case finding efforts	1 Supervisor to review and aggregate results
			Number of sputum collection posts established in the community		Hire and train lab technicians to conduct smear tests	Car and driver to transport sputum to the lab
					Hold community meetings to discuss & troubleshoot physical barriers to care	Laboratory equipment, tests, personnel

FIGURE 10.6 An example of a portion of a tuberculosis program's log frame. Note that compared to the logic model there is more detail on staffing, supply chain, outputs, and objectives.

The culture of quality improvement in impoverished countries is more recent.[50,51] The lack of material inputs (from sufficient drugs to adequate staffing) is an obstacle to providing quality health care, as is the lack of data systems. Given these limitations, a blame-free environment is an important foundation to build solidarity among team members. As health systems are strengthened, the drive to improve the quality of the services delivered is increasingly important.[51] In 2007, the WHO published a "Framework for Action"[18] as a guide to support quality improvement in impoverished countries. In a subsequent conference in 2008, health leaders from around the world identified quality improvement as a political and health care management imperative, a method to reduce waste of limited health resources, and an instrument for supporting capacity-building efforts. They also called for more evidence- and document-sharing between programs to promote quality improvement methods.[51] There are multiple methodologies used to improve quality, but a common set of principles underpins virtually all of the quality improvement methods. These include understanding delivery systems in a stepwise fashion, trying changes within each step, measuring the effect of a change, and a collaborative process for improving the system based on the findings.[52]

One commonly used method of quality improvement is the Plan-Do-Study-Act or PDSA cycle.[53] While PDSA cycles are not research per se, they begin with a hypothesis that "an intervention would work better *if*," and the "if" generates a plan for improvement. For example, there *would be more handwashing* by health professionals *if* there were hand sanitizer dispensers between every two beds instead of only at the end of the ward. The "do" part of this cycle, then, is to put dispensers between every two beds, and the "study" part is to measure the handwashing events. The "study" aspect is often done collaboratively, and stakeholders use a chart to show achievement of the goal over time. The "act" part of the cycle is to take the lessons learned from the intervention and further iterate them into the care delivery system. This technique is easy to teach, and many health care teams have found this helpful to inspire collaborative processes.[54] While there is a variation in the methodology used for quality improvement, all programs are based on the measurement of data and the development of action plans that are adequately resourced to have an impact. Programs are analyzed using log frames or logic models that, like the care delivery value chain, capture the interrelated steps of care.

Conclusion

This chapter discusses the importance of data in planning, monitoring, and evaluating global health delivery projects. Efforts to collect data in impoverished settings generally rely on paper-based systems. With the demand for reports from many vertical programs, the need for data leads to overwhelming paperwork and disruption of workflows. The movement to EMR systems is important as more complex care is given. Efforts to develop low-cost electronic systems are bearing fruit in many countries and programs. Data should be disaggregated to measure equity and to support program design that targets the vulnerable to achieve equitable outcomes. Choosing indicators that reflect equity is an important part of a rights-based agenda. In an effort to streamline and standardize measurements, a list of core health indicators were defined and are used in monitoring and evaluation models. Quality improvement is a growing imperative in global health and relies on good data systems.

References

1. Jamison DT, Bank W. *Disease control priorities in developing countries.* New York: Oxford University Press; 1993.
2. Lea RA. World development report 1993: "Investing in health." *Forum Dev Stud.* 1993;20(1):114–117.
3. Murray CJ, Lopez AD, Jamison DT. The Global Burden of Disease in 1990: Summary results, sensitivity analysis and future directions. *Bull World Health Org.* 1994;72(3):495–509.
4. WHO Ebola Response Team. Ebola virus disease in West Africa: The first 9 months of the epidemic and forward projections. *N Engl J Med.* 2014;371(16):1481–1495.
5. Heymann DL, Rodier G. Global surveillance, national surveillance, and SARS. *Emerg Infect Dis.* 2004;10(2):173.
6. Barzilay EJ, Schaad N, Magloire R, et al. Cholera surveillance during the Haiti epidemic: The first 2 years. *N Engl J Med.* 2013;368(7):599–609.
7. World Health Organization. *Global reference list of 100 core health indicators, 2015.* Geneva: World Health Organization; 2015.
8. Nunan M, Duke T. Effectiveness of pharmacy interventions in improving availability of essential medicines at the primary healthcare level. *Trop Med Intl Health.* 2011;16(5):647–658.
9. Blaya JA, Fraser HSF, Holt B. E-health technologies show promise in developing countries. *Health Aff (Millwood).* 2010;29(2):244.
10. Crisp NG, Donald PR. The "road to health" card and immunisation records. *S Afr Med J.* 1987;72(5):331.
11. Giglio J, R., Papazian J, B. Acceptance and use of patient-carried health records. *Med Care.* 1986;24(12):1064–1092.
12. Travis P, Bennett S, Haines A, et al. Overcoming health-systems constraints to achieve the millennium development goals. *Lancet.* 2004;364(9437):900–906.
13. Blumenthal D, Tavenner M. The "meaningful use" regulation for electronic health records. *N Engl J Med.* 2010;363(6):501–504.

14. Stephani V, Opoku D, Quentin W. A systematic review of randomized controlled trials of mHealth interventions against non-communicable diseases in developing countries. *BMC Public Health*. 2016;16.

15. Sacks JA, Zehe E, Redick C, et al. Introduction of mobile health tools to support Ebola surveillance and contact tracing in guinea. *Glob Health Sci Pract*. 2015;3(4):646.

16. Nguyen L, Bellucci E, Nguyen LT. Electronic health records implementation: An evaluation of information system impact and contingency factors. *Int J Med Inf*. 2014;83(11):79–796.

17. Nucita A, Bernava GM, Bartolo M, et al. A global approach to the management of EMR (electronic medical records) of patients with HIV/AIDS in sub-Saharan Africa: The experience of DREAM software. *BMC Med Informat Decision Making*. 2009;9:42.

18. World Health Organization. Everybody's business: Strengthening health systems to improve health outcomes. WHO's framework for action. 2007. Available from: http://www.who.int/iris/handle/10665/43918.

19. AbouZahr C, Boerma T. Health information systems: The foundations of public health. *Bull World Health Org*. 2005;83(8):578.

20. McCluskey PD. Partners' $1.2b patient data system seen as key to future. *The Boston Globe*. Jun 1, 2015. Available from: https://www.bostonglobe.com/business/2015/05/31/partners-launches-billion-electronic-health-records-system/oo4nJJW2rQy-fWUWQlvydkK/story.html. Accessed May 11, 2017.

21. OpenMRS. OpenMRS distribution program. 2016. Available from: http://openmrs.org/. Accessed May 11, 2017.

22. Baobab Health Trust. About us. 2017. Available from: http://baobabhealth.org/. Accessed May 11, 2017.

23. Ubuntu, Canonical Ltd. The Ubuntu story. 2017. Available from: https://www.ubuntu.com/about/about-ubuntu. Accessed May 11, 2017.

24. USAID. The demographic and health surveys program. USAID from the American People Web site. 2016. Available from: https://www.usaid.gov/what-we-do/global-health/cross-cutting-areas/demographic-and-health-surveys-program. Accessed Feb 7, 2017.

25. DHS Program. Demographic and health surveys. Available from: http://dhsprogram.com/. Accessed Feb 7, 2017.

26. CDC. *Developing evaluation indicators*. National Center for HIV/AIDS, Viral Hepatitis, STD, and TB Prevention, CDC. Washington, DC: Centers for Disease Control.

27. World Health Organization. Health impact assessment (HIA): Glossary of terms used. 2017. Available from: http://www.who.int/hia/about/glos/en/index1.html. Accessed Feb 7, 2017.

28. Styblo K, Rouillon A. Tuberculosis. *Health Policy Plan*. 1991;6(4):391–397.

29. World Health Organization. The stop TB strategy. 2010. Available from: http://www.who.int/tb/strategy/stop_tb_strategy/en/. Accessed Feb 7, 2017.

30. Volmink J, Matchaba P, Garner P. Directly observed therapy and treatment adherence. *Lancet.* 2000;355(9212):1345–1350.

31. World Health Organization. Compendium of indicators for monitoring and evaluating national tuberculosis programs. *Stop TB Partnership.* Geneva, Switzerland: World Health Organization; 2004. http://apps.who.int/iris/bitstream/10665/68768/1/WHO_HTM_TB_2004.344.pdf

32. WHO. Global tuberculosis control—surveillance, planning, financing, 2004. Available from: http://replace-me/ebraryid=10062380.

33. Orenstein EW, Basu S, Shah NS, et al. Treatment outcomes among patients with multidrug-resistant tuberculosis: Systematic review and meta-analysis. *Lancet Infect Dis.* 2009;9(3):153–161.

34. Farmer P. Managerial successes, clinical failures editorial. *Intl J TB Lung Dis.* 1999;3(5):365–367.

35. Obermeyer Z, Abbott-Klafter J, Murray CJL. Has the DOTS strategy improved case finding or treatment success? An empirical assessment. *PLoS One.* 2008;3(3):e1721.

36. UNICEF, WHO. Immunization summary, A statistical reference containing data through 2011. Geneva, Switzerland: UNICEF and the World Health Organization; 2013. https://www.unicef.org/immunization/files/EN-ImmSumm-2013.pdf

37. Ariadne Labs. Primary health care performance initiative. 2017. Available from: https://www.ariadnelabs.org/programsincubationprimary-health-care/. Accessed Apr 25, 2017.

38. PHCPI. Primary health care performance initiative. 2017. Available from: http://phcperformanceinitiative.org/. Accessed Mar 2, 2017.

39. Chen J, Rehkopf D, Waterman PD, et al. Mapping and measuring social disparities in premature mortality: The impact of census tract poverty within and across Boston neighborhoods, 1999–2001. *Am J Epidemiol.* 2006;163(11):S139.

40. García-Elorriaga G. *Practical and laboratory diagnosis of tuberculosis: From sputum smear to molecular biology.* 1st ed. Cham, Switzerland: Springer International Publishing; 2015.

41. Siddiqi K, Lambert M, Walley J. Clinical diagnosis of smear-negative pulmonary tuberculosis in low-income countries: The current evidence. *Lancet Infect Dis.* 2003;3(5):288–296.

42. Braveman P. Health disparities and health equity: Concepts and measurement. *Annu Rev Public Health.* 2006;27:167.

43. Reynolds HW, Sutherland EG. A systematic approach to the planning, implementation, monitoring, and evaluation of integrated health services. *BMC Health Serv Res.* 2013;13:168.

44. McQueen DV. Strengthening the evidence base for health promotion. *Health Promot Intl.* 2001;16(3):261–268.

45. Shojania K, Grimshaw J. Evidence-based quality improvement: The state of the science. *Health Aff.* 2005;24(1):138–150.

46. Guthrie P. US creates blame-free adverse event reporting. *CMAJ.* 2006;174(1):19.

47. Haynes AB, Weiser TG, Berry WR, et al. A surgical safety checklist to reduce morbidity and mortality in a global population. *N Engl J Med.* 2009;360(5):491–499.

48. de Vries EN, Prins HA, Crolla, Rogier M P H, et al. Effect of a comprehensive surgical safety system on patient outcomes. *N Engl J Med.* 2010;363(20):1928–1937.

49. Blumenthal D, Kilo CM. A report card on continuous quality improvement. *Milbank Q.* 1998;76(4):625–648.

50. Mate KS, Sifrim ZK, Chalkidou K, et al. Improving health system quality in low- and middle-income countries that are expanding health coverage: A framework for insurance. *Intl J Qual Health Care.* 2013;25(5):497–504.

51. Leatherman S, Ferris TG, Berwick D, Omaswa F, Crisp N. The role of quality improvement in strengthening health systems in developing countries. *Intl J Qual Health Care.* 2010;22(4):237–243.

52. Berwick, DM. *Curing health care: New strategies for quality improvement. A report on the national demonstration project on quality improvement in health care.* San Francisco, CA: Jossey-Bass; 1990.

53. Leis JA, Shojania KG. A primer on PDSA: Executing plan–do–study–act cycles in practice, not just in name. *BMJ Qual Saf.* 2016;26(7):572–577.

54. Anatole M, Magge H, Redditt V, et al. Nurse mentorship to improve the quality of health care delivery in rural Rwanda. *Nurs Outlook.* 2012;61(3):137–144.

PART FOUR

Toward the Right to Health

11

Universal Health Coverage

ENSURING HEALTHY LIVES AND PROMOTING
WELL-BEING FOR ALL AT ALL AGES

Key Points

- The concept of Universal Health Coverage (UHC) has been discussed for many years.
- Renewed calls for UHC are a natural outgrowth of the successes and remaining challenges of the movement for AIDS treatment access and the Millennium Development Goals.
- UHC is part of the Sustainable Development Goals.
- UHC has two objectives: equity in access to quality health services, and protection against financial risk.
- Several countries have made significant strides toward achieving UHC.
- To effectively deliver UHC in impoverished countries, donors and countries themselves will need to make investments in infrastructure, staffing, and supply chain that match the burden of disease.

Introduction

The achievements made toward the UN's Millennium Development Goals (MDGs) between 2000 and 2015 were remarkable.[1] Yet the complexities of meeting the MDGs and the uneven achievements between and within countries laid bare the need to build and strengthen health systems.[2] As discussed in Chapter 3, Sustainable Development Goal (SDG) 3 moves beyond the handful of targets set by the MDGs and seeks to "ensure healthy lives and promote well-being for all at all ages."[2] SDG 3 includes the MDGs' focus on reductions of child mortality (MDG 4) and maternal mortality (MDG 5) as well as increased coverage of AIDS, tuberculosis (TB), and malaria treatment (MDG 6). But SDG 3 goes further, adding other disease-related targets, including the reduction of mortality from noncommunicable diseases, the promotion of mental health, the prevention and treatment of substance abuse, and a decreasing number of deaths and injuries due to road traffic accidents. SDG 3 also focuses on geopolitical issues that go beyond country boundaries, including reducing the number of deaths and illnesses from pollution and contamination of air, water, and soil. Furthermore, it calls for a significantly increased health workforce to deliver the care that is needed to improve morbidity and mortality, respond to epidemic threats, and sustain long-term health systems.

Importantly, SDG 3 reinforces the promise of Universal Health Coverage (UHC) "including financial risk protection, access to quality essential health-care services and access to safe, effective, quality and affordable essential medicines and vaccines for all."[2] If the global community commits sufficient resources and aligns resources to support health systems to achieve UHC, disease-specific targets will also be met be met. UHC will not be acheived without an implementation strategy to fulfill the right to health. One of the most important lessons in the movement for AIDS treatment access is that practical, country-led, and adequately financed plans with targets are needed to fulfill the right to health. This chapter discusses the concept of UHC, reviews select country achievements in health delivery, and discusses the implementation challenges in achieving UHC.

Universal Health Coverage

The World Health Organization (WHO) defines UHC as a state in which "all people and communities can use the promotive, preventive, curative, rehabilitative, and palliative health services they need, of sufficient quality to be effective, while also ensuring that the use of these services does not expose the user to financial hardship."[3] The WHO further elaborates the definition of UHC in the following two objectives:

1. Equity *in access to quality health services*
   a. Everyone who needs services should get them, not just those who can pay for them.
   b. *The quality of health services should be good enough to improve the health of those receiving services.*
2. *People should be protected against financial-risk*, ensuring that the cost of using services does not put people at risk of financial harm.

Financing is critical. Even in wealthy countries, very large, sometimes called *catastrophic* health expenditures[4] result in impoverishment.[5] Because of this, an important focus of UHC is health financing addressed in Chapter 12.[6,7] This chapter focuses on the first component of UHC: equitable access and quality health care.

There is debate over the proper definitions of the terms "universal," "health," and "coverage."[8] Some authors suggest that universal coverage is the legal obligation of a government, as a signatory to international treaties, to provide health care as a right to all its citizens.[9] Embedded within the concept of universal coverage is equity, including reaching vulnerable and marginalized communities. This presupposes that special efforts must be made to cover these populations.

A number of philosophical and ethical theories discuss the distribution of resources in regards to health care and health equity. One of these constructs is *utilitarianism*. Utilitarianism proposes that appropriate actions are those that maximize utility.[10] In regards to health, this generally means providing the greatest good for the greatest number of people, usually with a fixed resource. This concept underpins selective primary health care and cost-effectiveness for priority setting that is based on fixed and meager resources. Another approach centers around the idea that the most vulnerable should be given special care if equity is to be achieved. In 1972, the Latin American movement of *liberation theology* emerged as a moral reaction to poverty, injustice, and profound societal inequality. This movement coined the term "preferential option for the poor"; the prioritization of the most vulnerable.[11] Many social programs throughout the world are based on the view that the vulnerable need special protection and assistance. For example, in the United States, poor women with young children are eligible for Medicaid[12]; in South Africa underserved communities are eligible for government grants designed to spur economic development.[13] *Communitarianism* is an ideology in which the community decides who is most at risk or in need of services.[14] This approach is used for microfinance in Bangladesh[15] and for health insurance in Rwanda.[16] In general, the achievement of UHC will require a progressive approach to seeking out and providing particular support to the most vulnerable.

Health itself has a very broad definition. As has been discussed earlier in this book, it is defined not only as the absence of disease but as a complete state of emotional and physical well-being.[17] In the UN General Assembly's drafting of the SDGs and UHC, it called for the "highest attainable standard of physical and mental health" as well as "work on the social determinants of health."[2] This notion of health is holistic and implicitly recognizes that vertical interventions and health sector-only solutions will not achieve UHC. Intersectional cooperation, such as between agriculture and health, education and health, and infrastructure and health, are all needed to address social forces.[18] Moreover, the health sector must be improved significantly in impoverished countries so that the highest attainable standard is equitable throughout the world.

In most impoverished countries, the starting point on the road to UHC is an under-resourced health system. Therefore, significant strengthening of the health system will be needed. In addition, to address adverse social determinants of health inequities, many countries have adopted a broader definition of health that requires intersectoral work.[19,20]

Achieving Equity and Covering the Disease Burden

In the past four decades, a progression from selective primary health care to the targeted interventions of the MDGs to UHC has occurred. To achieve coverage that is truly universal, equity must be at its root. Many international groups, including the World Bank, under the leadership of Partners In Health Founder Dr. Jim Kim since 2012, have advocated for measuring the achievement of UHC by evaluating the access to health care and health outcomes of the poorest segments of the population.[21] UHC assumes that people get the coverage they need for the conditions they have. This means providing care for conditions and problems that were previously neglected in the public health context, including surgery[22] and mental health services,[23,24] as well as the treatment of noncommunicable diseases[25,26] and cancer.[27] Adding these components to the weak health care delivery systems of impoverished countries will require plans to increase the number of facilities and the number and capacity of health workers. It will also require improved access to medicines, labs, and infrastructure. Despite the obvious challenges, UHC is now a development priority for middle-income and impoverished countries. While governments are forced to set priorities and make tradeoffs due to limited ability to finance care, human rights language is helpful in considering the idea of the "progressive realization"[28] of the right to health care in the achievement of UHC.[29]

All health systems make strategic decisions that are based on priorities.[30] Explicit priorities to assure access are important because equity can be embedded within the framework *a priori*. For example, a country can decide that because TB is a disease of the poor, is contagious, and has a known, standardized therapy, it will be prioritized over cancer. Cancer has many forms, many treatments, and is not explicitly a disease of the poor. Therefore the national health system carefully plan out the number of TB drugs needed to treat every case, the necessary staffing at each level of care and laboratory supplies for diagnosis and follow up. In contrast, cancer therapy may only be given at one site nationally, and drugs may only be available for a few causes of cancer.

This does not mean that cancer is not treated or that the government will not look for additional resources for cancer care. Cancer care is still part of the disease burden and therefore part of the ultimate achievement of UHC. As such, the government may develop a stepwise plan and advocate for resources that will increasingly address this important condition. However, the government in this example prioritizes one disease—TB—with a known disease burden, proven treatment, and a plan for decentralization over another one for the first step of decentralization and UHC. Without setting explicit priorities, ad hoc rationing becomes the norm. In that case, TB coverage would not prioritized in the budget process, leaving clinics understaffed and drugs stocked-out in the public system. The poor, who disproportionately suffer from this affliction, would get no care or poor care. Meanwhile, the government might invest in a modern cancer hospital with a fee-for-service model. Those with money could receive treatment for a variety of conditions, even with very expensive drugs. Ad hoc rationing is often driven by politically motivated priority setting and lacks clear plans to cover the vulnerable. The poor, those from rural areas, and people from marginalized groups are often excluded from any care while more affluent urban dwellers get more services.

Ethicists have weighed in on how priorities should be set in a way that causes the least harm. They argue that there are unacceptable tradeoffs, particularly substituting high-cost, complex interventions for a few in lieu of full coverage for life-saving interventions for all. In the article "Ethical Perspective: Five Unacceptable Trade-Offs on the Path to Universal Health Coverage" Norheim argues that there are five unethical tradeoffs:[31]

> *Unacceptable tradeoff I*: To expand coverage for low- or medium-priority services before there is near universal coverage for high-priority services. This includes reducing out-of-pocket (OOP) payments for low- or medium-priority services before eliminating OOP payments for high-priority services.
>
> *Unacceptable tradeoff II*: To first include in the universal coverage scheme only those with the ability to pay and not include informal workers and the poor, even if such an approach would be easier.
>
> *Unacceptable tradeoff III*: To give high priority to very costly services (whose coverage will provide substantial financial protection) when the health benefits are very small compared to alternative, less costly services.
>
> *Unacceptable tradeoff IV*: To expand coverage for well-off groups before doing so for worse-off groups when the costs and benefits are not vastly different. This includes expanding coverage for those with already high coverage before groups with lower coverage.

Unacceptable tradeoff V: To shift from OOP payment toward mandatory pre-payment in a way that makes the financing system less progressive.

While the logic of minimizing the harm may seem obvious, countries may be pushed by political considerations. For example, in all countries, wealthy and impoverished, a Ministry of Health or government may be forced to build a state-of-the-art facility in a capital city or in the hometown of a political leader. Such facilities are often geographically and financially inaccessible to the poor. Also, in every country, lobbyists or those who influence political process are dispro-portionately the voice of monied interests. These groups may have an outsized voice in the political process, thereby shaping decision-making within the health system.[32] An ethical framework of decision-making is helpful in crafting national plans and progressively increasing the availability of interventions needed to achieve UHC.

In addition to the difficult choices that are made every day, medical science is constantly evolving. New technologies slowly trickle down to impoverished countries and communities.[33] The equity gap between those who have access to the best treatment and those who do not is even greater when a new drug or diagnostic tool is developed (as was seen with HIV in the 1990s or hepatitis C in 2014).[34] It is important to consider technological advances in impoverished countries for both moral reasons of equity and because new technologies can sometimes be used to overcome access barriers.[33] The penetration of cell phones, for example, has allowed for a variety of improvements in health care, such as the rapid transmission of information for program evaluation or calling for emer-gency transport.[35] Some countries and UHC advocates are focused on the role of technologies in a deliberative process as opposed to waiting for new technologies to trickle down. The World Health Assembly in 2014 adopted tools to perform what they call a *health intervention and technology assessment* (HITA).[36] The con-cept of HITA and its contribution to UHC planning is to assess the benefit of a new technology (drug, diagnostic test, or procedure) based on impact and scal-ability. The impact on the health budget of a country is considered after assessing the potential benefit.

Some countries are moving toward UHC with remarkable speed. A vari-ety of wealthy countries, such as Canada, Australia, and the United Kingdom, have national programs that provide nearly full coverage to their citizens.[37,38] Notably several middle-income countries such as Costa Rica, Cuba, Mexico, Turkey, and Thailand have moved rapidly to cover a high proportion of their population.[39–42] Rwanda and Ethiopia are impoverished countries that have made great strides toward achieving UHC in many areas.[43,44] These countries have used ethical priority setting, the progressive expansion of services, and community participation.

Aligning Services with Disease Burden

To realize the right to health and actualize UHC, services must be available to address the disease burden. As explained in earlier chapters, often the utilization of services is quite low owing to two distinct problems. First, there are many barriers that limit access. Second, the provision of services is massively under-resourced. The UHC movement has focused on decreasing the so-called demand-side barriers, particularly user fees[45] and other costs incurred while seeking care.[46,47] Decreasing barriers to access is important. Yet the UHC movement has focused less on the second problem—the lack resources to provide quality services. The supply side, which is the provision of services, is critical to delivering consistent, high-quality care.

The movement for AIDS treatment provides an example for the delivery of universal coverage.[48] In 2005, universal access to HIV testing and treatment was a stated goal.[49] The UN and the US Centers for Disease Control (CDC) supported HIV surveillance programs.[50] With this data, governments and partners like the Clinton Health Access Initiative planned to scale up services. Standard protocols for numbers of visits and treatment regimens were mapped out based on the HIV burden. This mapping supported drug forecasting for antiretroviral therapy (ART) and for laboratory equipment to match the targets for yearly patient enrollment and maintenance on therapy.[51] The need for scale also drove national-level plans for workforce development and distribution.[52] This process—mapping the burden, aligning the supply chain, and ensuring an adequate number of health professionals—was the underlying formula that resulted in a massive international scale-up of HIV testing and treatment. The public sector's health centers and hospitals were strengthened in this period, and utilization of all services improved. To achieve delivery of UHC, the lessons learned from HIV can be used to align resources with the disease burden.

In impoverished settings, particularly in sub-Saharan Africa, the majority of care delivery is done through the public sector. Thanks to years of work from the Global Burden of Disease project, the Disease Control Priorities program, Demographic and Health Surveys (DHS), and other national and international surveillance projects, the disease burden in communities is largely known.[53–55] Given these available data, it is possible to map the disease burden and align staff, training, supply chain, and infrastructure to meet the need. Mapping has been done in countries like Mexico and Rwanda to support the movement toward UHC.[41,44]

Case Study: Partners in Health's UHC Matrix

The history of Partners in Health's (PIH) use of Global Fund monies for HIV to support public health centers in rural Haiti is outlined in Chapter 2 and Rwanda's national plan, supported by PIH, described in Chapter 3. In both cases, vertical AIDS money was leveraged to provide primary care, leading to dramatic increases in overall health service utilization. However, this overwhelmed the weak system. Initially, stock-outs of medicines were frequent, and there was also an urgent need to improve staffing and clinic infrastructure to meet the surge of utilization. Forecasting the supply chain was difficult due to increasing patient volumes. The attempt to meet the health needs of the entire community led PIH to use the lessons learned from AIDS treatment scale-up to link the expected disease burden in the catchment area of each clinic with the staff, medications, and infrastructure needed to achieve UHC.[56] This clinic-based work on the so-called supply side of service delivery was supported on by the demand side work of community health workers (CHWs) who mobilized the community, performed active case finding, and accompanied the vulnerable to clinics. This led to increased utilization of key services (antenatal care, infant vaccination, TB case finding).[57]

While this strategy of using HIV money to support primary care led to a marked increase in the utilization of primary care services, it was unclear if the care delivered addressed the entire disease burden. But in public clinics the denominator is known. Each public clinic has a defined catchment area. Therefore by using the available surveillance data like the demographic health surveys (DHS), the burden of disease for each clinic's population can be calculated. The expected number of pregnant women per year, for example, is based on the fertility rate and the number of women of childbearing age in the area. Once the total number of expected births per year is known, a plan for the number of midwives, delivery packs, and delivery beds can be created. This work to link the disease burden with the staff, supply, and infrastructure needed to deliver care led to the development of the Partners in Health-Universal Health Coverage (PIH-UHC) matrix.

The matrix is a simple model that uses available DHS or other data to estimate the disease burden for the clinic's catchment area. The benchmarks for full coverage of an intervention are called the *UHC target*. The UHC targets are estimated by using (1) the population living within a clinic's catchment area, (2) the known or estimated burden of disease of that population, (3) the number of visits expected for the ideal treatment of a condition, and (4) the standard amount of drugs or supplies needed to address the disease or condition. Number 3 and 4 are based on standard national and international guidelines and protocols. Within the tool, these targets are linked with the staffing, supplies, and infrastructure needed to deliver care and achieve universal coverage. Figure 11.1 shows the used of the tool with HIV in three clinics.

In 2006, PIH was invited to support HIV and health systems strengthening in the mountains of Lesotho, a country with a not only a very high HIV

HIV/AIDS Coverage and Care				Sources and Assumptions	
1.Demographics & Epidemiology	**Haiti-Lascahobas**	**Lesotho Nohana**	**Liberia-Pleebo**	**Data Sources (white) Calculations (gray)**	**Assumptions/Notes**
Catchment population	47,322	25,000	50,690	Site data	
% of adult population	66.0%	67.0%	56.0%	Country DHS surveys	Over 15 yrs. old
Estimated county ADULT HIV prevalence (%)	1.7%	22.7%	1.1%	UNAIDS 2015	
2. Case Finding: Expected Tests & HIV Positive Cases	**Haiti-Lascahobas**	**Lesotho Nohana**	**Liberia-Pleebo**	**Data Sources/Calculations**	**Assumptions/Notes**
Annual target of people who know their status	100%	100%	100%	UHC target	
Expected number of ADULTS in catchment who are HIV+	531	3802	312	Total catchment*adult HIV prevalence*% of pop. aged 15 yrs.	Over 15 yrs. old
Expected number of CHILDREN in catchment who are HIV+	42	304	25	Expected # of HIV+ adults*.08	Pediatric HIV infections estimated at around 8% of the adult burden of disease. UNAIDS 2015
Expected total number of HIV positive in the catchment	573	4106	337	Expected HIV+ adults+ expected HIV+ children	
3. Anti-Retroviral Treatment & Retention in Care	**Haiti-Lascahobas**	**Lesotho Nohana**	**Liberia-Pleebo**	**Data Sources/Calculations**	**Assumptions/Notes**
Estimated % of all HIV+ ADULTS eligible for ART	100%	100%	100%		Based on the new test-and-treat protocol
Expected # of HIV+ ADULTS on ART	531	3802	312	# of HIV+ adults*% on ART	
Expected # of HIV+ children on ART	42	304	25	=Expected HIV+ children	Universal coverage protocol for pediatric HIV
Expected total number of patients on ART	573	4106	337	Expected HIV+ adults on ART+ expected HIV+ children on ART	
Number of HIV clinic days offered per year	260	260	260	# clinic days per week*52 weeks per year	Assuming all of these facilities have HIV clinics open 5 days per week, 52 weeks in a year
Recommended average number of clinic visits per ART patient, annually	8	8	8	Site protocol	Assuming 8 visits per year for ART patients
Total patient visits expected per year	4587	32851	2698	Total ART patients*recommended clinic visits	Children and adults will have same number of clinic visits
Expected total patient visits expected per HIV clinic day	18	126	10	(Total ART patients * clinic visits per year)/# of clinic days	
4. Patient Outcome & Viral Suppression	**Haiti-Lascahobas**	**Lesotho Nohana**	**Liberia-Pleebo**	**Data Sources/Calculations**	**Assumptions/Notes**
Expected % of patients needing a viral load, annually	100%	100%	100%	UHC target	
Expected # of viral load tests per patient, annually	1.5	1.5	1.5	Site protocol	Some patients may come more often than the standard 1 test per yr.
Expected number of patients who need a viral load, annually	860	6160	506	Total ART patients* # of annual tests per patient * % of HIV patients needing a viral load	

FIGURE 11.1 Example of the PIH-UHC matrix for planning the HIV program in three clinics from Haiti, Liberia, and Lesotho. The total burden of HIV is calculated by using the total catchment area of each clinic and the adult HIV prevalence. This figure is then used to plan the staffing for clinics based on how many times per year the patient should be seen (from national protocols), how many patients a provider can see per visit. The supply chain is calculated based on the percent of HIV patients that will need monitoring or ART. The infrastructure—or number of rooms needed to see the patients in a dignified way is also mapped from the burden of disease.

prevalence but extremely high maternal mortality.[58] This high maternal mortality was due in part to a low rate of facility-based delivery and poor quality of maternity care. The facility-based delivery rate was low because Lesotho is a very mountainous country, and more than 20 percent of the population lives more than a two-hours' walk away from a health center. But, as is often the case, the demand-side barriers were only part of the equation. Clinics had an insufficient number of delivery beds, supplies, and trained maternity staff. Because of this few women came forward to deliver in the clinic and even if a woman did come to deliver at a facility, the quality of care was very poor. The PIH team created a value chain elaborating the important steps in reducing maternal mortality including the elements needed to bring women into facilities and provide good quality care. Using the lessons from Haiti, the PIH-UHC matrix was adapted to address high maternal mortality (1,155 per 100,000) and used to map the needs at seven PIH-supported government health centers in Lesotho.[59]

PIH reoriented each clinic using the PIH-UHC matrix. The number of pregnant women expected in each catchment area was calculated based on fertility rate and the number of women of childbearing age. Using these data, PIH estimated the number of daily deliveries that should occur in a clinic to map the staffing, supplies, and infrastructure needed for 100 percent coverage of facility-based delivery. PIH also built maternal waiting houses for women who lived more than two hours away from the health center. Women could stay in these facilities for up to one week prior to delivery.[59] Last, on the demand side, CHWs were trained and compensated to accompany pregnant women to four antenatal clinic (ANC) visits, to the facility for delivery, and to a postpartum visit. The maternal mortality reduction program was built on these supply-side improvements toward UHC targets and the demand-side work of CHWs to accompany women through the barriers they faced. Two years after the plan was implemented in the remote Bobete clinic, there was a more than threefold improvement in ANC coverage and facility-based deliveries (Figure 11.2).

Because of these important results, and in the face of backsliding health indicators elsewhere in the country (Figure 11.3),[60] the government of Lesotho invited PIH to support the reform of the health sector to achieve UHC at the primary care level. In 2014, the PIH-UHC matrix was used to plan health sector reform in Lesotho. Based on this process, the reform has achieved remarkable results. The matrix has been used in more than 70 primary care facilities to align staff, supply chain, and infrastructure to move toward full coverage of antenatal visits and facility-based delivery (Figure 11.4).

The PIH-UHC matrix has been expanded to cover other components of care delivery and triaging at public facilities. These components include antenatal care, facility-based delivery, TB case-finding, child health, and general outpatient services. Most primary care clinics in impoverished countries triage patients into five separate

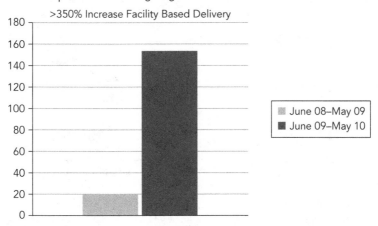

FIGURE 11.2 Graph shows the increase in facility based delivery in Bobete clinic after 2 years of using the PIH-UHC tool to map maternal health needs and align staff, supplies and infrastructure to meet the burden. At this time, CHWs were also trained to find and accompany pregnant women.

Source: Satti H, Motsamai S, Chetane P et al. Comprehensive approach to improving maternal health and achieving MDG 5: Report from the mountains of Lesotho. *PLoS One*. 2012;7(8):e42700.

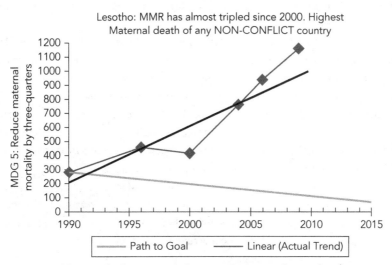

FIGURE 11.3 This graph shows Lesotho's increasing maternal mortality (2000–2010). Despite significant international assistance for HIV since 2000, Lesotho's maternal mortality rate has almost tripled, having the highest maternal death of any nonconflict country.

Data compiled from World Bank Data Base of Health and Nutrition. http://data.worldbank. org/data-catalog/health-nutrition-and-population-statistics

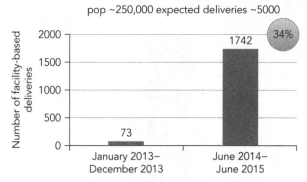

FIGURE 11.4 Aligning human resources, infrastructure, and supply chain with Universal Health Care. Facility-based delivery in Mohoele's Hoek District, Lesotho (2013–2015). The number of facility-based deliveries drastically increased once Partners in Health reoriented clinics to align with the expected number of pregnant women in the district using the PIH-UHC matrix.

Source: Partners In Health, Lesotho.

areas: (1) ANC, (2) labor and delivery, (3) infectious disease (for TB and HIV), (4) general care outpatient services, and (5) under-5 child health services. The targets developed using the PIH-UHC matrix are for aligning resources with anticipated burden in these four areas.

There are several limitations of this approach. First, the clinics in the PIH example are quite rural so there is little spillover from communities outside the catchment area. Target setting and alignment of resources is quite different in densely populated urban areas that draw patients from many places outside the defined catchment. Second, the matrix does not yet include mapping and planning for other important and common conditions, such as mental illness and noncommunicable diseases. However, these aspects are in development. Third, while this tool is very helpful for organizing and planning primary care, it does not yet include the important aspects of secondary and tertiary care, such as the need for surgery, referral for severe illness, or the treatment of cancer. UHC must include care for serious illness that is often life-threatening and also impoverishing to families. Last, the matrix—focused on utilization and delivery of services—does not yet focus on the quality or effectiveness of the services delivered.

Effective Coverage

The need to deliver high-quality care is an important aspect of UHC. In a seminal study from India, increased facility-based delivery was not associated with decreased maternal mortality because the quality of care in the facilities was not optimal.[61] A recent study from Tanzania[62] used patient and provider interviews as well as tracing important facility-level inputs (drugs, supplies, etc.) to assess the quality of services provided. Studies have also linked the quality of services to the frequency of care delivered (i.e., more experienced providers with more practice perform better).[63] Other studies have shown that sustained mentorship can improve the quality of services.[64] However, when inadequate clinical training is the norm and facilities are not properly equipped, training alone is insufficient to improve quality.[65] The provision of effective coverage requires significant inputs in multiple arenas.

As discussed elsewhere in this book, quality implicates everything from adequately trained and compensated staff to a robust drug supply chain and much more. The recent Ebola epidemic shed light on the need for health care system strengthening and the lack of quality in the care that is provided. One important article outlines the preconditions necessary for a health system to be resilient and respond to crises.[66] These preconditions include[66] (1) a global health network and international health systems fund, (2) legal and policy foundations to guide frameworks and establish accountability, (3) a strong and committed health workforce; and (4) strong management.

The authors describe five characteristics of a resilient health system that inherently implicate overall quality. These characteristics are that a health system is (1) aware of the health landscape of its people, (2) diverse and can address a broad range of health concerns and conditions, (3) self-regulating to avoid propagating instability, (4) integrated with intersectional fields and legislation, and, finally (5) adaptive to both a changing health landscape and changing political conditions.[66] These characteristics implicate health information systems and health data (Chapter 10), the need to address the burden of disease and deliver value to patient (Chapter 6), the need to develop a well-trained and adequately compensated health workforce (Chapter 7), and the need to address social determinants and barriers to care (Chapter 5). Delivering high-quality health care will improve the health of individuals and protect against epidemic threats. To that end, the WHO called for more research into measuring and improving the quality of health care.[67] The *WHO Bulletin* launched a specially themed issue entitled "Measuring Quality of Care in the Context of Sustainable Development Goal 3" in June 2017.[67]

Conclusion

The movement from selective primary health care to UHC demonstrates a global commitment to the progressive realization of the right to health. However, access to UHC is limited by barriers to care, inadequate provision of care, and poor-quality services. To deliver UHC, it is critical to align inputs in the health system with the burden of disease. Quality of care must also be improved. Steady, sufficient financing is needed to achieve the laudable goal of UHC.

References

1. United Nations. Millennium development goals report, 2015. Available from: http://www.un.org/millenniumgoals/2015_MDG_Report/pdf/MDG%20 2015%20rev%20(July%201).pdf. Accessed Jul 11, 2016.

2. United Nations. Sustainable development goals. 2016. Available from: http:// www.un.org/sustainabledevelopment/sustainable-development-goals/. Accessed Jul 11, 2016.

3. World Health Organization. WHO universal health coverage (UHC). WHO Media Centre Web site. 2015. Available from: http://www.who.int/mediacentre/ factsheets/fs395/en/. Accessed Nov 22, 2016.

4. Xu K, Evans DB, Kawabata K, Zeramdini R, Klavus J, Murray CJL. Household catastrophic health expenditure: A multicountry analysis. *Lancet.* 2003;362(9378):111–117.

5. Dickman SL, Himmelstein DU, Woolhandler S. Inequality and the health-care system in the USA. *Lancet.* 2017;389(10077):1431–1441.

6. Sachs JD. Achieving universal health coverage in low-income settings. *Lancet.* 2012;380(9845):944–947.

7. Jamison DT, Summers LH, Alleyne G, et al. Global health 2035: A world converging within a generation. *Lancet.* 2013;382(9908):1898–1955.

8. O'Connell T, Rasanathan K, Chopra M. What does universal health coverage mean? *Lancet.* 2014;383(9913):277–279.

9. Kirby M. The right to health fifty years on: Still skeptical? *Health Hum Rights.* 1999;4(1):6–25.

10. Roberts MJ, Reich MR. Ethical analysis in public health. *Lancet.* 2002;359(9311):1055–1059.

11. Gutierrez G. Option for the poor: Review and challenges. *Month.* 1995;28(1):5–10.

12. Paradise J, Lyons B, Rowland D. Low-income pregnant women, children and families, and childless adults. The Henry J. Kaiser Family Foundation Web site. 2015. Available from: http://kff.org/report-section/medicaid-at-50-low-income-pregnant-women-children-and-families-and-childless-adults/. Accessed Jun 1, 2017.

13. National Treasury. Neighbourhood development programme. National Treasury, Republic of South Africa Web site. 2017. Available from: http://ndp.treasury.gov. za/default.aspx. Accessed May 11, 2017.

14. Mooney G. "Communitarian claims" as an ethical basis for allocating health care resources. *Soc Sci Med.* 1998;47(9):1171–1180.

15. Bhatt N. Microenterprise development and the entrepreneurial poor: Including the excluded? *Pub Admin Dev.* 1997;4:371–386.

16. Lewandowski JL, Basinga P, Chin BL, et al. Towards universal health coverage: An evaluation of Rwanda mutuelles in its first eight years. *PLoS One.* 2012;7(6):e39282.

17. World Health Organization. *Chronicle of the World Health Organization.* Geneva: World Health Organization, 1947.

18. Evans DB, Marten R, Etienne C. Universal health coverage is a development issue. *Lancet.* 2012;380(9845):864–865.

19. World Health Organization. *World health report: Health systems financing; the path to universal coverage.* Albany: World Health Organization; 2010.

20. CSDH. *Closing the gap in a generation: Health equity through action on the social determinants of health.* Final Report of the Commission on Social Determinants of Health. Geneva: World Health Organization; 2008.

21. World Health Organization, World Bank. Tracking universal health coverage: First global monitoring report. Geneva, Switzerland: World Health Organization; 2015.

22. Meara JG, Greenberg SLM. Global surgery as an equal partner in health: No longer the neglected stepchild. *Lancet Glob Health.* 2015;3:S2.

23. Raviola G, Becker AE, Farmer P. A global scope for global health—including mental health. *Lancet.* 2011;378(9803):1613–1615.

24. Patel V, Prince M. Global mental health. *JAMA.* 2010;303(19):1976.

25. Srinath Reddy K. *Prevention and control of non-communicable diseases.* 6th ed. Oxford, UK: Oxford University Press; 2015.

26. Gupta N, Bukhman G. Leveraging the lessons learned from HIV/AIDS for coordinated chronic care delivery in resource-poor settings. *Healthcare.* 2015;3(4):215–220.

27. Farmer P, Frenk J, Knaul FM, et al. Expansion of cancer care and control in countries of low and middle income: A call to action. *Lancet.* 2010;376(9747):1186–1193.

28. OHCHR. *The right to health fact sheet no. 31.* Office of the United Nations High Commissioner for Human Rights. Geneva: World Health Organization; 2008.

29. Ooms G, Brolan C, Eggermont N, et al. Universal health coverage anchored in the right to health. *Bull World Health Org.* 2013;91(1):2. http://www.who.int/bulletin/volumes/91/1/12-115808/en/

30. Chalkidou K, Glassman A, Marten R, et al. Priority-setting for achieving universal health coverage. *Bull World Health Org.* 2016;94(6):462–467.

31. Norheim OF. Ethical perspective: Five unacceptable trade-offs on the path to universal health coverage. *Intl J Health Policy Mgmt.* 2015;4(11):711.

32. Norman J. Affordable care act gains majority approval for first time. 2017. Available from: http://www.gallup.com/poll/207671/affordable-care-act-gains-majority-approval-first-time.aspx.

33. Frost LJ, Reich MR. *Access: How do good health technologies get to poor people in poor countries?* Cambridge, MA: Harvard Center for Population and Development Studies; 2008.

34. Messac L, Prabhu K. Redefining the possible: The global AIDS response. In: Farmer P, Kim JY, Kleinman A, Basilico M, editors. *Reimagining global health, an introduction.* Berkeley: University of California Press; 2013.

35. Kahn JG, Yang JS, Kahn JS. "Mobile" health needs and opportunities in developing countries. *Health Aff (Millwood)*. 2010;29(2):252.

36. World Health Assembly. *Health intervention and technology assessment in support of universal health coverage*. Sixty-seventh World Health Assembly. Geneva, Switzerland: World Health Organization; 2014.

37. Hutchison B, Levesque J, Strumpf E, Coyle N. Primary health care in Canada: Systems in motion.(report). *Milbank Q*. 2011;89(2):256.

38. Mckee M, Balabanova D, Basu S, Ricciardi W, Stuckler D. Universal health coverage: A quest for all countries but under threat in some. *Value Health*. 2012;16(1):S39–S45.

39. George S. What Thailand can teach the world about universal healthcare. *The Guardian*. March 24, 2016. Available from: https://www.theguardian.com/health-revolution/2016/may/24/thailand-universal-healthcare-ucs-patients-government-political. Accessed Mar 7, 2017.

40. Atun R, Aydın S, Chakraborty S, et al. Universal health coverage in Turkey: Enhancement of equity. *Lancet*. 2013;382(9886):65–99.

41. Frenk J, González-Pier E, Gómez-Dantés O, Lezana MA, Knaul FM. Comprehensive reform to improve health system performance in Mexico. *Lancet*. 2006;368(9546):1524–1534.

42. Peltzer K, Stewart Williams J, Kowal P, et al. Universal health coverage in emerging economies: Findings on health care utilization by older adults in China, Ghana, India, Mexico, the Russian Federation, and South Africa. *Glob Health Action*. 2014;7.

43. Wang H, Ramana GNV. *Ethiopia—universal health coverage for inclusive and sustainable development: Country summary report*. New York: The World Bank; 2014.

44. Logie DE, Rowson M, Ndagije F. Innovations in Rwanda's health system: Looking to the future. *Lancet*. 2008;372(9634):256–261.

45. Yates R. Universal health care and the removal of user fees. *Lancet*. 2009;373(9680):2078–2081.

46. Gopalan S, Durairaj V. Addressing maternal healthcare through demand side financial incentives: Experience of Janani Suraksha Yojana program in India. *BMC Health Serv Res*. 2012;12:319.

47. Fernald LC, Gertler PJ, Neufeld LM. 10-year effect of oportunidades, Mexico's conditional cash transfer programme, on child growth, cognition, language, and behaviour: A longitudinal follow-up study. *Lancet*. 2009;374(9706):1997–2005.

48. World Health Organization. The 3 by 5 initiative. 2017. Available from: http://www.who.int/3by5/about/initiative/en/. Accessed Apr 18, 2017.

49. World Health Organization. *Towards universal access: Scaling up priority HIV/AIDS interventions in the health sector, progress report 2008*. Geneva: World Health Organization; 2008.

50. Rehle T, Lazzari S, Dallabetta G, Asamoah-Odei E. Second-generation HIV surveillance: Better data for decision-making. *Bull World Health Org*. 2004;82(2):121.

51. Galarraga O, O'Brien ME, Gutierrez JP, et al. Forecast of demand for antiretroviral drugs in low- and middle-income countries: 2007–2008. *AIDS*. 2007;21:S103.

52. Binagwaho A, Farmer PE, Nsanzimana S, et al. Rwanda 20 years on: Investing in life. *Lancet.* 2014;384(9940):371–375.

53. Ministry of Health and Social Welfare. Lesotho demographic health survey. Maseru, Lesotho: Ministry of Health [Lesotho]; 2014.

54. DCP3. DCP3: Disease control priorities, economic evaluation for health. www.dcp-3.org. Accessed Nov 1, 2016.

55. Murray CJ, Lopez AD, Jamison DT. The global burden of disease in 1990: Summary results, sensitivity analysis and future directions. *Bull World Health Org.* 1994;72(3):495–509.

56. World Health Organization. *Initial summary conclusions: Maximizing positive synergies between health systems and global health initiatives.* Geneva: World Health Organization; 2009.

57. Ivers LC, Jerome JG, Sullivan E, et al. Maximizing positive synergies between global health initiatives and the health system. In: *Interactions between global health initiatives and health systems: Evidence from countries.* Geneva: World Health Organization; 2009. http://www.who.int/healthsystems/publications/MPS_academic_case_studies_Book_01.pdf

58. Ministry of Health and Social Welfare, MOHSW/Lesotho and ICF Macro. *Lesotho demographic and health survey, 2009.* Maseru, Lesotho: Ministry of Health [Lesotho]; 2009.

59. Satti H, Motsamai S, Chetane P, et al. Comprehensive approach to improving maternal health and achieving MDG 5: Report from the mountains of Lesotho. *PLOS One.* 2012;7(8):e42700.

60. World Bank. *Health nutrition and population statistics.* New York: World Bank; 2017. http://data.worldbank.org/data-catalog/health-nutrition-and-population-statistics

61. Randive B, Diwan V, De Costa A. India's conditional cash transfer programme (the JSY) to promote institutional birth: Is there an association between institutional birth proportion and maternal mortality? *PLoS One.* 2013;8(6).

62. Larson E, Vail D, Mbaruku GM, Mbatia R, Kruk ME. Beyond utilization: Measuring effective coverage of obstetric care along the quality cascade. *Intl J Qual Health Care.* 2016;29(1):104–110.

63. Kruk ME, Leslie HH, Verguet S, Mbaruku GM, Adanu RMK, Langer A. Quality of basic maternal care functions in health facilities of five African countries: An analysis of national health system surveys. *Lancet Glob Health.* 2016;4(11):e855.

64. Anatole M, Magge H, Redditt V, et al. Nurse mentorship to improve the quality of health care delivery in rural Rwanda. *Nurs Outlook.* 2012;61(3):137–144.

65. Hongoro C, McPake B. How to bridge the gap in human resources for health. *Lancet.* 2004;364(9443):1451–1456.

66. Kruk ME, Myers M, Varpilah ST, Dahn BT. What is a resilient health system? Lessons from Ebola. *Lancet.* 2015;385(9980):1910–1912.

67. Akachi Y, Tarp F, Kelley E, Addison T, Kruk ME. Measuring quality-of-care in the context of Sustainable Development Goal 3: A call for papers. *Bull World Health Org.* 2016;94(3).

12

Health Financing

Key Points

- Health financing is a critical aspect of Universal Health Coverage (UHC).
- In 2000, the Commission on Macroeconomics and Health elucidated the link between health and development and called for bold global political and financial commitments to health.
- The gross domestic product (GDP), gross national income (GNI), and Gini coefficient are used to assess a country's economy and level of inequality.
- The Abuja Declaration spurred African governments to commit more of their government's GDP to health.
- There is a need for coordination among financing sources to reduce inefficiencies and fragmentation of care if UHC is to be achieved.

Introduction

Achieving Universal Health Care (UHC) is still aspirational in most places. Prior to the global health era, the interventions chosen for impoverished countries—by outside experts—were selected based on the notion that they could be sustained on the country's meager budget[1,2] and delivered by volunteers. While aspirations have improved, country budgets remain too small to pay for UHC and fulfill the right to health. Thus, one of the biggest challenges to achieving this goal is financing.[3] Rather than looking to user fees, the overall landscape of health financing must change. Large-scale improvements in health delivery are not only the responsibility of the individual nation-state, but the collective responsibility of all. This chapter addresses the macroeconomics of health financing. *Macroeconomics* is a term that describes the large-scale forces that impact an economy.[4] This chapter also highlights sources for health funding, challenges for impoverished countries, and novel concepts for financing health.

Macroeconomics and Global Health

At the dawn of the global health era, the Commission on Macroeconomics and Health (CMH) elucidated the linkages between health and development.[5,6] The report of this committee, published in 2001, called for bold action in the form of economic commitments from wealthy countries and political will from impoverished countries to achieve targets set by the UN's Millennium Development Goals (MDGs). Officers of the commission estimated that a minimum of $34 per capita per year was needed for primary health care. A commitment to financing and achieving the MDGs, they calculated, would save 8 million lives per year by the end of the decade. The Commission elaborated a nine-point set of recommendations that included (1) national-level coordination on poverty reduction and scaling up of essential health interventions; (2) increased in-country financing (i.e., a larger proportion of the country's own budget allocated toward health); (3) increased financial contributions from wealthy countries to impoverished ones, specifically in the form of grants as opposed to loans; (4) new funding mechanisms beyond the nation-state to nation-state (so-called bilateral) support that implicated the whole international community committing to health through pooled contributions; (5) international support of public goods—from drugs and commodities to disease surveillance tools; (6) support for development of disease-specific drugs for illnesses that affect the poor; (7) ensuring a low-cost supply of essential medicines in collaboration with the pharmaceutical industry; (8) employing safeguards to allow impoverished countries to get drugs that may be patent protected, and (9) addressing the macroeconomic constraints that had been placed on poor countries that impacted health (specifically neoliberal spending caps on public expenditures for health and education).

Prior to the CHM report, the poor state of health and health systems in impoverished countries were largely ignored by the economic development community. Economists and other development professionals assumed that health would improve with increased economic growth (Chapter 4). With this underlying assumption, failures of the health system were attributed to the mismanagement of resources or to patients' behavior and choices.[7] In contrast to this prevailing belief, the authors of the CHM wrote that health was central to development. The data showed that the high morbidity and mortality in impoverished countries was due to poverty. They concluded that impoverished countries could not pay for health care without significant external (donor) funding and called for budgetary rather than extra-budgetary support. *Budgetary support* means that donor funds are put directly into a country's health budget and under the control of the government.[8] This recommendation was a notable change from years of structural adjustment and its requisite shrinking of the public sector in favor of private-sector investments or *off-budget support*. By 2012, Professor Sachs and others re-evaluated their estimates for the cost of health care and determined that the delivery of primary health care alone would cost a minimum of $50–60 per capita per year.[9] Notably, primary health care is only one component of UHC; it does not include more complicated but necessary aspects of UHC such as access to hospitalization or surgery. A recent study estimated the cost of UHC at about $80 per capita per year.[10,11]

Global financial inputs must match the aspiration of UHC by 2030. Since the drafting of the CMH report, the financial inputs into global health have changed, particularly as the movement for AIDS treatment access challenged the notion of sustainability based on country budgets alone.[12] These shifts include (1) the significant movement to relieve the debt of impoverished countries,[13] (2) impoverished governments increasing the share of their gross domestic product (GDP) allocated for health,[14] and (3) new funds to support health pledged and distributed from wealthy countries to impoverished ones (predominantly for HIV, TB and malaria).[15]

Furthermore, philanthropic interest in health has grown, led by groups such as the Bill and Melinda Gates Foundation, the Open Society Institute, and the older Rockefeller and Ford Foundations.[16,17] Some countries have also started health insurance programs to decrease out-of-pocket spending at the time that illness occurs.[18,19] Finally, there is more focus on a government's planning and coordination of various sources of health financing (government, donor, insurance) to minimize the fragmentation of the health system. Despite these strategies, much more work is needed to finance UHC.

Assessing the Health Financing Landscape

Some health financing data are publicly available for all countries. A review of a simple set of data can illuminate the strengths and weaknesses of a country's ability to finance health. The first factor to consider when assessing a country's ability to finance health is the GDP. A country's GDP is a measure of the total dollar value of all goods and services produced in an economy during a given period, usually one year.[20] It refers to the size of the economy and can be calculated by either adding up total income (personal, corporate, tax, etc.) or total expenditure. GDP includes foreign direct investment and foreign ownership. A similar measure is the gross national income (GNI), which also measures the total dollar value of the economy but measures only domestic value-added production and ownership. In other words, the GNI reflects how much of the GDP is generated by and stays in a country. Luxembourg, for example, has a strong financial sector and a high GDP per capita. However, many of the people who work in Luxembourg commute into the country every day from neighboring countries; therefore their income does not stay in the country. Therefore, Luxembourg's GNI is lower than its GDP.[21] Economists use GNI as an indicator for stratifying countries to low-, middle-, and high-income. In 2017, the World Bank defined a low-income country (what this book terms "impoverished") as a country with a GNI per capita of less than $1,025. Middle-income countries have a GNI per capita of $1,026 to $12,475, and high-income countries have a GNI per capita of $12,476 or more.[20]

Once the GDP (or GNI) is known, it is important to understand the distribution of the wealth among the population within a country. The standard measure of inequality is called the *Gini coefficient*, named for its developer, Corrado Gini.[22] The United Nations Development Programme (UNDP) defines the Gini coefficient as the "deviation of the distribution of income among individuals or households within a country from a perfectly equal distribution."[23] A Gini coefficient of 0 reflects perfect income equality. A Gini coefficient of 100 reflects perfect inequality. In other words, if the Gini coefficient is high, there is more inequality between rich and poor. If the Gini coefficient is low, income distribution is more equitable.

A country's wealth is best evaluated when both the GDP and the Gini coefficient are taken into account. A country may have a relatively equitable distribution of wealth, but a very low GDP with which to provide services. For example, in 2010, Malawi had a per capita GDP of just $471 and a Gini coefficient of 46. The income distribution is fairly even, but the country is quite poor. In contrast, in 2012, Haiti had a per capita GDP of $767 and a Gini coefficient of 61.[24] Despite the higher per capita income in Haiti, wealth disparity is more significant than in Malawi. In wealthy countries, the Gini coefficient can be instructive as well. Norway had a per capita GDP of $87,646 in 2010 and a low Gini coefficient of 26.[24] In contrast, the United States had a per capita GDP of $48,374 in 2010 and a Gini coefficient of 40.5.[24] The United States has a much higher level of income inequality than Norway. Wealth inequality is correlated with health inequality due to unequal access to health services and the impact of negative social determinants of health (Table 12.1).[25]

Health Expenditure

Total health expenditure in impoverished countries generally comes from four sources. The first source is the *government health expenditure*. It is the percent of the total government budget (GDP or GNI) that is used for health. The second source is *external financing*. That is the percent of the total health expenditure that comes from donors. The third source is the percent of the total health expenditure that comes from *health insurance*. This source is very low in impoverished

Table 12.1 Comparison of selected country financial equality and health outcomes (2010–2012).

	GDP per Capita (Constant US$)	Gini Coefficient	% of GDP Spent on Health (Public Funds)	Life Expectancy
United States	49,941.50	41.1	8	78.8
Haiti	698.8	60.8	1	62
Malawi	471.1	46.1	6.3	56.8
Norway	88,584.90	25.9	7.8	81.5

Wealth inequality and government expenditure on health influence life expectancy.

Source: Data abstracted from World Bank. World development indicators. The World Bank Databank Web site. 2017. Available from: http://databank.worldbank.org/data/reports.aspx?source=world-development-indicators. Accessed Mar 29, 2017.

countries but may come from people buying insurance from private or government sources or it may come from employers provision of health insurance. The fourth source is *out-of-pocket expenditure*. It is the percent of the total health expenditure that is borne by the patient at the time of illness (Figure 12.1).

Government Health Expenditure

The government health expenditure is a necessary component of financing health yet in impoverished countries it is insufficient. In 2014, government expenditure on health ranged from $8 per capita per year in the Central African Republic to $4,541 per capita per year in the United States.[26] Wealthy countries that provide health care as a basic right (such as the United Kingdom, France, and Canada) finance health through tax revenues. The United Kingdom spent $3,272 per capita on health in 2014. Their famous National Health Service is financed through taxes.[26] Some middle-income countries like Thailand,[27] Turkey,[28,29] and Mexico[30,31] have changed the tax structure to finance improvements in health delivery with the goal of reducing catastrophic health expenditures[32] and supporting the achievement of UHC. Other countries, such as Botswana[33] and Venezuela,[34] have used revenues from state-owned natural resources to support health. In general, increased government expenditures on health are associated with positive population-based health outcomes.[35,36] Impoverished countries, however, have much lower GDPs from which to generate tax revenues and may not own their natural resources.[37] Such countries have far less potential for raising revenues through taxes or tariffs to pay for health.[38]

Nigeria: Total Health expenditure: $118 per capital (GDP $2671 per capita, Gini 48.8)

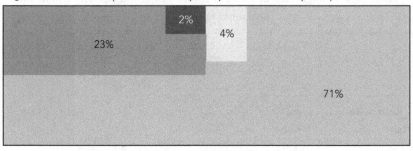

Honduras: Total Health expentiture: $212 GDP $2528.9 per capita, Gini 57

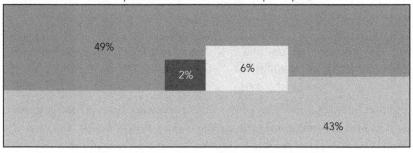

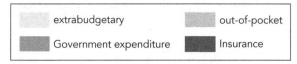

FIGURE 12.1 Figure shows different funding sources for health in Nigeria and Honduras countries with similar GDPs. While Honduras has higher wealth inequality, the government commits more of its resources to health and thus people have much lower out-of-pocket expenditure.

Source: Data abstracted from World Health Organization. NHA indicators. 2014. Available from: http://apps.who.int/nha/database/ViewData/Indicators/en. Accessed Mar 29, 2017.

In 2000, against the backdrop of underfunded public health systems, increased calls for donor funding of HIV treatment and the MDGs resulted in an international dialogue about what impoverished countries themselves should commit to health.[6] In 2001, the same year as the UN General Assembly Special Session on AIDS and the release of the CMH report, African heads of state met in Abuja, Nigeria. They pledged to spend at least 15 percent of their governments' annual budgets on health.[39,40] At that time, African Union countries spent an average of 2.2 percent of government expenditure on health,[26] which was equal to about $5–10 per capita per year. The exact figures ranged from $0.38 to $380 per capita.[14] Although countries have increased health spending in the years after the

Abuja Declaration, only five African countries—Rwanda, South Africa, Zambia, Madagascar, and Togo—reached the goal of committing at least 15 percent of government expenditure on health.[39]

The percent of government expenditure that is used for health is widely considered a signal of political will. High government expenditure on health is attractive donors. Rwanda is an example of a country in which health is high on the government's agenda. Because of the increased percentage of government expenditure that is allocated to health, donors are more willing to give aid and to coordinate their aid with the government's plans. Countries with a low percentage of expenditure on health are often considered too weak to coordinate aid, and donors may sidestep government planning. This fragments and further weakens the health system.

In some cases, civil society and social movements are pushing governments to increase health expenditure. In South Africa, TAC and other civil society groups pushed for equitable access to antiretroviral therapy (ART). In Brazil and Thailand, civil society groups pressured governments to increase spending on health.[41–43] In 2015, a group of medical students in Uganda, called Focus15ForHealth, led a campaign to pressure their government to commit 15 percent of the government's expenditure for health (Figure 12.2A, B).[44,45] There is also a growing international organization called Article 25 that aims to foster a global movement for the public provision of health care as a human right (Box 12.1).[46]

Impoverished governments may be committed to health and commit a significant percentage of their budget to delivering care. However, the absolute value of the money committed may be too low to improve the health of the population. In 2014, in Malawi, the government expenditure on health is about 6 percent. Because the country is so impoverished, that percentage amounts to only $15 per person per year.[26] A health budget this low results in low and erratic pay for health workers and leads to internal and external brain drain.[47] The Malawian health sector also experiences frequent stock-outs of drugs[48] and has little money for the maintenance and general operating costs of facilities.[49] In the district of Neno, Malawi, where Partners in Health works, the money sent to the district is less than $2 per capita per year. This money cannot even cover the hospital's electric bill. The tiny, remote district is dependent on donor aid simply to light the facilities.[49] This penury is not uncommon.[50]

External Financing and Its Impact

Donor money is a critical component to financing health systems in impoverished countries. In 2005, wealthy countries met at the G-8 Summit in Gleneagles, Scotland. At that time, wealthy countries committed to spending 1 percent of their GNI on overseas development assistance. As is often the case, only a few

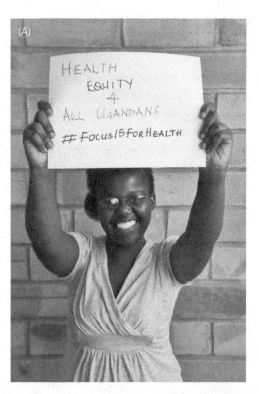

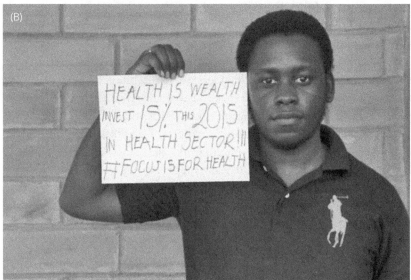

FIGURE 12.2 (A,B) Focus15ForHealth, a Ugandan student-led group advocating for increased government expenditure for health. Focus15ForHealth is advocating for the government to spend 15% of its annual expenditure on health.

Source: Michael Westerhaus.

BOX 12.1

Article 25

"Article 25 is building a people-powered movement to fight the global health crisis. We defend public health systems where they are threatened, hold the pharmaceutical industry accountable to ensure access to essential medicines, and transform the narrative on healthcare as a human right."[1] Named after the 25th Article of the Universal Declaration of Human Rights (UDHR): "[every person has] the right to a standard of living adequate for the health and well-being of himself and of his family,"[2] Article 25 is a non-profit organization founded in 2014 that advocates for the right to health. The group trains and supports people around the world to become activists for health equity. In October 2014, Article 25 held the first Global Day of Action for the Right to Health. This campaign brought together more than 15,000 people in 165 events across 65 countries.

1. Article 25. Available from: https://join25.org/. Accessed Mar 29, 2017.

2. United Nations General Assembly. *Universal declaration of human rights. Final authorized text.* New York: United Nations Dept. of Public Information; 1952.

---

countries met these pledges.[51] By 2016, the only countries that met the commitment were United Arab Emirates, Norway, and Luxembourg.[52] The United States only commits 0.2 percent of its GNI to overseas development assistance, most of which is not to assist impoverished countries for health. For geopolitical reasons, US overseas development assistance is highest in Afghanistan.[52,53]

Because of the history of impoverishment and the continued monetary policy that constricts public expenditures for health, impoverished countries desperately need external financing. Yet there are a myriad of obstacles facing in using aid effecting. One is the shortage of human resources. At the height of the AIDS crisis, the government of Malawi had to pass an emergency wage bill to hire nurses onto government payrolls, in direct contradiction with the externally imposed public sector spending caps.[54] Similarly, Uganda's first Global Fund grant was initially rejected by the government for fear that it would exceed their public-sector spending cap for health and would result in the loss of their World Bank loans.[55-58] Often donors support NGOs rather than public-sector institutions. This practice causes fragmentation of care delivery, poor care in public facilities, and internal brain drain of health care workers from public to NGO programs.[59] This rhetoric of shrinking the public sector is common in both impoverished and wealthy countries, as evidenced by the 2017 US congressional debate on repealing the Affordable Care Act or the debates about the United Kingdom's National Health Service.[60]

The most common reason cited to limit the size of the public sector comes from neoliberal theory and a preference for the private sector.[61] Another concept used to justify shrinking public expenditure is the fear of inflation. In post-World War II Holland, after an injection of cash into the public sector, inflation was seen. Because of this, the potential for inflation after large public expenditure is sometimes referred to as "Dutch disease."[62] The third reason used by donors for limiting their investment in the public sector is government corruption.[63] Transparency International is an anticorruption coalition that publishes reports on perceived corruption in each country.[64] Their 2016 report shows a high level perceived corruption in sub-Saharan African countries compared to the perception of corruption in North American and Western European countries.[64] This perception is likely based on a long history of racism, impoverishment, and the lack of systems for financial tracking. It also ignores the historical fact that many of the most brutal and corrupt dictators in Africa, such as Mobutu Sese Seko, were directly enriched by deals with the United States and financed by the World Bank.[65] The perception of corruption in impoverished countries ignores the billions of dollars of fraud committed in wealthy countries and the impact that such "white collar" crime has on the global economy. Take, for example, the fraud committed by banking executives that led to the US housing market crash and the global economic recession of 2008. Fraud committed by American bankers led to the loss of $16.4 trillion in household wealth between 2007 and 2009.[66] As is often the case, racial disparities in the impact of this crisis tracked the history of the United States. Home equity decreased 30 percent more for African-Americans than for white Americans.[67] Following the crash, 49 financial institutions paid only $190 billion in fines and settlements. Only one person was sentenced for the massive amount of fraud that sent the world into a recession.[68] More recently, in 2017, South Korean President Park was impeached for using her position to benefit close friends.[69] It is important to consider claims of corruption are most often leveled at impoverished countries in light of these much larger scandals.

Many rich countries, such as the United Kingdom and Canada, and middle-income countries, such as Mexico and Costa Rica, have large public expenditures on health. They achieve relatively equitable access and good health outcomes without significant inflation, evidence of corruption, or stifling economic growth. However, because of the entrenched avoidance of public-sector support, much of the aid to the health sector of impoverished countries does not directly support government health budgets.

Donor Coordination

In many impoverished countries, external financing makes up a significant proportion of the health budget. However, all external financing is not equal.

Governments prefer direct budget support. Direct budget support means that external financing is placed under the control of the government and may be used for any public expenditure. This promotes coordination of planning and delivery of health. However, a significant proportion of external financing is off-budget. This means it does not go directly into the health budget of the country but is managed separately, often by a nongovernmental organization (NGO). Governments try to harmonize off-budget money and programs to align with national plans, but may face difficulty if NGOs or donors have a different agenda than the government.

To support coordination of external assistance within the government framework, the new millennium also introduced country-driven poverty reduction strategy papers (PRSP) as part of the process to access foreign assistance.[63] The PRSP process promotes country leadership to develop a national strategy of poverty reduction—including investments in health, jobs, and education. The PRSP process focuses on the coordination of government expenditure, donor contribution, and the contribution of debt relief to the national budget.[70] PRSPs also incorporate civil society voices. Donor coordination is also seen with AIDS funds. Growing out of the AIDS movement's concept of the "three-ones,"[70] the Global Fund stipulated the creation of a country coordinating mechanism (CCM), which includes government and civil society groups.[71] Finally, in some countries, such as Rwanda, governments control the use of aid through strong national planning and guidelines.[72] Donor coordination in Rwanda includes a willingness on the part of the government to forgo aid if it does not fit with national priorities. There is strong evidence that donor coordination has a positive effect on health outcomes.[73,74]

In many countries, however, off-budget health work is still the norm and is performed by a set of poorly coordinated NGOs that are not accountable to the government. To address this issue, African health ministers and donors held a meeting in Paris in 2005.[73] The Paris Declaration on Aid Effectiveness called for results and mutual accountability in aid. The declaration, signed by 130 ministers and donors, represents a broad consensus on aid effectiveness. It called for aid-recipient countries to develop their own national development strategies and, most importantly, voiced the aspiration that donors would support national plans.[75] Whether well-coordinated or not, off-budget health support remains a significant factor to consider in analyzing the health financing landscape of a country. To this end, a large group of activists, public health professionals, and ministers of health from around the world drafted the Framework Convention on Global Health.[75] The Framework sets rigorous principles for aid coordination and supports long-term systems development to maximize the support for health in a given country (see Box 12.2).

BOX 12.2

Framework Convention on Global Health

In light of the growing number of international treaties and multinational collaborations in global health, the Framework Convention on Global Health is supported by a group of people from all sectors of public and global health who advocate for a coordinated effort with the mission of creating a right-to-health governance framework.[1] The part of the framework that relates to health financing calls for[2]:

1. Funding for universal health systems and the social determinants of health
2. Establishment of a national and global health financing framework with clearly delineated responsibilities to raise sufficient resources to achieve equitable and effective health systems, including public health functions such as ensuring clean water and nutritious food
3. Raising additional domestic and international resources for health and ensuring accountable and equitable use of these resources
4. Equitable distribution of financing within countries, including ensuring needed resources for underserved and marginalized communities and populations
5. Improving international health assistance harmonization and alignment with national health strategies, with mutual accountability particularly to affected populations

1. FCGH. FCGH platform. Platform for a Framework Convention on Global Health Web site. 2017. Available from: http://www.globalhealthtreaty.org/about-us/. Accessed Apr 27, 2017.

2. FCGH. Platform for a framework convention on global health: Realizing the universal right to health: Fundamental principles and joining the platform. Bangladesh: Global Health Treaty; 2014. http://www.globalhealthtreaty.org/docs/platform-for-an-fcgh-full.pdf

---

Out-of-Pocket Expenditures

Despite increased funding for health insufficient health financing pushes the burden of payment onto patients themselves (Table 12.2). Some examples of out-of-pocket expenditures include paying for a registration card, a user fee to access the clinic, as well as fees for a consultation, diagnostic tests, and medicines.[76–78] In addition, there are a variety of nonclinical out-of-pocket expenditures, such as transportation to clinic and lost wages. Whether within the system or hidden, out-of-pocket costs pose a significant barrier to

Table 12.2 Government and out-of-pocket expenditure on health in selected countries.

	Gini	GDP per Capita (Constant 2010 $US)	GNI per Capita (Constant 2010 $US)	Government Health Expenditure as % of GDP	Government Health Expenditure per Capita (Constant 2010 $US)	Out-of-Pocket Expenditure as % of Total Health Expenditure	Out-of-Pocket per capita (Constant 2010 $US)
Haiti (2012)	60.8	766.9	704.7	1	7	28	19
Luxembourg (2010)	30.9	103,267.30	76,825.40	7	6,838	10	763
Peru (2012)	45.1	5,519.20	5,171.30	3	182	36	102
Rwanda (2013)	50.4	631.8	620.2	3	18	28	13
Thailand (2013)	37.9	5,612.70	5,269.50	3	160	12	25
United States (2013)	41.1	49,941.50	50,507.70	8	4,058	11	979

Source: World Health Organization. NHA Indicators. 2014. Available at: http://apps.who.int/nha/database/ViewData/Indicators/en. Accessed Mar 29, 2017.

accessing health care for many. To achieve equity, it is important to minimize out-of-pocket expenditures because they impact the poor disproportionately.[79] Studies have shown that catastrophic expenses are most often incurred at the hospital level.[80] Catastrophic expenditures result in significant levels of impoverishment, with documented consequences even in wealthy countries. In the United States, one study estimates that 57.1 percent of cases of personal bankruptcy are due to medical bills.[32,81,82]

Out-of-pocket expenditures can be reduced in a variety of ways. An important step is to minimize financial barriers at the facility level.[83] Accordingly, an increasing number of governments are removing user fees (Table 12.3).[84] Sierra Leone has taken the step of assuring that maternal and child health services are free of charge. Signs are posted to remind patients that care is their right and that they should not be asked to pay (Figure 12.3).[39] After the 2014 Ebola epidemic, the government also offered free services to Ebola survivors, recognizing that this vulnerable group needed special support.[85] However, even after the removal of user fees, there may be additional costs for medicines. This is particularly true if government pharmacies are stocked-out of medicines which forces patients to turn to private pharmacies. With weak systems to forecast drugs and insufficient money for procurement, many of the services that are supposed to be free are still available only at a high cost.

Another method to alleviate out-of-pocket expenses for health is to offset the out-of-pocket costs with cash transfers. For example, studies document the positive impact of vouchers or cash to pay for transportation to ART clinic.[86] The use of cash to incentivize clinic utilization as a way to offset the out-of-pocket cost of care is called a *conditional cash transfer*.[87] Another example of a conditional cash transfer is Mexico's Oportunidades program, which provides a financial incentive to mothers if their children are vaccinated and receive age-appropriate medical follow-up.[88]

Health Insurance

Health insurance is another way to minimize the out-of-pocket cost of receiving care at the time a patient falls ill. Health insurance is based on the pooling of risk in a large group of people. If the pool of people who pay into the program is large enough, when a member of the pool falls ill, the funds are sufficient to cover the cost. For health insurance to work, the pool of people covered must include both the sick and the healthy. If too many people in the pool are sick, the payouts needed to cover health costs may exceed the money collected. This is why, in the United States, when the Affordable Care Act was passed, there was a conscious effort to enroll young people who are generally less likely to get sick.[89] Because poor people have a higher burden of disease and less money to commit to

Table 12.3 Some of the countries that have abolished user fees or provide formal exemptions.

Country (Year)	Maternal Health	Child Health	Total Population	Disease Categories
Benin	Free C-section	Under-fives	Primary Health Care and Secondary Health Care	Malaria, hemodialysis
Burkina Faso (2006)	Reduction of 80% for C-section and delivery fees	Neonatal care, 80% subsidy		
Burundi (2005)	Pregnant women and deliveries	Under-fives		
Cape Verde			There is also the basic Protection National Centre of Social Pension (9700 CNPS)[1]	
Congo (2010)	Pregnant women and deliveries			Free malaria treatment for those under 15 years
Côte d'Ivoire	Pregnant women	Under-fives		
Ghana (2008)	Pregnant women	Under-fives		
Guinea (2011)	Deliveries			
Kenya (2007)	Deliveries			
Lesotho (2008)			At Primary Health Care level	
Liberia (2007)			In late 2011, a user fee assessment was carried out with a view of reintroducing user fees by 2013	

(*continued*)

Table 12.3 Continued

Country (Year)	Maternal Health	Child Health	Total Population	Disease Categories
Madagascar (2008)	Free deliveries			
Malawi			Essential health care package free for all	
Mauritania				Malaria, HIV, tuberculosis, hemodialysis
Niger (2006)	Deliveries	Under-fives		
Senegal (2006)	Deliveries and free C-section		Students and people older than 60 years (SESAME programme)	
Sierra Leone (2010)	Pregnant women and lactating mothers	Under-fives		Malaria
Togo (2010)	Free C-section	Under-fives		Tuberculosis and leprosy
Uganda (2001)			All population	
Zambia (2006)			All in rural districts	

Source: WHO Africa. State of health financing in the African Region. Geneva: World Health Organization Regional Office for Africa; 2013.

insurance, pooling of risk is often very challenging if it is done only in communities that are predominantly poor.[90]

Rwanda has a well-known medical insurance scheme to support the poor. The Mutuelle de Santé program supports care at the primary and secondary levels and has a per-person, per-year enrollment cost.[19,73] The country is organized at the level of the *cellule* (a collection of villages). The cellule categorizes the population based on wealth quintiles and poorest quintile is enrolled in

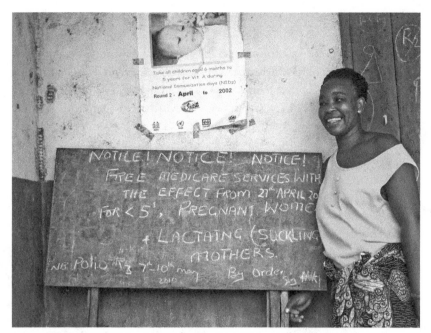

FIGURE 12.3 Free maternal health services at a clinic in Sierra Leone.

Source: Dodgeon S, Vowles Z, Lawrence N, Taqi RB, Edwards S. Sierra Leone's free healthcare initiative. Health Poverty Action; 2010. https://www.healthpovertyaction.org/wp content/uploads/downloads/2012/07/SierraLeoneFHIbriefingweb12.pdf

the *mutuelle* program free of charge.[91] Others pay on a sliding scale. When people fall ill, they pay a flat fee or co-pay instead of paying for consultation, medications, and diagnostic tests. Social insurance schemes that encourage enrollment of all and are supported through government and donor subsidies are considered progressive (more pro-poor). In contrast, voluntary or private insurance that favors the ability to pay is considered regressive. One of the challenges of the *mutuelle* program is the fact that the middle class and wealthy are insured through the private sector instead of through the government-run *mutuelle* program. With the lower health risk profile and larger contributions of wealthy people into the private sector, the insurance that covers sicker, poorer people had less money. Seeing this gap, the government of Rwanda has added both government revenues and taxes from the private insurance sector to the *mutuelle* program to assure that more money is available to cover the destitute sick. While such insurance schemes do help alleviate some of the cost of health care—particularly minimizing catastrophic expenditures—any fee is onerous to many.

Both Ghana and Nigeria also have interesting examples of national health insurance schemes (NHIS). In the postindependence era, both countries aspired to provide health care for their citizens and set up frameworks to enable health as a right. However, due to structural adjustment policies and dwindling health budgets in the 1980s, both countries were forced to forgo their NHIS.[18,92] Ghana reinstituted the NHIS in 2003, with benefits that covered about 95 percent of all common illnesses and conditions. Notably, these benefits do not cover ARTs, TB treatment, or mental health treatment because there are separate government agencies devoted to each of these illnesses. The scheme is divided into three insurance tiers: the district mutual, the private mutual, and the private commercial insurances. The only tier that receives direct government funding is the district mutual, as part of the government's poverty reduction strategy. Premiums are based on what people can pay, with a minimum annual contribution of $8 per person per year. The poorest and the elderly are exempt from this fee. By December 2009, the NHIS covered about 60 percent of the population. However, only about a third of the population contribute financially; the rest are exempt.[18] Nigeria's NHIS is also split into three tiers: formal sector, urban self-employed, and rural community. The formal sector scheme is implemented by health maintenance organizations (HMOs) and accredited providers. It is funded by employers and employees, who have a mandatory contribution. The other two schemes are run as nonprofits and are voluntary. By 2011, only 3.5 percent of the population that was self-employed or rural was covered.[92]

Nigeria has failed in covering their population while Ghana has made significant strides.[92] However, studies done in Ghana show that the likelihood of NHIS enrolment increases with increased education, income, and employment, which seems to suggest that the poorest and most vulnerable people are still being overlooked. Qualitative work also highlights that hospitals and health care administrators are not interpreting the legislation consistently. There are significant gaps in coverage of and access to care.[18] Nigeria, fares worse when it comes to the impact of its NHIS.[92] Studies show that while health outcomes are improving in the country, there are strong inequalities within the coverage of health insurance and access to health care. Furthermore, Nigeria's government expenditure on health did not change much between 2000 and 2010. Some reports indicate that the health insurance scheme actually had negative effects on out-of-pocket expenditure.[92]

Novel Financing

Eight men have more wealth than the poorest 3.6 billion people on the planet.[93] This shocking truth reflects a world economy that is unjust, unsustainable, and cruel to the poor.[93] In this setting, many have sought solutions to remediate global inequality, most notably Bill and Melinda Gates. Yet individual charity is not the solution to wealth inequality. Novel solutions to fund health, education, and other global social goods are needed. One example is the idea of the *Robin Hood tax* on financial transactions.[94] In 2011, more than 1,000 economists from 53 countries proposed this tax to the finance ministers of the G20 countries.[94] Another novel financing mechanism is called UNITAID. A key source of UNITAID funding is a *solidarity levy* a tax on airline tickets implemented by France, Cameroon, Chile, the DRC, Guinea, Madagascar, Mali, Mauritius, Niger, and South Korea.[95] UNITAID supports AIDS, TB, and malaria care and research. Yet proposed method of financing health is the newly proposed Financing Alliance, a group of health care providers and economists committed to helping governments design and fund community health programs. The Financing Alliance brings together corporations, investment banks, and private equity firms to develop new sources of capital for community health worker programs.[96]

Conclusion

UHC will not be achieved without financing. Health care is paid for by a mix of funds—government expenditure, donor financing, out-of-pocket expenditures, and health insurance. From the Paris Declaration on Aid Effectiveness of 2005[75] to the newly developed Framework Convention on Global Health,[97] there is a growing movement for the shared global responsibility to finance the right to health. Long-term financing is needed to break the constant cycle of underinvestment in health that cripples the delivery of health care in the most impoverished regions of the world.

References

1. Chen LC, Singh S, Victora CG. Sustainability of the world summit for children goals: Concepts and strategies. New York, NY: UNICEF; 1997.
2. Kim JY, Millen JV, Irwin A, eds. *Dying for growth: Global inequality and the health of the poor.* Monroe, ME: Common Courage Press; 2000.
3. Jamison DT, Summers LH, Alleyne G, et al. Global health 2035: A world converging within a generation. *Lancet.* 2013;382(9908):1898–1955.
4. Sims C. Macroeconomics and reality. *Econometrica.* 1980;48(1):1–48.
5. World Health Organization. *Investing in health: A summary of the findings of the commission on macroeconomics and health.* Geneva: World Health Organization; 2003.
6. Sachs J. Macroeconomics and health: Investing in health for economic development, report of the commission on macroeconomics and health. Geneva: World

Health Organization; 2001. http://www1.worldbank.org/publicsector/pe/PEAMMarch2005/CMHReport.pdf

7. Herbert B. Americans refusing to save Africans. *New York Times*. Jun 11, 2001. Available from: http://www.nytimes.com/2001/06/11/opinion/in-america-refusing-to-save-africans.html.

8. Antunes AF, Carrin G, Evans DB. *General budget support in developing countries: Ensuring the health sector's interest*. Department of Health Systems Financing Health Financing Policy. Geneva: World Health Organization; 2008.

9. Sachs JD. Achieving universal health coverage in low-income settings. *Lancet*. 2012;380(9845):944–947.

10. Rottingen John-Arne, Ottersen T, Ablo A, et al. *Shared responsibilities for health: A coherent global framework for health financing*. London: Chatham House, the Royal Institute of International Affairs; 2014.

11. Yates R. Estimate for UHC costs. May 3, 2017.

12. WHO Maximizing Positive Synergies Working Group. An assessment of interactions between global health initiatives and country health systems. *Lancet*. 2009;373(9681):2137–2169.

13. Giugale M. Does debt forgiveness work? Ask Africa. *The Huffington Post*. May 13, 2014. Available from: http://www.huffingtonpost.com/marcelo-giugale/does-debt-forgiveness-wor_b_5318764.html. Accessed Mar 28, 2017.

14. Organisation of African Unity. Abuja Declaration on HIV/AIDS, tuberculosis and other related infectious diseases. Geneva: United Nations; 2001.

15. Ravishankar N, Gubbins P, Cooley RJ, et al. Financing of global health: Tracking development assistance for health from 1990 to 2007. *Lancet*. 2009;373(9681):2113–2124.

16. Stone D. Private philanthropy or policy transfer? The transnational norms of the open society institute. *Policy Politics*. 2010;38(2):269–287.

17. Mccoy D, Chand S, Sridhar D. Global health funding: How much, where it comes from and where it goes. *Health Policy Plan*. 2009;24(6):407–417.

18. Barimah KB, Mensah J. Ghana's national health insurance scheme: Insights from members, administrators and health care providers. *J Health Care Poor Underserved*. 2013;24(3):1378–1390.

19. Makaka A, Breen S, Binagwaho A. Universal health coverage in Rwanda: A report of innovations to increase enrolment in community-based health insurance. *Lancet*. 2012;380:S2–S7.

20. World Bank. World bank country and lending groups. 2017. Available from: https://datahelpdesk.worldbank.org/knowledgebase/articles/906519-world-bank-country-and-lending-groups. Accessed Mar 29, 2017.

21. OECD Observer. GDP and GNI. 2000s. Available from: http://oecdobserver.org/news/archivestory.php/aid/1507/GDP_and_GNI.html. Accessed Apr 27, 2017.

22. Ceriani L, Verme P. The origins of the Gini index: Extracts from variabilit e mutabilit (1912) by Corrado Gini. *J Econ Inequal*. 2012;10(3):421–443.

23. UNDP. Income Gini coefficient. United Nations Development Programme—Human Development Report Web site. Available from: http://hdr.undp.org/en/content/income-gini-coefficient. Accessed Mar 29, 2017.

24. World Bank. World development indicators. The World Bank Databank Web site. 2017. Available from: http://databank.worldbank.org/data/reports.aspx?source=world-development-indicators. Accessed Mar 29, 2017.

25. Marmot MG, Stansfeld S, Patel C, et al. Health inequalities among British civil servants: The Whitehall II study. *Lancet*. 1991;337(8754):1387–1393.

26. World Health Organization. NHA indicators. 2014. Available from: http://apps.who.int/nha/database/ViewData/Indicators/en. Accessed Mar 29, 2017.

27. Prakongsai P. The equity impact of the universal coverage policy: Lessons from Thailand. *Adv Health Econ Health Serv Res*. 2009;21:57–81.

28. Baris E, Mollahaliloglu S, Aydin S. Healthcare in turkey: From laggard to leader. *BMJ*. 2011; 342(7797):579.

29. Atun R, Aydın S, Chakraborty S, et al. Universal health coverage in turkey: Enhancement of equity. *Lancet*. 2013;382(9886):65–99.

30. Frenk J, González-Pier E, Gómez-Dantés O, Lezana MA, Knaul FM. Comprehensive reform to improve health system performance in Mexico. *Lancet*. 2006;368(9546):1524–1534.

31. Atun R, de Andrade L, Monteiro O, Almeida G, et al. Health-system reform and universal health coverage in Latin America. *Lancet*. 2014;385(9974):1230–1247.

32. Xu K, Evans DB, Kawabata K, Zeramdini R, Klavus J, Murray CJL. Household catastrophic health expenditure: A multicountry analysis. *Lancet*. 2003;362(9378):111–117.

33. Health Policy Project. Health financing profile: Botswana. USAID, PEPFAR, Health Policy Project. Washington, D.C.: Health Policy Project; 2016.

34. Muntaner C, Benach J, Armada F. Venezuela's barrio adentro: An alternative to neoliberalism in health care. *Intl J Health Serv*. 2006;36(4):803–812.

35. Mays GP, Smith SA. Evidence links increases in public health spending to declines in preventable deaths. *Health Aff (Millwood)*. 2011;30(8):1585.

36. Nixon J, Ulmann P. The relationship between health care expenditure and health outcomes. *Eur J Health Econ*. 2006;7(1):7–18.

37. Rodney W. *How Europe underdeveloped Africa*. Washington DC: Howard University Press; 1982:85–89.

38. Cuddington JT. *Capital flight: Estimates, issues, and explanations*. Princeton, NJ: Princeton University Press; 1986.

39. WHO Africa. *State of health financing in the African region*. World Health Organization Regional Office for Africa. Geneva: World Health Organization; 2013.

40. World Health Organization. The Abuja Declaration: Ten years on. Geneva: World Health Organization; 2012. http://www.who.int/healthsystems/publications/abuja_report_aug_2011.pdf?ua=1

41. Ford N, Wilson D, Cawthorne P, et al. Challenge and co operation: Civil society activism for access to HIV treatment in Thailand. [Défi et coopération: Activisme de société civile pour l'accès au traitement du VIH en thaïlande. point de vue; retos y cooperación. Activismo de la sociedad civil para el acceso al tratamiento de VIH en tailandia; punto de vista.] *Trop Med Intl Health*. 2009;14(3):258–266.

42. Parker RG. Civil society, political mobilization, and the impact of HIV scale-up on health systems in Brazil. *JAIDS*. 2009;52:S51.

43. People's Health Movement. The Cape Town call to action. 2012. Available from: http://www.phmovement.org/en/pha3/final_cape_town_call_to_action. Accessed Mar 29, 2017.

44. Focus15ForHealth. #Focus15ForHealth. Tumblr Web site. 2015. Available from: https://focus15forhealth.tumblr.com/. Accessed May 18, 2017.

45. Westerhaus M. Uganda movement for health financing. March 22, 2017.

46. Article 25. Available from: https://join25.org/. Accessed Mar 29, 2017.

47. Mullan F. The metrics of the physician brain drain. *N Engl J Med*. 2005;353(17):1810–1818.

48. McCabe A. Private sector pharmaceutical supply and distribution chains: Ghana, Mali and Malawi. *Health Syst Outcomes: Pharmaceuticals*. Washington, D.C.: World Bank; 2009. http://documents.worldbank.org/curated/en/745621468270302773/Private-sector-pharmaceutical-supply-and-distribution-chains-Ghana-Mali-and-Malawi

49. Nazimera L. District health officer, Neno District Malawi. February 2014.

50. Humphreys G. Harnessing Africa's untapped solar energy potential for health: For a continent with abundant sunlight and poor electricity grid coverage, Africa makes very little use of solar power in the health sector. given recent initiatives, this may be set to change. *Bull World Health Org*. 2014;92(2):82.

51. United Nations. *Gleneagles 2005: Chairman's summary*. UN Millennium Project. New York: United Nations; 2005.

52. OECD. Net ODA. 2016. Available from: https://data.oecd.org/oda/net-oda.htm. Accessed Jun 1, 2017.

53. Bearak M, Gamio L. The U.S. foreign aid budget, visualized. *The Washington Post*. Oct 18, 2016. Available from: https://www.washingtonpost.com/graphics/world/which-countries-get-the-most-foreign-aid/. Accessed May 18, 2017.

54. Mccoy D, Bennett S, Witter S, et al. Salaries and incomes of health workers in sub-Saharan Africa. *Lancet*. 2008;371(9613):675–681.

55. Wendo C. Uganda stands firm on health spending freeze. *Lancet*. 2002;360(9348):1847.

56. Wendo C. Uganda and the global fund sign grant agreement. *Lancet*. 2003;361(9361):942.

57. Charles W. Ugandan officials negotiate global fund grants. *Lancet*. 2004;363(9404):222.

58. Ooms G, Schrecker T. Expenditure ceilings, multilateral financial institutions, and the health of poor populations. *Lancet*. 2005;365(9473):1821–1823.

59. Pfeiffer J, Johnson W, Fort M, et al. Strengthening health systems in poor countries: A code of conduct for nongovernmental organizations. *Am J Pub Health.* 2008;98(12):2134.

60. Norman J. Affordable care act gains majority approval for first time. 2017. Available from: http://www.gallup.com/poll/207671/affordable-care-act-gains-majority-approval-first-time.aspx.

61. Friedman M. *Capitalism and freedom.* 40th anniversary edition ed. Chicago, IL: University of Chicago Press; 2002.

62. Rajan RG, Subramanian A. Aid, Dutch Disease, and manufacturing growth. *J Dev Econ.* 2011;94(1):106.

63. Chong A, Gradstein M. What determines foreign aid? The donors' perspective. *J Dev Econ.* 2008;87(1):1–13.

64. Transparency International. Corruption perceptions index. Berlin Germany: Transparency International; 2017.

65. Ramsdell M. *When elephants fight.* 2015.

66. Isidore C. America's lost trillions. *CNN Money.* Jun 9, 2011. Available from: http://money.cnn.com/2011/06/09/news/economy/household_wealth/. Accessed May 26, 2017.

67. White GB. The recession's racial slant. *The Atlantic.* 2015.

68. Cohan WD. How wall street's bankers stayed out of jail. *The Atlantic.* 2015. https://www.theatlantic.com/magazine/archive/2015/09/how-wall-streets-bankers-stayed-out-of-jail/399368/

69. Sang-Hun C. South Korea removes President Park Geun-hye. *The New York Times.* Mar 9, 2017. Available from: https://www.nytimes.com/2017/03/09/world/asia/park-geun-hye-impeached-south-korea.html. Accessed Apr 27, 2017.

70. IMF. Poverty reduction strategy papers. 2016. Available from: http://www.imf.org/external/np/prsp/prsp.aspx. Accessed Mar 30, 2017.

71. The Global Fund. Country coordinating mechanism. 2017. Available from: https://www.theglobalfund.org/en/country-coordinating-mechanism/. Accessed Apr 27, 2017.

72. Brugha R, Donoghue M, Starling M, et al. The global fund: Managing great expectations. *Lancet.* 2004;364(9428):95–100.

73. Logie DE, Rowson M, Ndagije F. Innovations in Rwanda's health system: Looking to the future. *Lancet.* 2008;372(9634):256–261.

74. Meessen B, Soucat A, Sekabaraga C. Performance-based financing: Just a donor fad or a catalyst towards comprehensive health-care reform? *Bull World Health Org.* 2011;89(2):153.

75. OECD. The Paris declaration on aid effectiveness and the Accra agenda for action. Paris: Organisation for Economic Co-operation and Development; 2009.

76. Gostin LO, Friedman EA, Buss P, et al. The next WHO director-general's highest priority: A global treaty on the human right to health. *Lancet Glob Health.* 2016;4(12):e892.

77. Gostin LO. A framework convention on global health: Health for all, justice for all. *JAMA.* 2012;307(19):2087–2092.

78. FCGH Platform. Platform for a framework convention on global health (FCGH). Global Health Treaty Web site. 2016. Available from: http://www.globalhealth-treaty.org. Accessed Mar 30, 2017.

79. McIntyre D, Thiede M, Dahlgren G, Whitehead M. What are the economic consequences for households of illness and of paying for health care in low- and middle-income country contexts? *Soc Sci Med*. 2006;62(4):858–865.

80. Bonu S, Rani M, Bishai D. Using willingness to pay to investigate regressiveness of user fees in health facilities in Tanzania. *Health Policy Plan*. 2003;18(4):370–382.

81. Hayashi S. How health and homelessness are connected—medically. *The Atlantic*. 2016. https://www.theatlantic.com/politics/archive/2016/01/how-health-and-homelessness-are-connectedmedically/458871/

82. LaMontagne C. NerdWallet health finds medical bankruptcy accounts for majority of personal bankruptcies. Nerdwallet Web site. 2013. Available from: https://www.nerd-wallet.com/blog/health/managing-medical-bills/nerdwallet-health-study-estimates-56-million-americans-65-struggle-medical-bills-2013-2/. Accessed Mar 31, 2017.

83. Dhillon RS, Bonds MH, Fraden M, Ndahiro D, Ruxin J. The impact of reducing financial barriers on utilisation of a primary health care facility in Rwanda. *Glob Pub Health*. 2012;7(1):71–86.

84. Mukherjee J, Ivers L, Leandre F, Farmer P, Behforouz H. Antiretroviral therapy in resource-poor settings: Decreasing barriers to access and promoting adherence. *JAIDS*. 2006;43:S126.

85. World Health Organization. *WHO meeting on survivors of Ebola virus disease*. Geneva: World Health Organization; 2015.

86. Obare F, Warren C, Abuya T, Askew I, Bellows B. Assessing the population-level impact of vouchers on access to health facility delivery for women in Kenya. *Soc Sci Med*. 2014;102:183–189.

87. Galárraga O, Genberg B, Martin R, Barton Laws M, Wilson I. Conditional economic incentives to improve HIV treatment adherence: Literature review and theoretical considerations. *AIDS Behav*. 2013;17(7):2283–2292.

88. Rawlings LB, Rubio GM. Evaluating the impact of conditional cash transfer programs. *World Bank Res Observ*. 2005;20(1):29–56.

89. Kliff S. Five myths about "young invincibles." *The Washington Post*. Nov 26, 2013. Available from: https://www.washingtonpost.com/opinions/five-myths-about-young-invincibles/2013/11/26/7caa1dea-5208-11e3-9fe0-fd2ca728e67c_story.html?utm_term=.9f759b2983af. Accessed Apr 27, 2017.

90. Carrin G, Waelkens M, Criel B. Community-based health insurance in developing countries: A study of its contribution to the performance of health financing systems. *Trop Med Intl Health*. 2005;10(8):799.

91. Rosenberg T. In Rwanda, health care coverage that eludes the U.S. *The New York Times*. Jul 3, 2012. Available from: https://opinionator.blogs.nytimes.com/2012/07/03/rwandas-health-care-miracle/?_r=1. Accessed Apr 27, 2017.

92. Odeyemi IAO, Nixon J. Assessing equity in health care through the national health insurance schemes of Nigeria and Ghana: A review-based comparative analysis. *Intl J Equity Health*. 2013;12:9.

93. Oxfam. An economy for the 99 percent. Even it up. London: Oxfam; *Int J Equity Health*. 2013;12:9.

94. Stewart H. Robin Hood tax: 1,000 economists urge G20 to accept Robin tax. *The Guardian*. Apr 13, 2011. Available from: https://www.theguardian.com/business/2011/apr/13/robin-hood-tax-economists-letter. Accessed Apr 27, 2017.

95. UNITAID. UNITAID invests in better ways to prevent, diagnose and treat diseases. World Health Organization Web site. 2017. Available from: https://www.unitaid.eu/about-us/. Accessed May 12, 2017.

96. Finance Alliance for Health. Finance alliance for health. 2017. Available from: http://www.financingalliance.org/. Accessed Apr 19, 2017.

97. Gostin LO. A framework convention on global health: Health for all, justice for all. *JAMA*. 2012;307(19):2087–2092.

13

Governance

Key Points

- Governance is a key building block of the health system.
- The Ministry of Health (MOH) sets the national health strategy and supports its implementation. The MOH coordinates donors and partners to align actors with the national strategy. External influences can distort the Ministry's ability to govern.
- The Ministry of Finance allocates the budget for health. Both bilateral and multilateral donors influence the Ministry of Finance's allocation to health.
- International treaty obligations and international regulations are external influences that also impact the governance of health systems.
- Civil society can hold those with power accountable for health on local, national, and international levels through coordinated action.
- Global governance for health at a supra-national level is done through a series of formal and ad hoc agreements.
- In the global health era, governance for global health should address health inequalities and support the right to health.

Introduction

Governance is a key building block of a health system.[1] A government is responsible for the health of its people. Yet the power to govern is inextricably linked to resources. Because impoverished governments rely heavily on financial inputs from IFIs and other donors, governance of the health sector can be challenging. Other global forces such as trade, patents, and migration also impact governance for global health.[2-4]

There are a variety of definitions of governance.[5,6] This chapter uses the World Health Organization's (WHO) definition of governance: "[governance is] a political process that involves balancing competing influences and demands."[7]

This definition will be used to describe governance within the nation-state (governance for global health). The WHO's definition of governance includes five key principles[7]: (1) maintaining the strategic direction of policy development and implementation; (2) detecting and correcting undesirable trends and distortions; (3) articulating the case for health in national development; (4) regulating the behavior of a wide range of actors, from health care financiers to health care providers; and (5) establishing transparent and effective accountability mechanisms.

This chapter explores the governance of health from the perspective of the nation-state and examines the internal and external forces that influence national governance of the health sector (Figure 13.1). This chapter also introduces the evolving concept of global governance for health. Beyond the nation-state, global governance for health is weak and occurs through a variety of formal and ad hoc agreements.[8] The chapter also explains the different actors involved in global governance for health including international health and trade organizations, donors, nongovernmental organizations (NGOs), and the private sector.

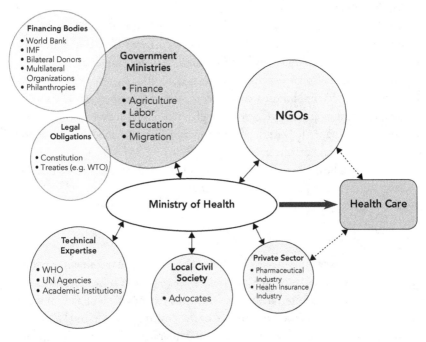

FIGURE 13.1 Global health governance from the perspective of the nation-state. There are a number of external forces that influence a Ministry of Health. Often, the Ministry is constrained in developing a strategy and implementing programs due to international treaties, donor priorities, and government budgets.

Governance of the Health Sector

In most countries, the Ministry of Health (MOH) is responsible for the governance of the health sector. The Minister of Health is generally a cabinet-level position appointed by the head of state or ruling party. The Minister is responsible for convening and coordinating health partners to develop and implement the national strategic plan. The central budget of the MOH covers the payroll of health workers and the procurement of drugs (for national drug stores). The central budget also covers the running costs of the Ministry. The second in command at the MOH is generally a Chief Medical Officer or Director General (DG). The DG is the strategic and technical expert at the MOH. Either the Minister or DG works with leaders of the government's programs such as primary health care; HIV, tuberculosis (TB), or malaria; child health; and women's health. When working in a country, it is important to know the structure of the leadership team and to know who is responsible for each program.

Based on neoliberal principles, governments are encouraged to decentralize budgets.[9] This is similar to the strategy promoted in the United States. In 2017, some US Republicans, in an attempt to dismantle the Affordable Care Act—a federal program—suggested giving block grants to states to cover health care costs.[10] Fiscal decentralization is spun as liberty, freedom, and choice for states or districts (Chapter 1). However, the purpose of decentralization is usually to shrink the federal budget. In the case of the US health care system, decentralization of health money through block grants directly enables massive tax cuts for the wealthy.[11] In most settings, money that is decentralized is often insufficient to provide health care. In addition, decentralization may worsen health inequalities between richer states or districts and poorer ones. The US Congressional Budget Office (CBO) analyzed the Republican's plan and predicted that block grants to states and other reforms to shrink the federal health budget would leave 24 million Americans without insurance and result in 44,000 deaths.[11]

In many impoverished countries, District Health Officers (DHOs) are the ranking public health officials at the district level and receive the decentralized funds. Like the Minister, the DHOs are responsible for convening and coordinating district-level health partners to develop and implement the district's health plans. District-level budgets may cover operations for the district hospital and its health centers (including funds for electricity, fuel for vehicles, and maintenance of facilities). Salaries are generally paid at the central level. Districts may also be responsible for purchasing the drugs they need from the national drug stores. Decentralized budgets are often insufficient to cover the running costs of the hospital, procurement of drugs, and more.

The MOH also works with other ministries in the government. The Ministry of Labor determines regulations pertaining to employment, both in the public and private sectors. Labor laws are very different from country to country and will impact both the local and international workforce. The connection between health programs and programs to address the social determinants of health are coordinated between the Ministry of Social Welfare and the Ministry of Health. Ministries of Social Welfare may provide support for vulnerable groups like orphans, the disabled, or children who head households. The partnership between these two sectors at the local and national levels may help to achieve health equity. In the global health era, the Ministries of Health and Education increasingly collaborate to address shortfalls in physicians, nurses, and other health professionals.[12]

Strategic Planning

In regard to the WHO's principles of governance, maintaining the strategic direction of policy development and implementation[7] is the role of the Minister of Health. A national strategic plan is developed about every five years. The Minister convenes partners in the country including donors (like the US Agency for International Development [USAID] or the World Bank), NGOs, and civil society to draft the strategic plan in a coordinated fashion. In impoverished countries, donors and well-funded NGOs may have an outsized voice in priority setting and national planning. While governance of the health sector is led by the MOH the government health budget of impoverished countries is often much lower than the money brought in by partners.[13]

For example, in 1998, the WHO, UNICEF, the UN Development Programme (UNDP), and the World Bank launched the Roll Back Malaria partnership. This partnership aimed to halve the number of malaria-related deaths by 2010.[14] At the time, the WHO did not have a comprehensive set of guidelines for treating malaria.[15] Based on scattered WHO reports, the Global Fund, one of the largest funders for malaria control, gave money to countries to use chloroquine as first-line malaria treatment.[15] However, the majority of people in Africa have malaria that is resistant to chloroquine, newer, artemisinin-based combination therapy (ACT) were known to be significantly more effective.[15] Despite overwhelming evidence that chloroquine could not sufficiently treat malaria in Africa, the WHO guidelines and the money from the Global Fund pushed governments to buy the useless drug.[14] Scholars and global health practitioners called the promotion of chloroquine medical malpractice and said that it was "terrible to waste lives and money."[14] Even when the WHO did change its guidelines to promote more effective drugs, the Global Fund continued to reject country proposals that included ACT. Kenya's malaria strategy was rejected for requesting ACT-based treatment in 2003.[15] That same year, the Global Fund spent $27.7 million on chloroquine in Africa, despite the fact that 64 percent of the time the treatment failed.[15] Many African governments knew that chloroquine was both ineffective and a waste of money. Armed with the knowledge that chloroquine was ineffective, and refusing to succumb to neoliberal policies, Zambia fought the norm. After heated debate, Zambia became the first country to provide ACT, free of charge, as first-line treatment for malaria in Africa.[16] The Zambian government eventually received $4 million from the Global Fund to purchase ACT.[17]

In addition to NGOs and donors, there are a myriad of public–private partnerships (PPPs) involved in global health. A PPP consists of two or more bodies, at least one of which is private (such as a corporation or NGO) and one public (the government). PPPs produce mixed results in global health. The African Comprehensive HIV/AIDS Partnerships (ACHAP) is an example of a well-known successful PPP.[18] In 2001, the pharmaceutical company Merck, along with the Harvard AIDS Institute and the Gates Foundation, partnered with the government of Botswana to form ACHAP and support the government's AIDS program. At that time, ART was not available in Africa. ACHAP supported the government by building clinics, training staff, and providing some antiretroviral drugs. The initial ACHAP partnership lasted for five years. It is widely credited with the success of Botswana's early efforts to scale-up ART.[19]

Some PPPs have less favorable results. The government of Lesotho (GOL) entered into a PPP with the private South African company NETCARE to build a tertiary-care hospital in Lesotho's capital.[20] Prior to the facility being built, if GOL employees needed complex health care, the GOL would pay for their care in South Africa. The GOL hoped to save money by treating complex conditions in Lesotho. The GOL took out a $200 million loan from the World Bank to fund the facility, which would be managed by NETCARE. The agreement has proved to be extremely expensive for the GOL. NETCARE charges the GOL for the care of its employees. More importantly, the debt that the GOL is paying on the World Bank loan is a significant portion of the overall health budget. The arrangement has distorted the GOL's ability to govern the health sector.[21] When very large corporations are involved in PPPs, governments may not have the power to correct undesirable trends and distortions or regulate the behavior of health care financiers.

However, there are examples of governments correcting distortions and stewarding resources within the Ministry's budget and among partners. For example, within its national health plan, the government of Rwanda provided specific support for orphans and vulnerable children (OVC) using HIV monies. In 2008, Rwanda's National AIDS Control Commission evaluated the funding streams and expenditures of a program called National Orphans and Vulnerable Children Spending Accounts (NOVCSA). The assessment found that nearly 80 percent of funds never reached the intended communities. Most of the funds were being spent on travel, reports, and overhead.[22] Using this study as evidence, the Rwandan Ministry of Health outlined a clear vision within the health plan for the support of OVC.[23] The Ministry then worked prospectively to coordinate the activities of all stakeholders involved in caring for OVC to comply with the national strategy.[22] This assured that the program reached the intended beneficiaries.

Organizations with a health mandate—particularly the WHO and UNICEF—play important roles in the strategic planning and policymaking of health in impoverished countries. Lacking technical expertise due to years of impoverishment, Ministries of Health rely on the guidelines made by WHO and UNICEF to support national strategic planning. Unfortunately, the development of guidelines generally lags behind the development of new science.

Strong governance on health is required in countries to assure that donor support is aligned with the national plan. The Paris Declaration on aid effectiveness[24] promoted principles of country ownership, alignment of aid with national strategic plans, harmonization of donors, and mutual accountability. To accomplish this, political will is needed at the highest level (head of state) to assure that all partners and donors are following the country's plan. Internationally, there is growing support for the coordination of health systems strengthening. A consortium of partners called UHC2030[25] supports the coordination of aid and technical assistance at the country level by strengthening government systems.

Coordination of Financing

Once the national strategic plan is drafted, the Ministry of Health develops a work plan and budget. The Minister then articulates the case for health in national development (also part of the WHO's governance framework) by presenting the plan and budget to the Ministry of Finance. Because impoverished countries rely heavily on external financing to support their national plans, coordinating the financing of the national health plan is an important aspect of the governance needed to achieve good health outcomes.

Financing may come from bilateral or multilateral donors. A *bilateral donor* is a government that gives support to another country. Political interets are inherent in government to government contracts. For example, USAID is a bilateral donor to many countries. All bilateral aid is not the same in terms of governance. Some donor countries provide direct budgetary support to a government for health. Other donors favor off-budget support that is controlled by NGOs. The United Kingdom's Department for International Development (DfID) is an example of a bilateral program that provides both direct budgetary support and off-budget support for health in impoverished countries. In the DfID's 2007–2011 country assistance plan to Malawi,[26] DfID pledged direct budgetary support to the Malawian government as well as off-budget support. DfID also pledged support through a multilateral channel by funding the United Nations Development Programme's efforts in the country. In contrast, bilateral aid from the United States, given through USAID, is most commonly off-budget and given to American NGOs. These NGOs may or may not coordinate with governments. Often the size of the US commitment may be larger than the health budget of the country itself.[27] This type of large-scale, off-budget support can challenge national sovereignty and distort the governance of health.

A *multilateral donor* is a group of two or more entities that pool resources--the Global Fund is an example of a multilateral donor. The Global Fund to Fight AIDS, TB, and Malaria is multilateral fund that receives voluntary contributions from wealthy countries and philanthropic organizations. The Global Fund to Fight AIDS, TB, and Malaria was chartered with aid coordination in mind. It calls for governance of grants through a novel structure called the country coordinating mechanism (CCM). The CCM is a multipartner group that includes the Ministry of Health, civil society groups, NGOs, and the private sector. The purpose of the CCM is to assure that those most affected by AIDS are decision-makers in creating national plans.[28] This structure is separate from the Ministry of Health. As such, it removes the locus of control of this large portion of the budget from the Ministry of Health. However, in many countries, Ministries of Health receive direct support from the Global Fund for the public provision of services.[28]

In many countries, the major source of external financing is the World Bank. The Bank, a multilateral donor, requires the country to draft a national poverty reduction strategy paper (PRSP) to receive loans or grants. The PRSP was introduced in 2000 to link economic development strategies explicitly with programs to reduce poverty. The guidelines for drafting the PRSPs include health indicators (Box 13.1).[29]

One of the requirements of the PRSP is to include a health strategy that addresses the most vulnerable as part of poverty reduction. The Minister of Health may give direct input into this process and include elements of the national strategic health plan within the PRSP. The Ministry of Finance, however, is often under relatively strict, neoliberal constraints imposed on the provision of public services. In several studies, the PRSPs were only weakly linked to health plans. One study reviewed the PRSPs of Haiti, Liberia, and Afghanistan, all of which

---

BOX 13.1

Poverty Reduction Strategy Paper Health-Specific Guidelines

PRSPs should include:

- The main **health outcomes** for the population
- Disaggregated health data for **income groups**
- Disaggregated health data for **geographic locations**
- Analysis of health outcomes based on **household, community and health system factors**
- **Understanding** of the underlying causes of health outcomes
- Health strategies which **reflect the needs of the poor**
- Health strategies with **aim to increase equity** within the health system

Source: Bartlett S. Poverty reduction strategy papers and their contribution to health: An analysis of three countries. *McGill J Med.* 2011;13(2).

---

have very poor and unequal health outcomes. The study found that these PRSPs did not explicitly elaborate a health strategy targeting the most vulnerable, yet the PRSPs were still approved.[29] The PRSP process is heavily weighted toward private-sector development. In the case of the PRSP, governance to advocate for health in development plans requires leadership from the head of state and international actors.

External Legal Frameworks

International laws and treaties also influence the health sector in impoverished countries. International treaties are put into the language of national law through the process of ratification. Once a treaty is ratified into law, the nation must uphold international treaty agreements. Chapter 2 highlighted the example of South Africa implementing national laws that violated World Trade Organization (WTO) treaty agreements.[3] Treaties and international agreements may implicate the social determinants of health as well. For example, the WTO treaty prohibits agricultural subsidies as they inhibit free trade.[30] Yet this prohibition was not enforced evenly. In the United States and Europe, the production of food is heavily subsidized by governments. Meanwhile, in impoverished countries, agricultural subsidies are prohibited by the WTO treaty and neoliberal policies.[31] The combination of these two external forces decreases the ability of small farmers in impoverished countries to compete with large agribusiness in wealthy countries. This has undermined of local production of food and caused severe food insecurity in some countries.[30] In Malawi, in 2005, after many years of famine conditions, then-President Bingu subsidized the price of fertilizer for peasant farmers. For local farmers, the policy was very helpful. On the global stage however, the World Bank threatened to cut off Malawi's loans for violating public-sector spending caps. Bingu went ahead with the program, and the results were remarkable: in just one year, Malawi went from being a recipient of food aid to an exporter of corn.[32-34] Concurrently, life expectancy in Malawi increased from 48 in 2005 to 55 in 2009, and under-five mortality decreased from 116 per 1,000 in 2005 to 95 per 1,000 in 2009.[35] These successes were not only due to increased food production but also to the treatment of AIDS, TB, and malaria. Clearly, as this case illustrates, external legal frameworks have a significant impact on a country's ability to govern health and impact its social determinants. Governance is intimately tied to resources, rules, and international policies.

Donor country laws also affect governance of global health. For example, the Trump administration has reinstated the United States' Mexico City Policy,[36] also known as the global gag rule. The policy was first ratified in 1984 by President Reagan and imposes stringent antiabortion rules on US-funded projects. Since that time, administrations have either repealed the law or reenacted it depending on the political party in control of the government. On January 23, 2017, Trump signed an executive order restricting family planning policies in a more far-reaching manner than even in the Reagan era. The order expands the previous prohibition on funding organizations that refer women for or mention abortions. It now covers all US global health departments and agencies (about $9.5 billion in 2016).[37] The global gag rule—a donor government's legislation—has a direct impact on health in impoverished countries. The WHO estimates that in sub-Saharan Africa unsafe abortions account for 68,000 maternal deaths per year.[38,39] Knowing these figures, restrictions in access to reproductive health services based on US politics are an example of the profound effect the laws and politics of donor countries have on global health. Often these impacts are felt most acutely at the grassroots level (i.e., a child who loses her mother).

Civil Society

Civil society—local, national, international activist groups, and local community members—can shape governance in global health. At the community level, civil society governance for health is widespread, if limited in scope. To steward the National Health Service in the United Kingdom, community health councils were launched in 1974.[40] Community councils for health have also been used in the United States and in other wealthy countries. Community participation is ever-present in impoverished countries, and the engagement of civil society is critical in assuring the right to health. In countries where the village structure is historically robust, community governance is done through traditional authorities (such as village headmen or chiefs). In other countries, it is done administratively through decentralized political structures, like the *cellule* in Rwanda.[41,42]

In regard to civil society's role in global health governance, the People's Health Movement wrote "Bottom-up (health) activism will continue to be an essential strategy for health equity."[43] While some civil society groups seek to strengthen existing organizations that govern global health,[44] others critique the top-down approach of the WHO and have called for a multistakeholder approach.[45] Civil society activism is needed to hold governments, transnational organizations, and companies accountable. Activism will be discussed in Chapter 14.

Global Governance for Health

Governments are responsible for respecting, protecting, and fulfilling rights. However, in a globalized world there are many external influences on health and on governance. Yet there is no formal architecture for the supra-national global governance of health. Some authors define global health as those health issues that "transcend national boundaries" and demand concerted global action.[5] For the health concerns that transcend national boundaries, such as the spread of infectious diseases, the increasing rates of air pollution–related disease, and the rise in cancer related to the transnational marketing of cigarettes, global governance for health is needed. Often this function is to protect the public health of the citizens of powerful countries from the spread of contagion. This need for global governance for health to protect the public health can be traced back to the 19th century. During that time, European powers attempted to control cholera outbreaks that spread along trade routes.[46] In 1903, 20 countries (including the United States and European powers) signed an agreement detailing guidelines for future outbreaks of cholera, plague, and yellow fever.[27] After World War I, the League of Nations developed the League of Nation's Health Organization (precursor of the WHO) to work in concert with large, nongovernmental health organizations such as the International Red Cross and the Rockefeller Foundation's International Health Board.[27]

Yet global governance is also needed to address health beyond epidemic control. After World War II, when the United Nations was formed, the WHO was created with the explicit mission of coordinating health globally.[47] The organization has a broad array of functions, including outbreak and disaster response, immunization campaign oversight, and the provision of technical assistance to national health programs. The WHO's technical assistance is in the form of drafting guidelines and supporting policy implementation. Centrally, the WHO also performs the prequalification process for drugs, updates the essential drug list, and supports disease surveillance.

UNICEF is another important UN organization involved in global governance for health. The organization was founded in 1946 as a response to the suffering of children in Europe in the aftermath of World War II. UNICEF is concerned with the welfare of children and, in this regard, focuses specifically on child survival programs.[48] UNICEF develops guidelines and supports the treatment of childhood conditions such as respiratory infections, malaria, malnutrition, and pediatric HIV.[49] UNICEF coordinates with Ministries of Health and supports NGOs to implement child survival projects. The organization has a unique role in global governance for health because it procures and distributes vaccines. In this role, UNICEF works closely with governments and with the Global Alliance for Vaccines and Immunizations (Gavi) to assure a sufficient vaccine supply.[50]

While both the WHO and UNICEF are involved in global governance for health, neither have any legal weight. Wealthy countries and corporations often shape global health interventions to advance their national security and market interests. Individuals and organizations focused on fairness and justice in a globalized world increasingly call for major changes to global governance for health. The 2014 Lancet Commission on Global Governance for Health issued a report[6] that stated that inequality in both health risks and outcomes is a ranking human rights problem for our times. The report affirms that health inequities are fundamentally unfair and immoral. Global governance for health is needed because the impacts of globalization often deepen the power differential between wealthy countries and impoverished ones. The Commission clearly concluded that political and financial power differentials that cause and perpetuate health inequities must be addressed. Global health practitioners and activists must continue to work to change harmful imbalances and move the global health balance toward justice and equity.

Conclusion

Governance of health is a key building block of health systems. At the national level, governments and Ministries of Health develop national policy and coordinate partners. The power of outside actors can profoundly impact the Ministry of Health's ability to govern. The Ministry of Finance must determine a national budget for health but is often under significant neoliberal constraints. Power differentials between monied interests and impoverished countries exacerbate health inequality.

In the global health era, global governance for health must shift toward fairness and justice both within countries and among countries.

References

1. World Health Organization. Everybody's business—strengthening health systems to improve health outcomes: WHO's framework for action. 2007. Available from: http://www.who.int/iris/handle/10665/43918.

2. Mullan F. The metrics of the physician brain drain. *N Engl J Med*. 2005;353(17): 1810–1818.

3. World Trade Organization. Understanding the WTO. Geneva: World Trade Organization; 2015. https://www.wto.org/english/thewto_e/whatis_e/tif_e/understanding_e.pdf

4. Lancet. Commissions from the Lancet journals: Essential medicines. 2016. Available from: http://www.thelancet.com/commissions/essential-medicines. Accessed Jan 17, 2017.

5. Kickbusch I, Szabo M. A new governance space for health. *Glob Health Action*. 2014;7(1):1–7.

6. Ottersen OP, Dasgupta J, Blouin C, et al. The Lancet Commission on Global Governance for Health. The political origins of health inequity: Prospects for change. *Lancet*. 2014;383(9917):630–667. http://www.thelancet.com/commissions/global-governance-for-health

7. World Health Organization. Health systems: Governance. 2017. Available from: www.who.int/healthsystems/topics/stewardship/en. Accessed May 17, 2017.

8. Gostin LO, Mok EA. Grand challenges in global health governance. *Br Med Bull*. 2009;90(1):7–18.

9. Bossert T. Analyzing the decentralization of health systems in developing countries: Decision space, innovation and performance. *Soc Sci Med*. 1998;47(10):1513.

10. Carroll AE. How would Republican plans for Medicaid block grants work? *The New York Times*. Feb 6, 2017.

11. Congressional Budget Office. American Health Care Act. Washington, DC: Congressional Budget Office, Nonpartisan Analysis for the U.S. Congress; 2017.

12. Frenk J, Bhutta ZA, Chen LC, et al. Health professionals for a new century: Transforming education to strengthen health systems in an interdependent world. 2010.

13. Fidler D. The challenges of global health governance. New York, NY: Council on Foreign Relations; 2010. https://www.cfr.org/sites/default/files/pdf/2010/05/IIGG_WorkingPaper4_GlobalHealth.pdf

14. Yamey G. Malaria researchers say global fund is buying "useless drug". *BMJ*. 2003;22(327):7425.

15. Attaran A, Barnes KI, Curtis C, et al. WHO, the global fund, and medical malpractice in malaria treatment. *Lancet*. 2004;363(9404):237–240.

16. Redditt V, ole-MoiYoi K, Rodriguez J, Weintraub R. Malaria control in Zambia. *Cases Glob Health Delivery*. Cambridge, MA: Harvard Business; 2012. http://www.globalhealthdelivery.org/files/ghd/files/ghd024_malaria_control_in_zambia.pdf

17. Sipilanyambe N, Simon JL, Chanda P, Olumese P, Snow RW, Hamer DH. From chloroquine to artemether-lumefantrine: The process of drug policy change in Zambia. *Malaria J*. 2008;7:25.

18. ACHAP. Welcome to ACHAP. African Comprehensive HIV/AIDS Partnerships Web site. 2017. Available from: http://www.achap.org/. Accessed Jun 1, 2017.

19. Ramiah I, Reich MR. Building effective public–private partnerships: Experiences and lessons from the African comprehensive HIV/AIDS partnerships (ACHAP). *Soc Sci Med*. 2006;63(2):397–408.

20. Webster PC. Lesotho's controversial public-private partnership project. *Lancet*. 2015;386(10007):1929–1931.

21. Marriott A. A dangerous diversion: Will the IFC's flagship health public-private partnership bankrupt Lesotho's ministry of health? Oxfam. 2014. https://www.oxfam.org/sites/www.oxfam.org/files/bn-dangerous-diversion-lesotho-health-ppp-070414-en.pdf

22. Binagwaho A. Chapter 15: Aid effectiveness: The experience of Rwanda. In: Beracochea E, editor. *Improving aid effectiveness in global health*. New York: Springer; 2015.

23. Republic of Rwanda. Vision 2020. Kigali, Rwanda: Republic of Rwanda; 2000. http://www.minecofin.gov.rw/fileadmin/templates/documents/NDPR/Vision_2020_.pdf

24. OECD. *The Paris declaration on aid effectiveness and the Accra agenda for action*. Paris: Organisation for Economic Co-operation and Development; 2009.

25. UHC2030. Healthy systems for universal health coverage—a joint vision for healthy lives. *uhc2030 International Health Partnership*. Geneva: World Health Organization and the World Bank; 2017. https://www.uhc2030.org/fileadmin/uploads/ihp/Documents/About_IHP_/mgt_arrangemts___docs/UHC2030_Official_documents/UHC2030_vision_paper_WEB2.pdf

26. DfID. DFID Malawi: Country assistance plan 2007–2011. *Draft for the Secretary of State Comment 5*. Lilongwe, Malawi: DFID: Department for International Developments [Malawi]; 2007. http://webarchive.nationalarchives.gov.uk/%2B/http%3A/www.dfid.gov.uk/consultations/malawi-cap.pdf

27. Clinton C, Sridhar DL. *Governing global health: Who runs the world and why?* New York, NY: Oxford University Press; 2017.

28. Brugha R, Donoghue M, Starling M, et al. The global fund: Managing great expectations. *Lancet*. 2004;364(9428):95–100.

29. Bartlett S. Poverty reduction strategy papers and their contribution to health: An analysis of three countries. *McGill J Med*. 2011;13(2).

30. Gonzalez CG. Institutionalizing inequality: The WTO agreement on agriculture, food security, and developing countries. *Columbia J Environ L.* 2002;27:491–633.

31. Riddell J. Things fall apart again: Structural Adjustment Programmes in sub-Saharan Africa. *J Mod Afr Stud.* 1992;30:53–68.

32. Denning G, Kabambe P, Sanchez P, et al. Input subsidies to improve smallholder maize productivity in Malawi: Toward an African green revolution (essay). *PLoS Biol.* 2009;7(1):e1000023.

33. Sachs JD. How Malawi fed its own people. *International Herald Tribune.* April 19, 2012. http://www.nytimes.com/2012/04/20/opinion/how-malawi-fed-its-own-people.html

34. Dugger CW. Ending famine, simply by ignoring the experts. *The New York Times.* Dec 2007. Available from: http://www.nytimes.com/2007/12/02/world/africa/02malawi.html. Accessed May 17, 2017.

35. World Bank. World development indicators. The World Bank Databank Web site. 2017. Available from: http://databank.worldbank.org/data/reports.aspx?source=world-development-indicators. Accessed Mar 29, 2017.

36. Cincotta RP, Crane BB. Public health: The Mexico City Policy and U.S. family planning assistance. *Science (New York, N.Y.).* 2001;294(5542):525.

37. Starrs AM. The Trump global gag rule: An attack on US family planning and global health aid. *Lancet.* 2017;389(10068):485–486.

38. World Health Organization. *Unsafe abortion: Global and regional estimates of incidence of unsafe abortion and associated mortality in 2000.* 4th ed. Geneva: World Health Organization, Department of Reproductive Health and Research; 2004.

39. Ronsmans C, Graham WJ. Maternal mortality: Who, when, where, and why. *Lancet.* 2006;368(9542):1189–1200.

40. Klein R. *The politics of consumer representation: A study of community health councils.* London: Centre for Studies in Social Policy; 1976.

41. Rosenberg T. In Rwanda, health care coverage that eludes the U.S. *The New York Times.* Jul 3, 2012. Available from: https://opinionator.blogs.nytimes.com/2012/07/03/rwandas-health-care-miracle/?_r=1. Accessed April 27, 2017.

42. Baum F, Sanderson C, Jolley G. Community participation in action: An analysis of the south Australian health and social welfare councils. *Health Promot Intl.* 1997;12(2):125–134.

43. De Vos P, Schuftan C, Sanders D, et al. Commission on global governance for health: Just another report? *Lancet.* 2014;383(9926):1379–1380.

44. Lee K. Civil society organizations and the functions of global health governance: What role within intergovernmental organizations? *Glob Health Govern.* 2010;3(2). http://www.ghgj.org/Lee_CSOs.pdf

45. Sridhar D, Gostin LO. Reforming the World Health Organization. *JAMA.* 2011;305(15):1585–1586.

46. Loughlin K, Berridge V. *Global health governance: Historical dimensions of global governance*. Discussion paper no. 2. Geneva: Dept. of Health & Development World Health Organization, Centre on Global Change and Health, London School of Hygiene and Tropical Medicine; 2002.
47. World Health Organization. *Chronicle of the World Health Organization*. Geneva: World Health Organization; 1947.
48. UNICEF. About UNICEF. 2017. Available from: https://www.unicef.org/about-us. Accessed May 17, 2017.
49. Watkins K, Quattri M, Dooley T, et al. State of the world's children, 2016. A fair chance for every child. United Nations Children's Fund (UNICEF). 2016. Available from: http://statistical.proquest.com/statisticalinsight/result/pqpresultpage.previewtitle?docType=PQSI&titleUri=/content/2016/4020-S2.1.xml. Accessed May 17, 2017.
50. UNICEF. Supplies and logistics. 2017. Available from: https://www.unicef.org/supply/index_immunization.html. Accessed May 17, 2017.

14

Building the Right to Health Movement

ACTIVISM, ADVOCACY, AND SOCIAL CHANGE

Key Points

- Activism works.
- Social movements are made up of constituencies that come together with a shared purpose.
- Many successes in the fight for health justice and health equity are linked to movements, both in the US and globally.
- The achievement of Universal Health Care (UHC) and the realization of health care as a human right require growing a social movement.

Introduction

The world is not okay. Many readers of this book have chosen to study global health because of a realization that globalization shaped by the neoliberal project of capitalism has left billions behind in its wake. Delivery of health care to the world's poor is one way to work toward global justice and fight for a world in which human rights are globalized. Health care can be a tool for social change if the delivery of care is rooted in the knowledge of structural violence and strives to achieve equity. Today, the status quo is that the poor get sick and die at an alarming rate. Tuberculosis (TB) currently kills as many people as a jumbo jet crashing every hour, AIDS kills more than 3,000 people every day, and daily, 16,000 children before their fifth birthday.[1–3] Almost all of these premature deaths occur in communities throughout the world that were devastated by slavery and colonialism.

Race- and class-based ideologies are institutionalized through national and international policies throughout the world. Structural violence kills people. The lack of effective health care relegates a billion people to suffering, pain, and premature death. In reference to the systematic denial of the human right to health, Dr. Martin Luther King Jr. famously said, "Of all the forms of inequality, injustice in health is the most shocking and inhuman."[4] To overcome health inequities rooted in racism, impoverishment, structural violence, and injustice, nothing short of a global movement will succeed in achieving Universal Health Coverage (UHC) and realizing the right to health. Dr. King famously paraphrased the theologian Theodore Parker when he stated that "the arc of the moral universe is long but it bends toward justice."[5] Although health care is not considered a right by most US politicians, in speaking about the fight to expand health care coverage in the United States, President Barack Obama recognized that "[the arc] does not bend on its own. It bends because we bend it, because we put our hand on that arc and we move it in the direction of justice, and freedom, and equality, and kindness, and generosity. It does not happen on its own."[6] With the understanding that justice requires action, a new generation of global health practitioners and activists must fight for the right to health.

In order to achieve health equity, the structures created to perpetuate injustice must recognized and dismantled. Collective work is needed if we are to achieve health equity in the fight for global justice. The delivery of life-saving care depends on moving away from narrowly defined health interventions that are built on the notion of a first-, second-, and third-world. In rejecting three worlds and fighting for one, justice must be the starting point for global health delivery. The right to health is universal. Strategies and tactics to realize this right must be rooted in undoing the systems that create noxious inequalities. Stronger health systems are needed. They require a larger and stronger cadre of health workers, community health workers, robust supply chains, sufficient infrastructure, and systems of monitoring and evaluation. In addition, innovation in delivery is needed to rapidly bring the fruits of modern medicine to those who are suffering. To accomplish this and achieve UHC, continued activism and advocacy are required. It is therefore imperative that civil society demands health equity and supports leaders who demonstrate the political will to fight for health as a human right. Activists must also pressure governments, multilateral organizations, and foundations to expand financing for this global goal. This chapter introduces the concept of social movements. It highlights the strategies and tactics used by successful and ongoing movements that seek global health equity and justice. The chapter also presents concrete examples for action that can be used to help build and support the movement needed to realize the universal right to health care.

What Is a Social Movement?

We exist in a world shaped by people who came before us. Those who fight and have fought oppression fundamentally change the world and make it more just. Throughout human history, people have come together in the struggle to improve life. To quote famed community organizer Marshall Ganz, "social movements are based on the human tradition of interdependent struggle."[7] They use the resources and talents of people as power to advance justice against the forces of oppression.[8] Movements for justice, like the movement to abolish the transatlantic slave trade,[9] the American civil rights movement to end racial segregation, the African National Congress' struggle against apartheid in South Africa,[10] and ACT UP's struggle for the development of new AIDS drugs were built on long-standing traditions of organizing against oppression and toward human rights.[11] It is within this tradition that the burgeoning global movement for the right to health is taking place.

A social movement is a form of collective action in which individuals unite around a shared social or political goal and act together to achieve their shared purpose. Organizing is necessary for a community with shared purpose to achieve their goals. During the civil rights movement in the United States, a community of oppressed people and their allies came together to achieve the shared purpose of ending racial segregation. Different parts of the community organized into constituencies that supported different angles of the movement. The National Association for the Advancement of Colored People (NAACP), founded in 1909, primarily focused on lobbying and litigation for change.[11] The fight for employment justice was led by the National Urban League, founded in 1910.[12] The Black Panthers were initially formed to fight police brutality and impunity in Oakland in 1966.[13] The Southern Christian Leadership Coalition (SCLC), founded by Dr. King, taught Gandhian tactics of nonviolence to others in the movement.[14] Individual members of these constituencies often took individual actions to fight for civil rights with the support of the movement: from children who led the way in the desegregation of schools to adults who registered to vote.[16,15]

Movements, however, do not simply occur. They are shaped by constituencies that organize and develop strategies to change social structures. The continuous adaptation of strategy is needed to respond to new and shifting conditions. Social change requires targeted pressure over time. Movements do not create change in a linear fashion, although they may seem to in retrospect. In reality, constituencies form and disband, political opportunities rise and evaporate. Extremely serious setbacks occur. Despite these uncertainties, the practice of developing an organizing strategy and using a set of tactics to demand change can achieve remarkable results.

Strategy and Tactics

There are lessons from around the world about how to develop an organizing strategy. In addition, there are many tactics used to bring about change. The practice of making change through strategic organizing and tactical action can be taught and learned. This section will heavily reference the groundbreaking work of Marshall Ganz, the well-known community organizer who worked with the Mississippi Summer Project for voting rights in 1964 and alongside Cesar Chavez and Dolores Huerta of the United Farm Workers from 1965 to 1981.[16] Ganz teaches organizing at the Harvard University's Kennedy School of Government. He and his team support many movements around the world.

The first step in organizing is to create a constituency. The constituency is a group of people who come together for a shared purpose. They work to create a strategy or theory of change and use specific actions or tactics to achieve their goal.[7]

Ganz's organizing strategy includes:

1. The messaging of shared purpose through public narrative
2. The creation of a knowledge base about the problem
3. The analysis and choice of targets for action through the process of power-mapping
4. The analysis of the constituency's resources
5. The translation of collective resources into power
6. The learning of different ways to act to bring about change (tactics)
7. The setting of goals and measuring of outcomes (change is measurable)
8. The collaboration with overlapping constituencies to combine power in coalitions[7]

The first questions a constituency faces are "What is our shared purpose? What problems do we face? What change is needed?" By coming together around a shared purpose and shaping a collective public narrative, a constituency takes the first steps toward achieving its goal.[7] The group then builds the knowledge base necessary to fully understand where the problem comes from and what forces maintain the status quo. A group must then identify the actors or institutions to be targeted to affect change. Ganz says, "targeting is figuring out precisely how to focus limited resources on doing what is likely to yield the greatest result."[7] This is done through the practice of what Ganz calls *power mapping*, which involves asking the following questions: "Who has a stake in our problem? What or who has political power over our problem? Which targets are movable?" By answering these questions, a constituency can understand both how its problem is situated within a network of power and who, within the network of power, controls the problem.[7]

A constituency must then analyze what resources it has. Resources include all forms of potential power, from physical capacity to scientific knowledge to artistic skills to proximity to power to fearlessness. The strategic use of resources generates power for the movement. The collective power of the group is channeled into action through tactics. Someone might have a big house that can be used for meetings. A group might have access to an elected official and can arrange a meeting. An artist might be interested in making an installation for the movement. Successful social movements employ a wide variety of tactics coordinated around the shared purpose.[7]

Tactics for change include protests, sit-ins, civil disobedience, meeting with policymakers, writing and delivering petitions, and communicating the problem through the media. Calling the offices of government representatives is a tactic that has been widely used in the United States to influence policy decisions. In democratic countries where officials depend on voters to keep their job, elected officials are important targets for generating the political will necessary to achieve social change. Economic tactics such as financial divestment, boycotts (refusing to buy a commodity), and calling for sanctions (blocking trade with a group or government) are used by activists to demonstrate the combined economic power of their constituency. Tactics are often organized into campaigns to leverage the most power possible at a critical point in time.[7]

An Organization for Social Change: Universities Allied for Essential Medicines

Student activists for global health equity powerfully operationalized a movement for social change. In the beginning of the global health era, American students who cared about global health equity formed an important constituency within the right to health movement. One group organized around the belief that essential medicines should be available to all. Specifically, they believed that university-based drug discovery ought to be part of the public commons. Prior to their work, even if drugs were developed with public funds at universities, patent protections established by private companies to maximize profits would place drugs out of reach for billions of people. In 2001, a group of students came together as a constituency to launch a campaign at Yale University to fight for lower prices for the important AIDS drug d4T (stavudine). The preclinical research for stavudine was done at Yale and the university held a portion of the patent. The group built their knowledge base around the extremely high price of antiretroviral therapy (ART), the challenges around intellectual property laws, and the significance of the preclinical development of the drug at Yale. Members

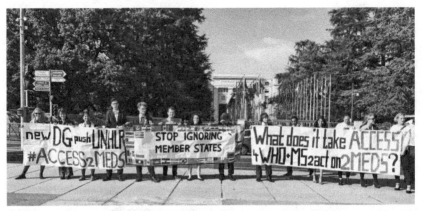

FIGURE 14.1 Universities Allied for Essential Medicines (UAEM) members demonstrate at the 70th World Health Assembly, May 2017.
Photo courtesy of Universities Allied for Essential Medicines.

had a variety of resources that they brought to the fight. Some were law students who could understand patent laws, and others were students who were willing to protest. They also had collective political power as students of the university. The students worked in coalition with other activist groups to combine power. Together, they protested, wrote letters, and met with administrators to get Yale to end the patent protection of d4T. Under this pressure, Yale released d4T from its patent obligations. d4T was the first ART available to be produced as a generic drug, and the price dropped 30-fold.[17] It became a cornerstone of the global scale-up of ART. The Yale student group founded the organization Universities Allied for Essential Medicines (UAEM). UAEM now has chapters at university campuses throughout the United States and around the world.

The fight for d4T was the first campaign in what UAEM saw as a broader strategy to expand access to essential medicines. In the years that followed, UAEM continued to adapt its strategy. To expand the global knowledge base about access to essential drugs, UAEM now publishes a University Report Card that evaluates top research universities on their contributions to global access to medicines.[18] Additionally, UAEM has used the expertise of its constituency to propose alternative drug research and development strategies.[19] UAEM's tactics continue to include direct actions. Its members hold protests at specific times and locations to target policymakers. A recent direct action of UAEM targeted the 2017 World Health Assembly and called on delegates and the Director General of the World Health Organization (WHO) to support discussions on the UN High Level Panel on Access to Medicines Report[20] (Figure 14.1). UAEM members also influence high-level meetings on drug development and access to medicines. The organization actively pressured Johns Hopkins University to license a promising new TB drug (sutezolid) to the Medicines Patent Pool, a UN-backed organization that enables generic drug manufacturing, rather than to a private company.[21-23] Under pressure from UAEM and other allies, Johns Hopkins University licensed sutezolid to the medicines patent pool.[24,25] Through these methods, students play a critical role in the right to health movement.

The Movement for the Right to Health

A global constituency is growing around the shared purpose of delivering on the rights-based promise of high-quality health care for all. Achieving this goal will require changes in local, national, and global policies that dictate the flow of resources. Many constituencies are organizing at the grassroots level across the world. Multiple organizations and actors bring a wide range of resources to create the power and tactics needed to broker change. Scholars are leveraging specific technical knowledge to generate scientific and economic evidence in support of UHC. Activists in impoverished countries have called for increased government expenditure on health.[26] The People's Health Movement (PHM) is working globally to coordinate grassroots struggles around the right to health and to educate people about their rights.[27] PHM has used the Indian constitution as a framework for litigation around the right to health.[28] Groups like UAEM are working to hold the WHO accountable for expanding access to essential drugs.[20] AIDS activists including the Treatment Action Campaign (TAC), Treatment Action Group (TAG), ACT UP, AIDS Support Organization (TASO), and Gay Men's Health Crisis (GMHC) continue to pressure governments, pharmaceutical companies, and multilateral organizations to increase support to achieve universal coverage of ART. The US-based grassroots lobbying group RESULTS is working to pressure the US government to continue its commitments to global health, particularly the support of the Global Fund and the President's Emergency Plan for AIDS Relief (PEPFAR), and to increase the United States' share of overseas development assistance for health.[29]

These constituencies have the shared purpose of achieving health as a human right. Much of the knowledge base on the root causes of health inequalities and the strategies needed to scale up care are known. The objective of this movement is to generate long-term, sustained funding to deliver on the right to health. Power mapping reveals several movable targets that hold the power to change global health financing. Targets include wealthy countries, which must commit more resources; for-profit pharmaceutical companies, which must allow for the development of generic medicines; and the international financial institutions

(IFIs), which must support public expenditure on health. The resources of the constituency that strives to achieve health as a human right are vast and include a willingness to protest, access to policymakers, scientific knowledge, experience in care delivery, and an understanding of development economics. These resources are being translated into power by many activists today. Many forms of activism are under way to demand health as a human right. On the 2016 US presidential election campaign trail, activists demanded that candidates pledge to continue and even expand PEPFAR.[30] Even candidate Trump did.[31-34] Films like *How to Survive a Plague* (by David France)[35] and *Bending the Arc* (by Cori Stern)[36] raise awareness about the movement for AIDS treatment access and the right to health.

Despite the fledging stage of the movement for health care as a right, measurable change has already occurred. The World Bank, for example, is now under the leadership of Dr. Jim Y. Kim, a medical anthropologist and one of the founders of Partners In Health. The very institution that constrained public sector spending is now lead by someone who understands the both grass roots and public sector challenges of health delivery. Under Kim's leadershiping, the World Bank and the Global Fund have committed $24 billion toward achieving UHC in Africa.[37] Novel financing helped to create the first new drugs for TB in decades which were developed explicitly for use in impoverished settings.[38] The new TB drugs are currently being used in a multicountry trial to demonstrate efficacy and expand access. The trial and expansion of access is funded by UNITAID (Chapter 12).[38] The expansive goal of UHC is now an explicit target of the UN's Sustainable Development Goals (SDGs) launched in 2016.

Yet continued advocacy is needed. Advocacy directed toward policymakers is key to leveraging needed resources. The involvement of students who want to join the constituency that is fighting for the right to health adds power to the movement. This can be done through a variety of tactics including protests, engagement with policymakers, publishing letters in local and national news outlets, attending town hall meetings, demanding pledges from candidates, and calling representatives. Members of the constituency that cares about health as a human right should also run for office and occupy positions of power. Everyone needs to vote and advocate for candidates who support the right to health. Importantly, passionate students and other constituents will need to build relationships and spread the word to family, friends, and a new generation. Widespread education is a key component of a successful movement for social change.

Boxes 14.1, 14.2, and 14.3 on direct action tactics provide a starting point for anyone wanting to join the movement for the Right to Health.

1. Look up your Congressional representatives online or call the Capitol Switchboard at 202-224-3121 to connect to the offices of your senators and representatives.
2. You will be connected to your representative or a staff member in your representative's office. During the call, tell them about your stance on the issue you care about. Staff members track calls and provide a summary to the representative. Every call counts.

   You may use a call script like the following one:

   "My name is [name] and I'm a constituent of [representative's name]. I'm calling in support of [e.g., increased funding for PEPFAR, the "Improving Access to Affordable Prescription Drugs Act," the "Reach Every Mother and Child Act"] and would ask [representative] to support this effort through [e.g., a public statement or co-sponsoring or voting for the bill]. Thank you for taking my call."

3. Call again tomorrow and ask family and friends to join you to amplify your power.

BOX 14.2

Meeting with US Members of Congress

1. Call the district or Washington DC office of your representative to set up a meeting with your representative or staff members. You can bring allied constituents to the meeting.
2. During the meeting, be sure to explain your purpose: the problem facing your constituency.
3. Make concrete requests, if possible: e.g., "please write a public statement of support" or "please co-sponsor this bill."
4. Thank the representative or office staff for their time, and leave behind any useful materials. Grassroots advocacy groups dedicated to an issue will often have "leave-behinds" available for this purpose.
5. Follow-up after your meeting with phone calls, emails, or further meetings to build a relationship with your representative and achieve your goals.

BOX 14.3

Writing Letters to the Editor Using the EPIC Format

What is a Letter to the Editor? A Letter to the Editor (LTE) is a brief statement expressing your opinion, generally in response to current events or a recently published article. LTEs are a chance to talk about an issue that's important to you and what can or should be done about it. You can use LTEs to target specific politicians or ask your audience to take particular action.

Why Letters to the Editor? LTEs are quick to write, relatively easy to have published, and appear in the most widely read section of the paper: the editorial page. Politicians and government agencies routinely clip and circulate letters to the editor to understand what is important and urgent to their constituents.

How to Frame LTEs: Use the EPIC format:

*E*ngage audience: Respond to recent news, relate issues to your community, or draw from your personal experience to capture your audience's attention.

*P*roblem statement: Present the issue you care about.

*I*nform on the solution: Make it clear that the problem you presented is solvable! Present a solution and explain why you know it will work (or how it has worked in the past).

*C*all to action: Call your readers to action: "Will you call Representative X and ask them to vote for Y?" This can show lawmakers that their constituents are interested and put pressure on them to take action.

Follow-up: Follow-up is critical to maximizing the political impact of your published letter! Send a copy to your representative and to their aides, and bring a copy the next time you visit their office.

Case Studies of Social Movements for Health Equity and Health Justice

The Fight for Justice for Haitians Affected by the Cholera Epidemic: 2010–2017

> The way this hit my son, he woke up one morning, went to get water. He got back and was not sick. Suddenly he started shaking. We tried some home remedies, then diarrhea began. We rented a motorbike to get him to a hospital quickly. They started an IV, then another one. On the third and final one, he died. He died.[39]

A United Nations peacekeeping force was sent to Haiti in 2004 to quell civil unrest.[40] By 2010, the force included 454 peacekeepers from Nepal. The Nepali battalion's housing compound was located on the banks of Haiti's Artibonite River. The UN's ill-designed and hastily constructed outhouses dumped untreated sewage into the Artibonite river, the main water source for millions of Haitians who live without access to municipal water.[40] Cholera is endemic in Nepal—which means that a percentage of the population may asymptomatically carry the bacteria. Haitians, however, were never exposed to cholera. Thus, when sewage containing the cholera bacteria was dumped in the river, the attack rate of cholera was high, and it felled people quickly. The first Haitians to get sick with cholera lived near the peacekeepers' compound.[40] The disease is preventable if clean water and sanitation exists, yet given the profound impoverishment of Haiti, cholera spread from person to person rapidly. Cholera is also treatable with fluids and antibiotics. But the same impoverishment and structural violence that led to the country's lack of municipal water and sanitation[41] also meant there was little public provision of health care. The first cases of cholera were found in the St. Nicolas Hospital in St. Marc, Haiti. Luckily, this public facility had been strengthened by Zanmi Lasante's team by leveraging HIV monies (Chapter 3), beginning five years earlier. The hospital therefore had doctors, nurses, labs, and medicines. Because of health system strengthening in St. Marc, lives were saved with treatment. However, across the country, treatment was scarce. Between a lack of health care and the ongoing lack of water and sanitation, a massive cholera epidemic rocked the country. By 2016, cholera had killed more than 11,250 Haitians and sickened more than 880,000. The current cholera epidemic in Haiti is one of the most severe in modern times.[42]

The UN denied all responsibility for the spread of cholera in Haiti for almost six years.[42] Activism was crucial in the fight for justice in Haiti. Citizens, health professionals, lawyers, and policymakers in Haiti, the United States, and around the world worked to organize a social movement to seek justice from the UN for the victims of the cholera epidemic. The strategy they used tracked along the organizing framework already discussed.

Brian Concannon, an American lawyer and the Executive Director at the Institute for Justice and Democracy in Haiti (IJDH), describes how a large coalition of stakeholders and activists worked together to apply pressure on the UN in the quest for justice (Figure 14.2).[43] The various actors outlined in Figure 14.2 each played an important role in the overall social movement. The shared purpose of the movement was to realize justice for the cholera victims—including compensation for the victims of cholera, a formal apology from the UN, and financing to build comprehensive water and sanitation infrastructure in the country that would save 3,000 lives a year and eliminate the devastating cholera epidemic.[42] The movement believed that this work would also serve to transform UN accountability so that, in the future, the organization would respond to harm done by its employees or operations—or, more importantly, have better oversight and do less harm.[43] The knowledge base for this important movement had several key areas. First, scientists and doctors from Haiti and around the world provided epidemiological evidence through genetic testing to show that the cholera strain sickening Haitians was the same strain that was endemic in Nepal.[44] Second, legal scholars developed a knowledge base to understand how to challenge to the UN's immunity. Last, the biosocial knowledge related to the needs of the Haitian people who were affected by cholera was built through accompaniment of the affected. The power to remediate this injustice lay mainly at the feet of the UN, but through power mapping UN member states who were friendly to the cause were also seen as potential targets. The resources for this epic battle of Haitian citizens versus the UN were, in fact, numerous. The Haitian people themselves are well organized and familiar with protest.[45] The legal effort in Haiti was spearheaded by award-winning human rights lawyer, Mario Joseph, Managing Attorney at the Bureau des Advocats Internationaux (BAI) (Figure 14.3). Joseph and his staff took the testimonies of thousands of victims to enter into evidence of harm. On the US side, lawyers Beatrice Lindstrom and Brian Concannon[46] used their legal expertise of human rights and international and US law to develop a plan for how and where the case could be tried. The tactics that were employed by the consortium of constituencies included protests in Haiti and in the United States[47]; opinion pieces in Haitian, American, and European newspapers[48,49]; full-length new stories on television and radio; videos and photography[39]; a movie about an affected child; and a legal case. In November 2011, BAI and IJDH filed 5,000 claims against the

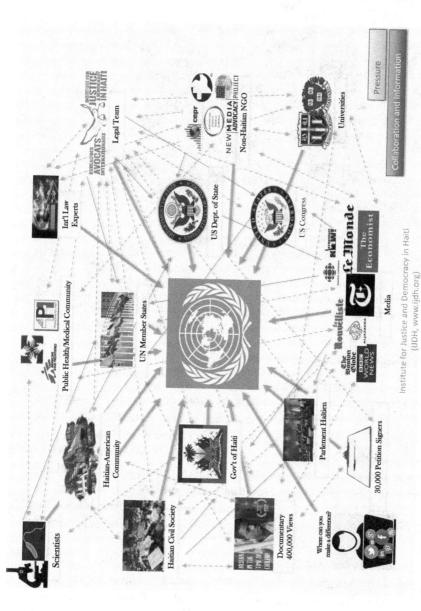

FIGURE 14.2 Institute for Justice and Democracy in Haiti (IJDH) activism map. This map shows the various actors and stakeholders who played a role in fighting for justice in Haiti after the introduction of cholera by UN peacekeeping forces.

Source: Courtesy of Brian Concannon, Institute for Justice & Democracy in Haiti.

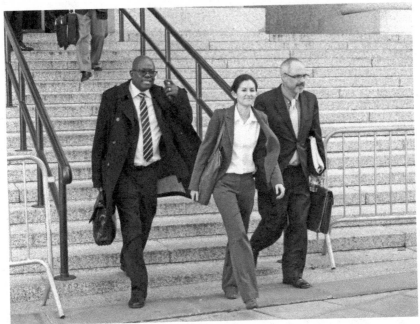

FIGURE 14.3 Photo of lawyers from the Institute for Justice and Democracy in Haiti (IJDH) and the Bureau des Avocats Internationaux (BAI) filing the case on behalf of cholera victims against the United Nations for bringing cholera to Haiti. From the left: Mario Joseph (BAI), Beatrice Lindstrom (IJDH), and Brian Concannon (IJDH) leaving the New York federal court.
Photo courtesy of Edgar Lafond/Haiti Liberté.

UN in a New York federal court, seeking the installation of a national water and sanitation system, compensation for individual victims of cholera, and a public apology. In 2013, the UN High Commissioner for Human Rights Navi Pillay publicly called for the UN to claim responsibility and to be held accountable for the cholera epidemic.[50] This was a monumental achievement of activists in building the political will necessary to reverse the position of the UN. The case against the UN brought by Lindstrom, Concannon, and Joseph was considered but not formally tried. However, the threat of the legal case tipped the scales and pressured the UN into issuing an apology.

On December 1, 2016, Secretary-General of the United Nations Ban Ki-moon publicly apologized for the UN's role in the cholera epidemic and introduced the UN's "New Approach to Cholera in Haiti."[51] This approach pledged $200 million to combat cholera with funding for vaccines and treatment and another $200 million for material support and direct payments to cholera victims. In his statement, the Secretary-General said:

> On behalf of the United Nations, I want to say very clearly: we apologise to the Haitian people. We simply did not do enough with regard to the cholera outbreak and its spread in Haiti. We are profoundly sorry for our role. . . . Eliminating cholera from Haiti, and living up to our moral responsibility to those who have been most directly affected, will require the full commitment of the international community and, crucially, the resources necessary. The United Nations should seize this opportunity to address a tragedy that also has damaged our reputation and global mission. That criticism will persist unless we do what is right for those affected. In short, UN action requires Member State action.

The movement for justice and the right to health, water, and sanitation for Haitians demonstrated the success of organizing strategy and tactics to win a massively unbalanced fight. It highlights the critical power imbalances that influence efforts in the fight for justice. When the cholera epidemic first began in 2010, the UN, backed by the United States, completely denied claims for accountability and claimed immunity for its disastrous actions.[43] The UN was powerful enough to brush away claims for justice. However, the movement, driven by local voices, a legal battle, and scientific evidence, leveraged the collective power of its constituencies to shift power from the UN toward civil society. The transnational coalition was able to collaborate by harnessing the resources of social media and low-cost communications to shift power and achieve victories of social justice.[43]

Seasoned activists know that there are few such moments when measurable goals are so suddenly and clearly achieved. Victories are important to celebrate. Yet when justice is the goal, the work of bending the arc must continue. In the case of the UN and cholera, the story is far from over. According to a UN General Assembly report, the Secretary-General's plan fit into a longer 10- to 15-year plan that had already been developed to implement clean water and sanitation facilities in Haiti.[43,51] In the months that followed the promise of reparations, the UN has yet to raise funds for these projects. Cholera continues apace in Haiti, and clean water and sanitation are distant promises.[52,53] The movement must return to the strategy of organizing, develop a knowledge base about which countries may be willing to foot this bill, discern who the targets should be for the next set of actions, and decide which resources can be brought to bear through strategic tactics to achieve the next steps toward justice.

Fight Against the Repeal of the Affordable Care Act: 2017

A powerful example of a social movement for the right to health is the recent success of collective activism against the US Republican party's repeated attempts to repeal the Affordable Care Act (ACA or "Obamacare") in 2017 and cut Medicaid funding. The House replacement bill, the American Health Care Act (AHCA),[54] the US Senate's Better Care Reconciliation Act (BCRA), the Obamacare Repeal Reconciliation Act (ORRA), and Health Care Freedom Act (known as "skinny" repeal), all failed to pass.[55] Each of these bills would lead to more than 16 million people losing their health insurance, as scored by the independent Congressional Budget Office.[56] The loss of health insurance and the closure of clinical facilities leads to increased mortality. Medicaid coverage includes the poor, children, the disabled, and the elderly. The Affordable Care Act expanded Medicaid and allowed over twenty million people to have health insurance for the first time.[57] It has been a lifesaving program. The two major proposals, the AHCA and the BCRA, aimed to cut Medicaid spending and government assured insurance subsidies by hundreds of billions of dollars over time, in part to provide major tax cuts for the wealthiest Americans. Furthermore, the bills were crafted in complete secrecy, without even a single public hearing on the effects of legislation that would dramatically affect hundreds of millions of people's lives and one-sixth of the economy.

"Obamacare repeal and replace," a longtime political slogan, was overcome by the collective power of millions of people who made their voices heard in opposition to this effort. The Republican-led House and Senate pushed forward bills shaped by the wealthiest Americans who have an outsized voice in politics through lobbying and campaign financing. Yet people in all 50 states took action in their towns and in D.C. to fight against these bills. Millions attended town halls, called their Senators' offices, showed up at local events with Senators, marched on D.C., and protested with sit-ins, sleep-ins, die-ins and other forms of civil disobedience that led to an historic number of arrests. This movement was led by patients, parents, caregivers, nurses, doctors, faith leaders, and other organizers. Organizers who previously protested with ACT UP and many heroes from AIDS treatment activism were arrested again for civil disobedience in protest of these bills, which would have devastating effects for people living with AIDS in the US. The grassroots disability rights organization, ADAPT, led nationwide sit-ins that captured the attention of the American people, as people with severe disabilities put their bodies on the line to save their health care and the health care of millions.[57] Housing Works and Center for Popular Democracy led repeated and historic civil disobedience actions in the Senate office buildings, keeping the terrible bill in the forefront of news coverage and speaking to the American public with tens of millions of people viewing the protest on television in a single evening and coverage in major national news outlets as well as local press. Indivisible, MoveOn, and Planned Parenthood supporters organized national protests with thousands of people. Allied groups including Democracy Spring, the Little Lobbyists, Repairers of the Breach, GlobeMed Alumni, RESULTS, and PIH Engage, participated in lobbying visits and direct actions Figure 14.4.[58]

Activists flipped the votes that ended repeal efforts. People thanking Senator Susan Collins (ME) at a 4th of July parade helped her remain an outspoken champion against efforts to repeal the ACA and cut Medicaid.[59] Senator Lisa Murkowski (AK) stood strong in voting no because a woman undergoing treatment for cancer shared her story. Murkowski said, "It's these types of stories that remind me that no, the importance of a timeline is not nearly as important as getting this right."[60] Senator Jerry Moran (KS), a staunch conservative, voted no after he held a town hall where not even a single person was in favor of the BCRA and where he heard about the potential effects of rural hospitals closing.[61] Senator Dean Heller (NV) voted no on the BCRA because of similar pressures.

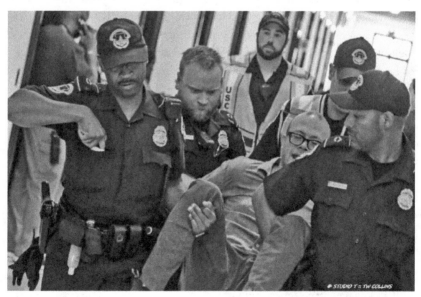

FIGURE 14.4 Photo of protester being removed from the Senate Office building, Washington DC, July 2017. Courtesy Todd Collins

The cumulative effects of these actions on the public's views of health care were tremendous and have created a fundamental social change. People's personal stories, videos of arrests at sit-ins, and anger at town halls circulated across print, online, and television news coverage. The public support of this bill fell to record lows, with only 12% of the American public supporting the BCRA bill.[62] A vast majority wanted the Republicans to work in a bipartisan manner on health care.[63] Through the process, the public became educated on importance of Medicaid, of government support for expanding insurance coverage including the expansion of Medicaid. Public approval of the ACA swung from a majority against to a majority for. By July, 62% of people polled believed that it is the responsibility of the federal government to make sure that all Americans have health care coverage, up from 52% in March.[64]

Activism has changed the entire national dialogue around health care has changed dramatically, with millions of people for the first time speaking out for health care as a right and for a change in the current system that does not deliver on that promise. More Americans are now calling for a Medicare-for-all system that delivers health care while saving trillions of dollars on health care spending.[65,66]

Conclusion: Toward the Right to Health

Activism was essential in causing the paradigm shift from prevention to care delivery that gave birth to the global health era. Further activism will be necessary to change the global double standard that implicates who lives and who dies. High-quality health care is necessary for all. To achieve this goal, we must fight for health systems that can address the entirety of burden of disease, improve the social determinants of health, deliver high-quality equitable care, and build capacity, infrastructure, and systems for the long term. This chapter highlights advocacy and the impact that social movements have in advancing the realization of human rights. Through organizing a social movement, change is possible, even when the odds seem historically, politically, and legally stacked in favor of the status quo. By analyzing case studies, it is clear that strategies and tactics can turn human resources, talents, and capacities into power and successfully move the world closer to achieving the right to health.

Much more needs to be done. There are many ways that readers of this book can help. A good starting point is joining existing chapters or beginning new chapters of organizations active in the movement for the right to health:

PIH Engage: http://engage.pih.org
RESULTS: http://www.results.org

UAEM: http://uaem.org/
Article 25: https://join25.org/
Student Global AIDS Campaign: http://www.studentglobalaidscampaign.org/
GlobeMed: http://globemed.org/

Global health equity depends on increased funding from the United States, particularly for the key programs of PEPFAR and the Global Fund. Global issues, such as an international fund for the achievement of UHC and innovative financing, such as the Robin Hood tax, UNITAID, and the Financing Alliance, all need support. Activism works. It is with the recognition of gross injustices in world history and the tools of organizing that a difference will be made in the fight for justice and health as a human right. As the South African antiapartheid activist Stephen Biko once urged: "We have set out on a quest for true humanity, and somewhere on the distant horizon we can see the glittering prize. Let us march forth with courage and determination."[67]

References

1. World Health Organization. Children: Reducing mortality. 2016. Available from: http://www.who.int/mediacentre/factsheets/fs178/en/.
2. UNAIDS. Latest statistics on the AIDS epidemic. 2016. Available from: http://www.unaids.org/en/resources/fact-sheet.
3. Saunders MJ, Evans CA. Fighting poverty to prevent tuberculosis. *Lancet Infect Dis.* 2016;16(4):395.
4. Munro D. America's forgotten civil right—healthcare. Forbes Web site. 2015. Available from: https://www.forbes.com/sites/danmunro/2013/08/28/americas-forgotten-civil-right-healthcare/#6599c0236599.
5. NPR. Theodore Parker and the "moral universe." 2010. Available from: http://www.npr.org/templates/story/story.php?storyId=129609461.
6. Time Magazine. Obama's speech urging Congress to do "what they believe deep in their hearts is right." 2017. Available from: http://time.com/4770353/barack-obama-profile-courage-speech-transcript/.
7. Ganz M. Organizing notes, charts, questions. Marshall Ganz Web site. 2016. Available from: https://projects.iq.harvard.edu/ganzorganizing/trainers-workshop.
8. Ganz M. *Organizing: People, power, change organizer's handbook.* Cambridge, MA: Harvard University; 2014. http://d3n8a8pro7vhmx.cloudfront.net/themes/52e6e37401925b6f9f000002/attachments/original/1423171411/Organizers_Handbook.pdf?1423171411
9. Hochschild A. *Bury the chains.* Boston, MA: Mariner Books; 2006.
10. Mandela N. *Long walk to freedom: The autobiography of Nelson Mandela.* Boston, MA: Back Bay Books; 1995.

11. Appiah A, Gates HL. *Africana: The Encyclopedia of the African and African American experience.* 2nd ed. New York: Oxford University Press; 2005.

12. Moore JT. *A search for equality: The National Urban League, 1910–1961.* University Park: Pennsylvania State University Press; 1981.

13. Allen RL. *Black awakening in capitalist America: An Analytic History.* 1st ed. Garden City, NY: Doubleday; 1969.

14. Southern Christian Leadership Conference (SCLC). Stanford King Encyclopedia Web site.

15. Nelson S. *Freedom summer.* PBS; 2014. http://www.pbs.org/wgbh/americanexperience/films/freedomsummer/

16. Ganz M. Marshall Ganz CV. 2016. Available from: http://marshallganz.com/files/2016/07/Marshall-Ganz-CV-July-2016.pdf.

17. UAEM. 2001. Available from: http://www.uaem.org/. Accessed Jan 18, 2017.

18. UAEM. University report card: Global equity in biomedical research. 2015. Available from: http://globalhealthgrades.org/.

19. UAEM Reroute Report: A map of the alternative biomedical R&D landscape. 2016. http://altreroute.com/

20. Quigley F. Listen to civil society: Medicines for people, not Profit—Dr. Chan. *Health Hum Rights J.* 2017. Available from: https://www.hhrjournal.org/2017/05/listen-to-civil-society-medicines-for-people-not-profit-dr-chan/.

21. Medicines Patent Pool. http://www.medicinespatentpool.org/about/.

22. UAEM. Coalition calls on Johns Hopkins University to ensure accessibility of tuberculosis drug. 2015. Available from: http://uaem.org/press/press-releases-statements-by-uaem/coalition-calls-on-johns-hopkins-university-to-ensure-accessibility-of-tuberculosis-drug/.

23. Mirabella L. Public health advocates call on Johns Hopkins to make TB drug widely available. 2015. Available from: http://www.baltimoresun.com/business/bs-bz-hopkins-tb-drug-protest-20150903-story.html.

24. UAEM Press Release. Public health groups welcome Johns Hopkins University and Medicines Patent Pool agreement for development of promising new TB drug. 2017. Available from: http://www.tbonline.info/posts/2017/1/25/public-health-groups-welcome-johns-hopkins-univers/#.

25. Basey M, Stone C. Students unite for open innovation and global access to tuberculosis drug sutezolid. *Lancet Glob Health Blog.* 2017. http://globalhealth.thelancet.com/2017/04/03/students-unite-open-innovation-and-global-access-tuberculosis-drug-sutezolid

26. Mukherjee J, personal communication with Westerhaus M. Uganda movement for health financing. 2017.

27. PHM. Health for all now! People's Health Movement Web site. 2017. Available from: http://www.phmovement.org/.

28. PHM. NHRC-JSA regional public hearings on health rights related to public and private healthcare sectors. 2016. Available from: http://phmindia.org/public-hearing-on-right-to-health/. Accessed May 15, 2017.

29. RESULTS 2015 annual report. Washington D.C; 2015. http://www.results.org/about/2015_annual_report/.

30. C-SPAN. Trump's PEPFAR commitment: C-SPAN video. 2015. Available from: https://www.c-span.org/video/?c4555530/trumps-pepfar-commitment.

31. Jaffe S. US global health leadership hangs on election result. *Lancet.* 2016;388(10055):1969.

32. McNeil D. Trump administration puts the US at a crossroad for global health aid. *New York Times.* Dec 19, 2016.

33. NPR. Gharib M. From AIDS to Zika: Trump on global health and humanitarian aid. 2016. Available from: http://www.npr.org/sections/goatsandsoda/2016/11/09/501425084/from-aids-to-zika-trump-on-global-health-and-humanitarian-aid

34. Seymour N. Trump's biggest impact: Global health financing. 2017. Available from: http://thehill.com/blogs/congress-blog/healthcare/313191-trumps-biggest-impact-global-health-financing.

35. France D, Richman TW, Walk TH, et al. *How to survive a plague* (film). New York: Sundance Selects/MPI Media Group; 2013.

36. Davidson K, Kos P. *Bending the arc* (film). USA. Brooklyn, NY: Impact Partners; 2017.

37. World Bank. Partners launch framework to accelerate universal health coverage in Africa; World Bank and Global Fund commit $24 billion. 2016. Available from: http://www.worldbank.org/en/news/press-release/2016/08/26/partners-launch-framework-to-accelerate-universal-health-coverage-in-africa-world-bank-and-global-fund-commit-24-billion.

38. EndTB. endTB partnership launches clinical trial to target toughest strains of tuberculosis. 2017. Available from: http://www.endtb.org/news/endtb-partnership-launches-clinical-trial-target-toughest-strains-tuberculosis.

39. *Fight the outbreak: Cholera in Haiti the United Nations.* Brooklyn, NY: Vimeo; 2012. https://vimeo.com/39599088

40. Katz JM. UN admits role in cholera epidemic in Haiti. *The New York Times.* Aug 17, 2016. Available from: https://www.nytimes.com/2016/08/18/world/americas/united-nations-haiti-cholera.html?_r=0. Accessed May 21, 2017.

41. Varma MK, Satterthwaite ML, Klasing AM, et al. Woch Nan Soley: The denial of the right to water in Haiti. *Health Hum Rights.* 2008:67–89.

42. IJDH. Cholera accountability. 2017. Available from: http://www.ijdh.org/advocacies/our-work/cholera-advocacy/. Accessed May 21, 2017.

43. Mukherjee J. Personal communication with Concannon B. Cholera in Haiti and IJDH. 2017.

44. Frerichs RR, Keim PS, Barrais R, Piarroux R. Nepalese origin of cholera epidemic in Haiti. *Clin Microbiol Infect.* 2012;18(6):E163.

45. Hallward P. *Damming the flood: Haiti, Aristide, and the politics of containment.* New York: Verso; 2007.

46. IJDH. Team. 2017. Available from: http://www.ijdh.org/about/team/. Accessed May 21, 2017.

47. Haiti cholera victims protest against UN. *Jamaica Observer*. Sep 13, 2016. Available from: http://www.jamaicaobserver.com/news/Haiti-cholera-victims-protest-against-UN.

48. Ivers L. A chance to right a wrong in Haiti. *New York Times*. Feb 22, 2013. Available from: http://www.nytimes.com/2013/02/23/opinion/a-chance-to-right-a-wrong-in-haiti.html.

49. Piarroux R. The U.N.'s responsibility in Haiti's cholera crisis. *New York Times*. Sep 7, 2016. Available from: https://www.nytimes.com/2016/09/08/opinion/the-uns-responsibility-in-haitis-cholera-crisis.html.

50. Daniel T. UN official makes rare case for compensation for Haiti cholera victims. *Huffington Post*. 2013. Available from: http://www.ijdh.org/2013/10/topics/health/un-official-makes-rare-case-for-compensation-for-haiti-cholera-victims/. Accessed May 21, 2017.

51. United Nations General Assembly. *A new approach to cholera in Haiti*. Geneva: United Nations; 2016. http://www.ijdh.org/wp-content/uploads/2016/12/Dec-1-UN-Report-A_71_620-E.pdf

52. Editorial. Haiti is still waiting on promised UN help for cholera epidemic. *Boston Globe*. Mar 27, 2017. Available from: http://www.bostonglobe.com/opinion/editorials/2017/03/26/haiti-still-waiting-promised-help-for-cholera-epidemic/wJg7J1EwnpM6Wra1xfqqGL/story.html?s_campaign=bostonglobe%3Asocialflow%3Atwitter. Accessed May 21, 2017.

53. Gladstone R. After bringing cholera to Haiti, UN can't raise money to fight it. *New York Times*. Mar 19, 2017. Available from: https://mobile.nytimes.com/2017/03/19/world/americas/cholera-haiti-united-nations.html?emc=edit_tnt_20170319&nlid=3007060&tntemailo=y&_r=0&referer=. Accessed May 21, 2017.

54. Wikipedia. American Health Care Act of 2017. https://en.wikipedia.org/wiki/American_Health_Care_Act_of_2017. Accessed Aug 1, 2017.

55. Eilperin J, Sullivan S, Snell K. Senate rejects measure to partly repeal Affordable Care Act, dealing GOP leaders a major setback. *Washington Post*. July 28, 2017. https://www.washingtonpost.com/powerpost/senate-gop-leaders-work-to-round-up-votes-for-modest-health-care-overhaul/2017/07/27/ac08fc40-72b7-11e7-8839-ec48ec4cae25_story.html. Accessed Aug 1, 2017.

56. Congressional Budget Office. H.R. 1628 Better Care Reconcilliation Act. https://www.cbo.gov/publication/52849. Accessed Aug 1, 2017.

57. Stein P. Disability Advocates Arrested During Health Care Protests at McConnell's Office. *Washington Post*. July 22, 2017. https://www.washingtonpost.com/local/public-safety/disability-advocates-arrested-during-health-care-protest-at-mcconnells-office/2017/06/22/f5dd9992-576f-11e7-ba90-f5875b7d1876_story.html. Accessed Aug 1, 2017.

58. Leonhardt D. The Americans Who Saved Health Insurance. *New York Times*. Aug.1, 2017. https://www.nytimes.com/2017/08/01/opinion/obamacare-trumpcare-citizen.html. Accessed Aug 1, 2017.

59. Weigel D. At parades and protests, GOP lawmakers get earful about health care. *Washington Post*. Jul 4, 2017. Available from: https://www.washington-post.com/powerpost/at-parades-and-protests-senators-get-earful-about-health-care/2017/07/04/ab675938-5de2-11e7-9fc6-c7ef4bc58d13_story.html?utm_term=.156455a0c4ac. Accessed Aug 1, 2017.

60. Brooks J. Murkowski rejects 'quick' fix for health care. *Juneau Empire*. Jun 1, 2017. Available from: http://juneauempire.com/news/2017-06-01/murkowski-rejects-quick-fix-health-care. Accessed Aug 1, 2017.

61. Hackman M. GOP Senator Is Urged to Oppose Health Bill at Town Hall. *Wall Street Journal*. Jul 6, 2017. Available from: https://www.wsj.com/articles/gop-senator-urged-to-oppose-health-bill-at-town-hall-1499383026?mod=e2twp. Accessed Aug 1, 2017.

62. Page S, Kinery E. Poll: Only 12% of Americans support the Senate health care plan. *USA Today*. Jun 28, 2017. Available from: https://www.usatoday.com/story/news/politics/2017/06/28/suffolk-poll-obamacare-trump-senate-health-care-plan/103249346/. Accessed Aug 1, 2017.

63. Blanton D. Fox News Poll: 74 percent want GOP to reach out to Democrats on health care. *Fox News Politics*. Jul 19, 2017. Available from: http://www.foxnews.com/politics/2017/07/19/fox-news-poll-74-percent-want-gop-to-reach-out-to-democrats-on-health-care.html. Accessed Aug 1, 2017.

64. Associated Press. Americans' Views on Replacing the ACA. *AP-NORC Center for Public Affairs Research*. Available from: http://www.apnorc.org/PDFs/July%20 2017%20Health%20Care/July%20Omnibus%20Topline_FINAL.pdf. Accessed Aug 1, 2017.

65. Kiley J. Public support for 'single payer' health coverage grows, driven by Democrats. *Pew Research Center FactTank*. Jul 23, 2017. Available from: http:// www.pewresearch.org/fact-tank/2017/06/23/public-support-for-single-payer-health-coverage-grows-driven-by-democrats/. Accessed Aug 2, 2017.

66. Gambino L. Bernie Sanders pushes universal health plan in wake of Republican repeal failure. *Guardian*. Aug 2, 2017. Available from: https://www.theguardian.com/us-news/2017/aug/02/bernie-sanders-universal-healthcare-medicare-single-payer. Accessed Aug 2, 2017.

67. Biko S. *I write what I like: Selected writings*. Chicago, IL: University of Chicago Press; 2015.

Exercises

Exercise 1 (Health system impoverishment, Chapter 1)

In 1997, Ethiopia's population was approximately 58 million people. Based on World Bank estimates, the prevalence of tuberculosis (TB) in the country was 472 cases per 100,000 people, there were 28,000 maternal deaths per year, life expectancy was only 50, and 162 children out of every 1,000 born died before the age of five years.[1] Furthermore, there were more than 500,000 cases of malaria in 1996, and only 55 percent of children between 12 and 23 months received standard childhood immunizations; 65.7 percent of the population was undernourished.[1] An international study found an HIV prevalence is 9.4 percent.[2]

You are the Minister of Health. Your job is to choose and implement health interventions to combat the main conditions that cause ill health and premature death.

1. Make a list of your health care priorities (irrespective of price).
2. Describe who will deliver the interventions and how.
3. Use Table A.1 to determine the approximate cost of your chosen interventions.
4. Readjust the priorities to fit the budget envelope (see Figure 1.6 from chapter 1 for Ethiopia's budget for health per capita per year).
5. Discuss what impact the budget will have on
    a. patients
    b. health workers
    c. Ethiopia's economy

This exercise paints a stark picture of the reality faced by many governments in impoverished countries. Between 1995 and 2000, the government of Ethiopia had between $2 and $3 to spend on health services for each person in the country. Considering the costs outlined in Table A.1, it was possible to cover some services (such as vitamins and

Table A.1   Estimated cost of interventions.

Intervention	Cost (USD)
Primary Health Care drugs	$2 per person
Measles, mumps, and rubella vaccination	$1.30 per person
Diphtheria and tetanus vaccination	$0.07 per person
Polio vaccination	$0.13 per dose, minimum 3 doses required
Standard 6 months non-multidrug resistant tuberculosis treatment (rifampicin, isoniazid, and pyrazinamide)	$55.45 per person
Permethrin impregnated rectangular bednet, cost per year (Binka, Mensah, and Mills 1997, 229-239)	$2.40 per household
Trained midwife, materials for facility based delivery (estimate Partners In Health)	$60 per person
Emergency Obstetrical care: blood, antibiotics, access to operating room, surgeon, anaesthesia (estimate Partners In Health)	$200 per person
Standard 1-year HIV medication (ART)	$10,000 per person per year
Reduced osmolarity ORS per patient	$0.13 per child per event

Source: Aggregated data from International Drug Price Indicator Guide, https://www.msh. org/resources/international-drug-price-indicator-guide Accessed August 2017 unless otherwise stated.

vaccines). However, any health system investments—infrastructure, human resources, ambulance systems—were impossible. The scenario described in this exercise parallels the reality of many countries in the 1970s, '80s, and '90s. Crippled by colonial impoverishment, debt from World Bank loans, and structural adjustment programs, nations often found themselves without sufficient funds to build strong health systems.

Exercise 2 (Advocacy to expand mental health treatment, Chapters 2 and 14)

Mental health and mental illness is moving to the forefront in global health. Due to increased detection efforts, effective therapy, and advocacy, the burden and importance of treating mental illness is apparent. Recent studies found a 50-fold increase in "patient care episodes" for mental health in the United States between 1955 and 2000.[3] In his book, *The Invisible Plague: The Rise of Mental Illness from 1750 to the Present*, Dr. Edwin Torrey described mental illness as an epidemic.[4] This epidemic continues to grow; suicide is now the second leading cause of death for 10- to 24-year-old men around the world.[5] However, despite both the increase in mental illness and its burden on both quality of life and mortality, few people seek care due to lack of treatment options and stigma.

Using the work of AIDS activists as inspiration, discuss what measures you would take to organize a movement around mental health. How would you decrease stigma? How would you bring this issue to the forefront of global health? Who would you lobby for increased funding and research? What steps should be taken to address the global mental health epidemic?

Exercise 3 (Linking HIV funding to health system strengthening, Chapter 3)

Figure A.1 compares Rwanda's and Lesotho's progress toward MDGs 4 and 5. In Lesotho, between 2000 and 2015, little improvement was made in maternal mortality and child mortality. Lesotho is a small highland country with a population of just under 2 million. More than 60 percent of the country is mountainous, and villages are only accessible by foot or on horseback. These geographic characteristics create a challenge for health care delivery because most of the population has to travel great distances to reach health centers.[6]

Consider that you are the Health Minister of Lesotho in 2005. The government has a health budget of $24 per capita, and external sources contribute an additional $8 per capita.[7] The 2005 prevalence of HIV was 22.8 percent, of whom only 3 percent were receiving antiretroviral therapy (ART). There was a maternal mortality ratio of 939 per 100,000 live births, an infant mortality rate of 88.1 per 100,000 live births, an under-five mortality rate of 123.4 per 1,000, and a TB death rate of 80 per 100,000 people.[7] Due to these dire health outcomes, the Global Fund disbursed almost $8 million earmarked for HIV/AIDS to Lesotho in 2005.[8]

As Health Minister, how would you leverage this Global Fund money to strengthen the health system? Where would you invest and what interventions would you put into place to increase access to primary health care, increase the quality of the health care provided, and address the HIV/AIDS burden?

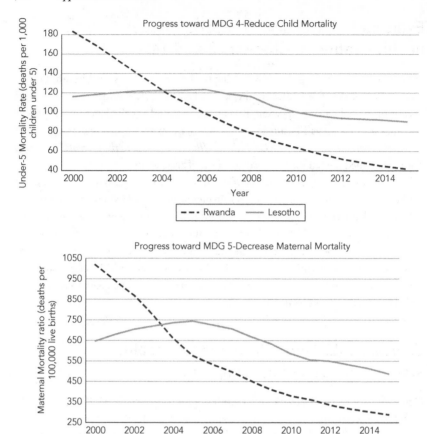

FIGURE A.I Comparison of Rwanda's and Lesotho's progress toward Millennium Development Goals (MDG) 4 and 5 (child and maternal health). Rwanda actively pursued a health systems approach. Lesotho struggled to meet MDG targets.

Source: Data adapted from World Bank. Health nutrition and population statistics. 2017. http://data.worldbank.org/data-catalog/health-nutrition-and-population-statistics

Exercise 4 (Understanding the burden of disease, detecting and outbreak, Chapter 4)

At one hospital in rural Haiti in 2010, an experienced public health physician noted that several adults admitted to the hospital died rapidly of dehydration and watery diarrhea, something that she had never seen before. Because of this new phenomenon, an outbreak investigation was launched and cholera was identified. See Table A.2 for data on cholera case loads from October 20, 2010, to October 20, 2012. Using this information:

Table A.2 Cholera surveillance during the Haiti epidemic.

Region	Cases	Hospitalizations	Deaths	Estimated Population (2009)
All	604,634	329,697	7436	9,923,243
Centre	62,722	30,795	686	678,626
Port-au-Prince	164,423	72,296	1065	875,978
Sud	30,560	18,599	317	704,760
Nord	57,370	51,642	877	970,495

Source: Barzilay EJ, Schaad N, Magloire R, et al. Cholera surveillance during the Haiti epidemic: The first 2 years. *N Engl J Med.* 2013;368(7):599–609.

1. Which measure is most pertinent in this data, prevalence or incidence of cholera?
2. Using your answer to Question 1, calculate the prevalence or incidence of the total population:
    a. Which region had the highest mortality rate from cholera during this time frame?

Exercise 5 (Social forces and diabetes care, Chapter 5)

Diabetes prevalence in the United States has increased dramatically over the past few decades. In 2011, 28.1 million Americans had diabetes.[9] Figure A.2 shows the prevalence of diabetes in the United States by county. One county with a high prevalence of diabetes is Kleberg, Texas. Kleberg has a population of 31,000 people: 4 percent identify as African-American, 72 percent as Hispanic, and 21 percent as Caucasian; 13 percent of the population is older than 65 years. The median yearly household income is around $37,000; 22.8 percent of people live in poverty, and 23.7 percent of the population under the age of 65 does not have health insurance.[10]

In contrast, Flathead, Montana, is a county with a moderate prevalence of diabetes. Flathead is home to about 96,000 people, of whom 17.7 percent are 65 or older. About 0.4 percent of the population identifies as African-American, 2.7 percent as Hispanic, and 92.9 percent as Caucasian. The median yearly household income is almost $47,000, and 13.6 percent of the population lives in poverty; 16.7 percent of the population under 65 is without health insurance.[10]

Discuss and contrast potential social forces that might influence the prevalence of diabetes in these two counties.

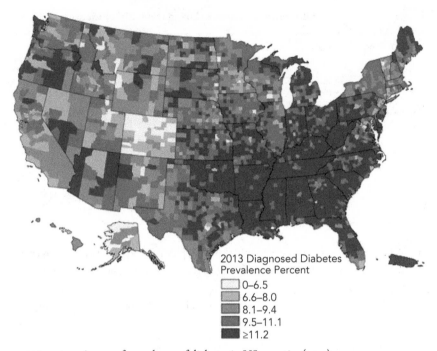

FIGURE A.2 A map of prevalence of diabetes in US counties (2013).

Centers for Disease Control and Prevention. Diabetes Home. Available from: https://www.cdc.gov/diabetes/data/county.html. Accessed Jan 3, 2017.

Exercise 6 (The care delivery value chain for TB, Chapter 6)

Despite the offer of free TB diagnosis and treatment in every country, the disease is not yet adequately managed. Referring to the case presented in chapter 6 and Figure 6.2, discuss how you would plan for a holistic care delivery value chain for TB in a rural, impoverished setting.

Exercise 7 (Human resources for maternal health, Chapters 3 and 7)

Lesotho is a small, mountainous country completely surrounded by South Africa. Like many impoverished countries, Lesotho struggled to meet Millennium Development Goal (MDG) targets. In 2008, the maternal mortality was among the highest in the world at 964 maternal deaths per 100,000 live births, an increase from 237 deaths per 100,000 live births in 1990.[11] As such, in 2009, Partners in Health (PIH) was awarded a grant to work with the Ministry of Health on a program for Universal Health Care (UHC) for maternal care.

You are a member of the PIH team. Use the following information to predict the number of health care professionals needed for antenatal clinic visits and delivery in the Bobete Health Center located in the mountainous Thaba-Tseka district. The health center serves a catchment area of 25,000 people: 23 percent are women of childbearing age. There is a birth rate of 29/1,000 people annually. Assume that 4.4 percent of the women are pregnant in a given year, and assume that the births are evenly distributed throughout the year. Using a target of one midwife per five births, how many midwives will need to be employed per day to cover all the births?

Assume that each pregnant woman comes for four antenatal check-ups. If the antenatal clinic is open twice a week, and each nurse can see 16 patients in a day, how many nurses will need to be scheduled per day to cover all antenatal check-ups? What strategies would you use to address the inadequate supply of health workers?

(More information and background can be found at Satti H, Motsamai S, Chetane P, et al. Comprehensive approach to improving maternal health and achieving MDG 5: Report from the mountains of Lesotho. *PLoS One*. 2012;7(8):e42700.)

Exercise 8 (Community health workers delivering child health interventions, Chapter 8)

Despite the emphasis on child mortality over the past decade, many countries still struggle to reduce child deaths. Leading causes of under-five mortality are pneumonia, malaria, and diarrhea. There are low-cost methods of prevention and treatment for these causes. Liberia had an under-five mortality rate of 76.3 per 1,000 live births in 2013, one of the highest rates in the world. In Liberia, only 55.7 percent of children with a fever are treated with antimalarials.

A catchment area in Liberia has 55,000 people: 20 percent of these people are under five years of age. There is one health center and 24 community health workers (CHWs). What interventions would you implement to address the undiagnosed and untreated malaria in Liberia?

(For more information, see Johnson AD, Thomson DR, Atwood S, et al. Assessing early access to care and child survival during a health system strengthening intervention in Mali: A repeated cross sectional survey. *PLoS One*. 2013;8(12):e81304.)

Exercise 9 (Hepatitis C supply chain, governance, and financing Chapters 9, 12 and 13)

Egypt with the highest prevalence rate of Hepatitis C in the world with estimates of 5–15% of the population carrying the virus and 15–85% of whom will develop progressive liver disease.[12] Hepatitis C can cause liver disease decades after a person is infected with the virus. The massive expansion of Hepatitis C in Egypt was initially due to contaminated injections used by the government during mass antischistosomal treatment in the 1960s and 1970s supported by the WHO. The virus then continued to spread from person-to-person through contact with blood. Because the program was led by the government of Egypt, the country has taken responsibility for providing universal access to treatment. Initially this treatment required an injectable agent (called interferon) and an antiviral medicine. The injections were associated with significant side effects and many people needed to be hospitalized. However, the cost of the drugs is over $80,000 US per treatment and the health budget of the country is less than $600 US per capita per year for a population of 91 million.

1. Calculate the disease burden and the cost of treatment.
2. Hep C is the second leading cause of death but other interventions are cheaper, how would you prioritize this treatment.
3. Discuss what avenues the government of Egypt might use (advocacy, concessional pricing, TRIPS flexibilities, donor support) to assure access to this new treatment and provide universal coverage that would stop transmission of this blood-borne disease.
4. Make your case to the international community.

Exercise 10 (Developing a logic model for CHW-led case detection of malnutrition, Chapters 8 and 10)

Malnutrition is a severe and fatal condition for children under the age of five years in impoverished countries. One way that severe wasting is diagnosed is by measuring children's mid-upper arm circumference (MUAC). In 2009, the World Health Organization (WHO) recommended treatment of all children with a MUAC of below 11.5 cm.

Nutrition programs often use CHWs to identify children who suffer from malnutrition (using MUAC) and treat them with ready-to-use therapeutic food (RUTF). RUTF is a peanut-based mixture of milk powder, vitamins, and minerals. The advantage is that it does not need to be mixed with water, thereby mitigating the risk of bacterial infection, and it does not need to be refrigerated.

Design a logic model for this CHW-based malnutrition program, from case-finding to treatment to follow-up of a child. Identify what resources or inputs your program would need, and develop indicators for inputs, processes, outputs, outcomes, and impact.

Table A.3 Health nutrition and population statistics (2017).

Input	Thailand (2000)	Thailand (2015)
Total population	62,693,322	67,959,359
Adult population, aged 15–64 (% of total)	69.5%	71.8%
HIV prevalence (total number of cases)	620,000	430,000
ART coverage (% people living with HIV)	0%	65%

ART, antiretroviral therapy.

Source: Data adapted from World Bank. Health nutrition and population statistics, 2017.

Exercise 11 (Achieving Universal Health Coverage, Chapter 11)

Using Figure 6.3 from chapter 6 and information from Table A.3, calculate the inputs needed to provide universal coverage of HIV treatment in Thailand in 2000 and 2015. What do you think accounted for the rise in ART coverage from 2000 to 2015? What strategies could be utilized to further increase HIV treatment and move toward universal coverage of HIV?

References

1. World Bank. Health nutrition and population statistics. 2017. http://databank.world-bank.org/data/reports.aspx?source=health-nutrition-and-population-statistics

2. Mekonnen Y, Sanders E, Messele T, et al. Prevalence and incidence of, and risk factors for, HIV-1 infection among factory workers in Ethiopia, 1997– 2001. *J Health Pop Nutrit*. 2005;23(4):358.

3. Whitaker R. Anatomy of an epidemic: Psychiatric drugs and the astonishing rise of mental illness in America. *Ethical Hum Psychol Psychiatry*. 2005;7(1):35,104.

4. Torrey EF. *The invisible plague: The rise of mental illness from 1750 to the present*. Rutgers University Press. Piscataway, NJ: 2003.

5. Pitman A, Krysinska K, Osborn D, King M. Suicide in young men. *Lancet*. 2012;379(9834):2383–2392.

6. Satti H, Motsamai S, Chetane P, et al. Comprehensive approach to improving maternal health and achieving MDG 5: Report from the mountains of Lesotho. *PloS One*. 2012;7(8):e42700.

7. World Bank. World development indicators. 2017. Available from: http://data-bank.worldbank.org/data/reports.aspx?source=world-development-indicators. Accessed Mar 29, 2017.

8. The Global Fund. Lesotho. 2017. Available from: https://www.theglobalfund.org/en/portfolio/country/?loc=LSO&k=01ae2dc3-49f1-48b7-b9fb-2be348d15051. Accessed May 5, 2017.

9. CDC. *National diabetes statistics report, 2014*. Atlanta, GA: National Center for Chronic Disease Prevention and Health Promotion, Division of Diabetes Translation; 2014.

10. US Census Bureau. Population estimates, July 1, 2015 (V2015). 2015. Available from: //www.census.gov/quickfacts/. Accessed Nov 7, 2016.

11. Hogan MC, Foreman KJ, Naghavi M, et al. Maternal mortality for 181 countries, 1980–2008: A systematic analysis of progress towards Millennium Development Goal 5. *Lancet*. 2010;375(9726):1609–1623.

12. Elgharably A, Gomaa AI, Crossey MM, Norsworthy PJ, Waked I, Taylor-Robinson SD. Hepatitis C in Egypt—past, present, and future. *Int J Gen Med*. 2017;10:1–6. doi:10.2147/IJGM.S119301

APPENDIX 2

Additional Resources

Introduction: Why Global Health Delivery

Farmer P, Kim JY, Kleinman A, Basilico M. *Reimagining Global Health: An introduction.* Berkeley: 2013.

Harvard University. Global health case studies from a biosocial perspective (free online course). edX Web site. https://www.edx.org/course/global-health-case-studies-biosocial-harvardx-sw25x-0#.

Cases in global health delivery. http://www.globalhealthdelivery.org/case-collection.

Packard RM. *A History of Global Health: Interventions into the lives of other peoples.* Baltimore: 2016.

Harvard University. Lessons from Ebola: Preventing the next pandemic (free online course). edX Web site. https://www.edx.org/course/lessons-ebola-preventing-next-pandemic-harvardx-ph557x.

Chapter 1: The Roots of Global Health Inequity

Black S. *Life and Debt.* [Documentary Film]. 2001.

Peck R. *Lumumba.* [Documentary Film]. 2001.

Hochschild A. *King Leopold's Ghost: A story of greed, terror, and heroism in colonial Africa.* Boston: Houghton Mifflin; 1998.

Hochschild A. *Bury the Chains: Prophets and rebels in the fight to free an empire's slaves.* Boston: 2005.

Johnson CR. *Middle Passage.* New York, NY, USA: Plume; 1991.

Fanon F. *The Wretched of the Earth.* New York, NY, USA: Grove Press; 1963.

Farmer P. *The Uses of Haiti.* 2nd ed. ed. Monroe, Me. 2003.

Hickel J. *The Divide: A brief guide to global inequality and its solutions.* London: 2017.

Sartre J, Brewe S. *Colonialism and Neocolonialism.* Florence: Taylor and Francis; 2001.

Chossudovsky M. *The globalization of poverty and the new world order.* Global Outlook; 2003.

Freire P. *Pedagogy of the oppressed.* New York, NY: Bloomsbury; 2000.

Morrison T. *Beloved.* Reprint Edition. New York: Vintage; 2004.

Elkins C. *Imperial Reckoning: The untold story of Britain's gulag in Kenya.* New York, NY: Henry Holt and Company; 2005.

James, CLR. *The Black Jacobins: Toussaint L'ouverture and the San Domingo revolution.* New York: Vintage Books; 1963.

Fanon F. *Black Skin, White Masks.* New York, NY, USA: Grove Press; 1967.

Fanon F. *A Dying Colonialism.* New York, NY: Grove Press; 1994.

Nkrumah K. *Consciencism: Philosophy and ideology for decolonization.* New York, NY: Monthly Review Press; 1964.

Pakenham T. *The Scramble for Africa: White man's conquest of the dark continent from 1876–1912.* New York, NY, USA: Avon Books; 1992.

Rodney W. *How Europe Underdeveloped Africa.* Bogle-L'Ouverture Publications. United Kingdom: 1972.

Washington BT. *Up From Slavery.* New York, NY: Dover Publications; 1995.

Du Bois, WEB. *The Souls of Black Folk.* New York, NY: Dover Publications; 1994.

Said E. *Orientalism.* 1st Vintage Edition. New York: Vintage; 1979.

Douglass F. *My Bondage and my Freedom.* New Haven, CT: Yale University Press; 2014.

Douglass F. *Narrative of the Life of Frederick Douglass, an American Slave.* New York, NY: Penguin; 1982.

Galeano E. *The Open Veins of Latin America.* New York, NY: Monthly Review Press; 1997.

Keshavjee S. *Blind Spot: How neoliberalism infiltrated global health.* Oakland, California: University of California Press; 2014.

Chapter 2: Reversing the Tide: Lessons from the Movement for AIDS Treatment Access

France D, Richman TW, Walk TH, et al. *How to Survive a Plague.* New York, NY: Sundance Selects : MPI Media Group; 2013.

France D. *How to Survive a Plague: The inside story of how citizens and science tamed AIDS.* First edition. New York: 2016.

Farmer P. *Aids and Accusation: Haiti and the geography of blame.* Berkeley; 2006.

Verghese A. *My Own Country: A doctor's story.* Vol 496. Vintage; 1994.

Lewis S. *Race Against Time.* Toronto: House of Anansi Press; 2005.

Behrman G. *The Invisible People: How the U.S. has slept through the global AIDS pandemic, the greatest humanitarian catastrophe of our time.* 1st ed. New York, NY: Free Press.

Individual Members of the Faculty of Harvard University. Consensus statement on antiretroviral treatment for AIDS in poor countries. *Topics in HIV Medicine.* 2001;9(2):14–26.

Sontag S. *Illness as metaphor and AIDS and its metaphors.* New York, NY: Picador; 2001.

Demme J. *Philadelphia.* [Film]. Culver City, California: TriStar Pictures; 1993.

Kushner T. *Angels in America: A gay fantasia on national themes.* Los Angeles, California; 1991.

Chapter 3: The Millennium Development Goals and Sustainable Development Goals

United Nations. Millennium development goal report, 2015. http://www.un.org/millenniumgoals/2015_MDG_Report/pdf/MDG%202015%20rev%20(July%201). pdf. Updated 2015.

Lawn J, Cousens S, Zupan J. Neonatal survival 1–4 million neonatal deaths: When? Where? Why? *Lancet.* 2005;365(9462):891–900.

Walton D, Farmer P, Lambert W, Leandre F, Koenig S, Mukherjee J. Integrated HIV prevention and care strengthens primary health care: Lessons from rural Haiti. *J Public Health Policy.* 2004;25(2):137–158.

Mukherjee JS, Barry DJ, Satti H, Raymonville M, Marsh S, Smith-Fawzi MK. Structural violence: A barrier to achieving the millennium development goals for women. *Journal of Women's Health.* 2011;20(4):593–597.

Chapter 4: Global Health and the Global Burden of Disease

Murray CJ. Quantifying the burden of disease: The technical basis for disability-adjusted life years. *Bulletin of the World Health Organization.* 1994;72(3):429–445.

Omran AR. The epidemiologic transition: A theory of the epidemiology of population change. *The Millbank Memorial Fund Quarterly.* 49(4):509–538.

Chapter 5: Social Forces and Their Impact on Health

Biehl JG, Petryna A. When People Come First: Critical studies in global health. Princeton University Press; 2013.

Farmer P. Infections and Inequalities: The modern plagues. Berkeley; 1999.

Mukherjee J. Hungry Bengal: War, famine and the end of empire. Oxford: Oxford University Press; 2015.

Ivers LC, Cullen KA. Food insecurity: Special considerations for women. The American journal of clinical nutrition. 2011;94(6):1744S.

Sen A. Development as Freedom. Knopf: New York; 1999.

Paton A. Cry, the Beloved Country. New York: C. Scribner's Sons; 1948.

Fadiman A. The Spirit Catches You and You Fall Down: A Hmong child, her American doctors, and the collision of two cultures. Farrar, Straus and Giroux; 2012.

Zinn H. A People's History of the United States. HarperCollins; 2005.

Alexander M. The New Jim Crow: Mass incarceration in the age of colorblindness. New York, NY: The New Press; 2012.

Stevenson B. Just Mercy: A story of justice and redemption. New York, NY: Spiegel & Grau; 2015.

Biehl JG. Vita: Life in a zone of social abandonment. Berkeley: University of California Press; 2005.

Pasternak J. Yellow Dirt: An American story of a poisoned land and a people betrayed. New York, NY: Free Press; 2010.

Farmer P, Connors M, Simmons J. Women, Poverty and AIDS. 2nd ed. Monroe, ME: Common Courage Press; 2007.

Pipher M. Reviving Ophelia: Saving the selves of adolescent girls. 1st ed. New York, NY: Penguin Group; 2005.

Sen A. Poverty and Famines: An essay on entitlement and deprivation. Re-print ed. New York, NY: Oxford University Press; 1983.

Peele J. Get Out. [Film]. Universal City, California: Universal Pictures; 2017.

Peck R. I Am Not Your Negro. [Documentary]. Dallas, TX: Magnolia Pictures; 2017.

Haney B. Price of Sugar. [Documentary]. Waltham, MA: Uncommon Productions; 2007.

Chapter 6: Giving Care, Delivering Value

Kleinman A. The art of medicine caregiving as moral experience. *Lancet*. 2012;380(9853):1550–1551.

Sontag S. *Regarding the Pain of Others*. 1st ed. New York, NY: Picador; 2004.

Orwell G. *Marrakech*. *The Complete Works of George Orwell*. http://www.george-orwell.org/Marrakech/0.html.

Orwell G. *The Road to Wigan Pier*. CreateSpace Independent Publishing Platform; 2014.

Chapter 7: Human Resources for Health

Republic of Rwanda. Vision 2020. 2000.

Hongoro C, McPake B. How to bridge the gap in human resources for health. *The Lancet*. 2004;364(9443):1451–1456.

Binagwaho A, Kyamanywa P, Farmer PE, et al. The human resources for health program in Rwanda—A new partnership. *N Engl J Med*. 2013;369(21):2054–2059.

Chapter 8: Community Health Workers

Palazuelos D, Ellis K, DaEun Im D, et al. 5-SPICE: The application of an original framework for community health worker program design, quality improvement and research agenda setting. *Global Health Action.* 2013.

Dahn B, Woldemariam AT, Perry H, et al. *Strengthening primary health care through community health workers: Investment case and financing recommendations.* World Health Organization; 2015.

Werner D, Thuman C, Maxwell J. *Where There is no Doctor: A village health care handbook.* Hesperian Foundation; 1992.

Farmer P, Léandre F, Mukherjee JS, et al. Community-based approaches to HIV treatment in resource-poor settings. *The Lancet.* 2001;358(9279):404–409.

Rich M, Miller A, Niyigena P, et al. Excellent clinical outcomes and high retention in care among adults in a community-based HIV treatment program in rural Rwanda. *Jaids-Journal Of Acquired Immune Deficiency Syndromes; JAIDS.* 2012;59(3):E42.

Satti H, Motsamai S, Chetane P, et al. Comprehensive approach to improving maternal health and achieving MDG 5: Report from the mountains of Lesotho (comprehensive maternal health program in Lesotho). 2012;7(8):e42700.

Newman P, Flores Navarro H, Palazuelos L, et al. Evaluation of a community health worker intervention to improve adherence to therapy for non-communicable disease in Chiapas, Mexico. *Annals of Global Health.* 2015;81(1):210.

Chapter 9: Evolution in Drug Access

Chaudhuri S. The WTO and India's pharmaceuticals industry: Patent protection, TRIPS, and developing countries. New York: Oxford University Press; 2005.

Forman L, Kohler JC, eds. Access to Medicines as a Human Right: Implications for pharmaceutical industry responsibility. Toronto, Buffalo, London: University of Toronto Press; 2012.

Meirelles F. The Constant Gardener. [Film]. Universal City, California: Focus Features; 2005.

Chapter 10: Monitoring, Evaluation, Disease Surveillance, and Quality Improvement

Gawande A. The Checklist Manifesto: How to get things right. 1st ed. ed. New York, NY; 2010.

AbouZahr C, Boerma T. Health information systems: The foundations of public health. (policy and practice: Theme papers). Bull World Health Organ. 2005;83(8):578.

Banerjee AV. Chapter 3—low-hanging fruit for better (global) health? In: Duflo E, ed. Poor Economics: A radical rethinking of the way to fight global poverty. New York: PublicAffairs; 2011.

Chapter 11: Universal Health Coverage— Ensuring healthy lives and promoting wellbeing for all at all ages

Wolff J. *The Human Right to Health*. 1st ed. New York: W.W. Norton & Co; 2012.

Sachs JD. Achieving universal health coverage in low-income settings. *The Lancet*. 2012;380(9845):944–947.

Jamison DT, Summers LH, Alleyne G, et al. Global health 2035: A world converging within a generation. *The Lancet*. 2013;382(9908):1898–1955.

O'Connell T, Rasanathan K, Chopra M. What does universal health coverage mean? *The Lancet*. 2014;383(9913):277–279.

Kirby M. The right to health fifty years on: Still skeptical? *Health Hum Rights*. 1999;4(1):6–25.

Kruk ME, Myers M, Varpilah ST, Dahn BT. What is a resilient health system? Lessons from Ebola. *The Lancet*. 2015;385(9980):1910–1912.

Ooms G, Brolan C, Eggermont N, et al. Universal health coverage anchored in the right to health. 2013.

Chalkidou K, Glassman A, Marten R, et al. Priority- setting for achieving universal health coverage/définition des priorités pour parvenir à la couverture sanitaire universelle/establecimiento de prioridades para conseguir una cobertura sanitaria universal. *Bulletin of the World Health Organization*. 2016;94(6):462–467.

Norheim OF. Ethical perspective: Five unacceptable trade- offs on the path to universal health coverage. *International Journal of Health Policy and Management*. 2015;4(11):711.

Chapter 12: Health Financing

Stuckler D. The Body Economic: Why austerity kills, and what we can do about it. 1st ed. New York, NY: Basic Books; 2013.

Chapter 13: Governance

Gostin LO. *Public Health Law and Ethics*. 2nd ed. Los Angeles, California: University of California Press.

Perkins JM. *Confessions of an Economic Hit Man*. 1st ed. ed. San Francisco, Calif.: Berrett-Koehler; 2004.

Frenk J, Moon S. Governance challenges in global health. *N Engl J Med.* 2013;368(10):936–942.

Bearak M, Gamio L. The U.S. foreign aid budget, visualized. *The Washington Post.* Oct 18, 2016. Available from: https://www.washingtonpost.com/graphics/world/which-countries-get-the-most-foreign-aid/. Accessed May 18, 2017.

Klein N. *The Shock Doctrine: The rise of disaster capitalism.* Penguin Books. London: 2008.

Abbott J, Achbar M. *The Corporation*. [Film]. New York, NY: Zeitgeist Films; 2004.

Chapter 14: Building the Right to Health Movement: Activism, Advocacy, and Social Change

Davidson K, Kos P. *Bending the Arc.* USA; 2017.

Ganz M. *Why David Sometimes Wins: Leadership, organization, and strategy in the California farm worker movement.* New York, NY: Oxford University Press; 2009.

Bratt P. *Dolores.* [Documentary].

Martin JP. *25 Human Rights Documents.* New York, NY: Columbia University: Center for the Study of Human Rights; 2001.

King ML, Jr. Letter from a Birmingham Jail. Stanford King Institute: 1963.

Walls DS. *Community Organizing (Social Movements).* 1st ed. Malden, MA: Polity; 2014.

Branch T. *Parting the Waters: America in the King years 1954–63.* Re-print ed. New York, NY: Simon & Schuster; 1989:143–205.

King Jr. ML. *The Drum Major Instinct. A Knock at Midnight: Inspiration from the great sermons of Reverend Martin Luther King, Jr.* New York, NY: Warner Books; 2000.

King Jr. ML. *Why We Can't Wait.* New York, NY: Signet Classics; 2000.

Thoreau HD. *Walden and Civil Disobedience.* New York, NY: Signet Classics; 2012.

The Ballot or the Bullet. Malcolm X Speaks: Selected speeches and statements. New York, NY: Grove Press; 1994.

Mandela N. I Am Prepared to Die. Nelson Mandela Foundation Web site. http://db.nelsonmandela.org/speeches/pub_view.asp?pg=item&ItemID=NMS010&txtstr=prepared%20to%20die. 1964.

Bell MS. *All Souls' Rising.* 1st ed. New York: Pantheon Books; 1995.

Bell MS. *Master of the Crossroads.* 1st ed. New York: Pantheon Books; 2000.

Bell MS. *The Stone that the Builder Refused.* 1st ed. New York: Pantheon Books; 2004.

Index

Page references for figures are indicated by *f*, for tables by *t*, and for boxes by *b*.